Drug Therapy for Gastrointestinal and Liver Diseases

Edited by

MICHAEL JG FARTHING DSc(Med), MD, FRCP, FMedSci
Executive Dean
Faculty of Medicine
University of Glasgow
Glasgow
UK

ANNE B BALLINGER MD, MRCP
Senior Lecturer in Medicine and Honorary Consultant Gastroenterologist
Digestive Diseases Research Centre
St Bartholomew's & The Royal London School of Medicine & Dentistry
London
UK

MARTIN DUNITZ

© 2001 Martin Dunitz Ltd, a member of the Taylor & Francis group

First published in the United Kingdom in 2001
by Martin Dunitz Ltd, The Livery House, 7–9 Pratt Street, London NW1 0AE

Tel.:	+44 (0) 20 74822202
Fax.:	+44 (0) 20 72670159
E-mail:	info.dunitz@tandf.co.uk
Website:	http://www.dunitz.co.uk

A CIP record for this book is available from the British Library.

ISBN 1 85317 733 4

Distributed in the USA by
Fulfilment Center
Taylor & Francis
7625 Empire Drive
Florence, KY 41042, USA
Toll Free Tel: 1-800-634-7064
Email: cserve@routledge_ny.com

Distributed in Canada by
Taylor & Francis
74 Rolark Drive
Scarborough
Ontario M1R G2, Canada
Toll Free Tel: 1-877-226-2237
Email: tal_fran@istar.ca

Distributed in the rest of the world by
ITPS Limited
Cheriton House
North Way, Andover
Hampshire SP10 5BE, UK
Tel: +44 (0)1264 332424
Email: reception@itps.co.uk

Composition by Wearset, Boldon, Tyne and Wear

Printed and bound in Great Britain by Biddles Ltd, Guildford and King's Lynn

Contents

Contributors

Paul LR Andrews BSc, PhD
Department of Physiology, St George's
Hospital Medical School, London, UK

Anne B Ballinger MD, MRCP
Digestive Diseases Research Centre,
St Bartholomew's & The Royal London
School of Medicine & Dentistry, London, UK

Matthew R Banks BSc, MBBS, MRCP
St Bartholomew's & The Royal London
School of Medicine & Dentistry, London, UK

Eleanor Barnes MRCP
Centre for Hepatology, Royal Free and
University College Medical School, Royal
Free Campus, London, UK

William Bernal MBBS, MRCP
Institute of Liver Studies, Kings College
Hospital, Denmark Hill, London, UK

Arnaud Bourreille MD
Department of Gastroenterology and
Hepatology, CHU Hôtel-Dieu, Nantes
University, Nantes, France

Michael Camilleri MD
Enteric Neuroscience Program,
Gastroenterology Research Unit, Mayo
Medical School, Mayo Clinic and Mayo
Foundation, Rochester, MN, USA

Elizabeth Carty MRCP
Digestive Diseases Research Centre,
St Bartholomew's & The Royal London
School of Medicine & Dentistry, London, UK

Roger WG Chapman MD, FRCP
Department of Gastroenterology, The John
Radcliffe, Headington, Oxford, UK

John ML Christie BM, MRCP
Wycombe Hospital, Queen Alexandra Road,
High Wycombe, Bucks, UK

Bernard Coulie MD, PhD
Global Experimental Therapeutics and
Human Pharmacokinetics, Janssen Research
Foundation, Belgium

David Cunningham MD, FRCP
Gastrointestinal and Lymphoma Units,
Department of Medicine, Royal Marsden
Hospital, Sutton, Surrey, UK

Geoffrey M Dusheiko FRCP
Centre for Hepatology, Royal Free and
University College Medical School, Royal
Free Campus, London, UK

Àngels Escorsell MD
Liver Unit, IMD, Hospital Clínic, University
of Barcelona, Barcelona, Spain

Peter D Fairclough MD, FRCP
St Bartholomew's & The Royal London
School of Medicine & Dentistry, London, UK

Michael JG Farthing DSc(Med), MD, FRCP, FMedSci
Faculty of Medicine, University of Glasgow,
Glasgow, UK

Jean Paul Galmiche MD, FRCP
Department of Gastroenterology and
Hepatology, CHU Hôtel-Dieu, Nantes
University, Nantes, France

Ralph RSH Greaves MD, MRCP
Whipps Cross Hospital, London, UK

Stefan Kahl MD
University of Magdeburg, Department of
Gastroenterology, Magdeburg, Germany

Michael JS Langman FMedSci
Department of Medicine, Queen Elizabeth
Hospital, Birmingham, UK

Peter Malfertheiner MD
University of Magdeburg, Department of
Gastroenterology, Magdeburg, Germany

Erik AJ Rauws MD
Academic Medical Centre, Amsterdam, The
Netherlands

Juan Rodés MD, FRCP
Liver Unit, IMD, Hospital Clínic, University
of Barcelona, Barcelona, Spain

Gareth J Sanger BSc, PhD, DSc
Department of Neurology Research,
GlaxoSmithKline Pharmaceuticals, Harlow,
Essex

Carmelo Scarpignato MD, DSc(Hons), PharmD(h.c.),
FCP, FACG
Laboratory of Clinical Pharmacology, School
of Medicine and Dentistry, University of
Parma, Parma, Italy

Guido NJ Tytgat MD, PhD
Department of Gastroenterology, Academic
Medical Centre, Amsterdam, The
Netherlands

Justin S Waters MD, FRCP
Gastrointestinal and Lymphoma Units,
Department of Medicine, Royal Marsden
Hospital, Sutton, Surrey, UK

George Webster MRCP
Centre for Hepatology, Royal Free and
University College Medical School, Royal
Free Campus, London, UK

Julia Wendon MBChB, FRCP
Institute of Liver Studies, Kings College
Hospital, Denmark Hill, London, UK

Preface

The treatment of gastrointestinal and liver disease has been revolutionized in the past two decades by a variety of factors including a better understanding of the cause of some common disorders, new drug development and new forms of biotherapy such as the use of monoclonal antibodies to target specific pathways involved in intestinal inflammation. The first potent acid inhibitory drug, cimetidine, an H_2 receptor antagonist was introduced in 1976 and many of us thought that this was the end of peptic ulcer disease and reflux. Soon to follow were the proton pump inhibitors which had even greater efficacy, the discovery of *Helicobacter pylori* and the introduction of triple therapy heralded yet another major advance in the treatment of ulcer disease which has clearly changed the natural history of this disorder.

Similarly, the recognition of the importance of the bioactive amine, 5-hydroxytryptamine in gastrointestinal function promoted the development of a range of agonists and antagonists with enormous therapeutic potential. The $5\text{-}HT_3$ receptor antagonists now play a major role preventing chemotherapy-induced emesis and may also find a place in the management of functional disorders including irritable bowel syndrome.

The aetiology of non-specific inflammatory bowel disease in the gut continues to elude us but since the introduction of cortisone about 50 years ago there have been major advances in the development of anti-inflammatory therapy including locally active steroids, new delivery systems for 5-amino salicylic acid and the widespread use of immunosuppressive drugs such as azathioprine. The development of anti-TNF-α antibodies was a landmark in the treatment of intestinal inflammation clearly showing that inhibition of a single pro-inflammatory cytokine can have a major effect on the inflammatory cascade and in the treatment of disease refractory to standard therapy. Although this approach may not survive in the long term it does prove the principle that targeted anti-cytokine therapy works in clinical practice.

Major advances have been made in the treatment of viral hepatitis with emergence of increasingly effective anti-viral regimens for both Hepatitis B and Hepatitis C virus infections. However, many challenges remain for the future including the development of more active agents to modify gastrointestinal mobility and visceral sensation, agents to limit damage in acute pancreatitis and drugs which can be used clinically to modify liver fibrosis.

Drug Therapy for Gastrointestinal and Liver Diseases aims to provide an up-to-date account of evidence-based treatment in gastrointestinal and liver disorders. Each chapter provides a brief summary of the pathophysiology of the disease, the rationale for drug intervention and appropriate treatment regimens as indicated by current knowledge. Also included is a drug list which summarizes mode of action, and other aspects of clinical pharmacology where appropriate, drug doses, common adverse affects and drug interactions. We anticipate that this book will be a useful clinical manual for both generalists and specialists and be a valuable resource for students and researchers in the health sciences who need to broaden their knowledge of clinical therapeutics of gut and liver disease.

Michael JG Farthing
Anne B Ballinger
March 2001

1

Drug therapy of gastro-oesophageal reflux disease

Jean Paul Galmiche, Arnaud Bourreille, Carmelo Scarpignato

INTRODUCTION

Gastro-oesophageal reflux disease (GORD) is a common disorder caused by retrograde flow of gastric contents through an incompetent gastro-oesophageal junction. It encompasses a wide range of clinical pictures from 'endoscopy-negative disease' (i.e. symptoms without lesions at endoscopy) to severe oesophagitis and complications.[1] The prevalence of heartburn, the most typical symptom together with regurgitation, is extremely high, affecting roughly 10–20% of adults at least weekly.[2] Moderate to severe symptoms, however, are present in only 1–4% of cases. In fact, many subjects in whom heartburn and/or regurgitation occur intermittently do not seek medical help and treat themselves with over the counter-medication such as antacids and, more recently, H_2-receptor antagonists.

In contrast, the prevalence of oesophagitis is far lower, probably affecting about 2% of the general population and no more than 30–50% of patients referred to an endoscopy unit because of symptoms suggestive of GORD. Moreover, most patients with mucosal breaks at endoscopy have mild-to-moderate oesophagitis (non-circumferential lesions). On the contrary, severe oesophagitis or complications such as strictures or deep ulcers are rare, especially in young subjects. Intestinal metaplasia of the distal oesophageal mucosa is also considered a severe complication of GORD but other factors are also implicated in its pathogenesis. Metaplasia is frequently detected if systematic biopsies are taken from the cardia but classic Barrett's oesophagus (i.e. columnar-lined oesophagitis extending 3 cm or more) is present in less than 10% of patients in whom endoscopy is performed for reflux symptoms. Barrett's oesophagus, although frequently asymptomatic and not always associated with the macroscopic changes of oesophagitis, is a premalignant condition, increasing by 30 to 40 times the risk of adenocarcinoma of the oesophagus. Malignant progression evolves through a well-identified sequence metaplasia to dysplasia and, finally, carcinoma.

During the last decade, major advance has been made in the treatment of GORD,[3,4] which has been revolutionized by the development of proton pump inhibitors (PPIs). Nevertheless, despite this dramatic improvement to our therapeutic armamentarium, it should be emphasized that none of the drugs available currently for anti-reflux therapy are able to cure the disease, which is frequently (but not always) a chronic relapsing disorder. Although not life-threatening, recent studies[5] have shown that GORD can impair severely the quality of life of the patient, even in the absence of lesions of oesophagitis (endoscopy-negative GORD).

PATHOPHYSIOLOGY OF GORD AND TARGETS FOR ANTI-REFLUX DRUG THERAPY

Although GORD is *primarily* a motility disorder that is characterized by impairment of the physiological barrier at the gastro-oesophageal junction, the pathogenesis (Fig. 1.1) of reflux symptoms and oesophagitis is multifactorial.[6] The most important factors include:

- Motility disturbances of the lower oesophageal sphincter and proximal stomach
- The role of acid and pepsin secretion
- The defence mechanisms of the oesophagus (i.e. the clearance function and the resistance of the oesophageal mucosa itself)
- The perception of the various stimuli elicited by the contact of the oesophageal mucosa with the refluxed material[6,7]

Most reflux episodes occur during transient relaxations of the lower oesophageal sphincter (TLOSRs) when resting lower oesophageal sphincter (LOS) pressure is normal. In patients with GORD, both the absolute number of TLOSRs and the proportion of relaxations associated with acid reflux seem to be increased compared with healthy subjects with physiological amounts of acid reflux. Unfortunately, none of the currently used prokinetic drugs, is able to modify the underlying abnormal motor pattern observed in GORD. TLOSRs are elicited through a vagovagal reflex triggered by distension of mechanical receptors located in the wall of the proximal stomach, especially in the subcardiac area. In pharmacological experiments conducted in humans or in animals, a variety of drugs are able to decrease the rate of TLOSRs induced by a meal or gastric distension with air (Table 1.1). These compounds hold promise for more rationale drug therapy in the future but, at present, their use in clinical practice is hampered by the occurrence of non-specific side-effects, such as the development of sedation in relation to the central action of morphinomimetic compounds.

Besides abnormal motility, the key role of acid and pepsin aggression on oesophageal mucosa has been confirmed largely by the impressive benefit of acid suppression achieved

by PPIs in GORD. Non-acid components of the gastric refluxate can also contribute to the pathogenesis of reflux oesophagitis. Hence, bile acids can potentiate the noxious effect of acid and pepsin, resulting in more severe mucosal injury. In most cases, however, acid and non-acid components act synergistically at low pH rather than at alkaline pH (making pH-monitoring an inappropriate tool for the investigation of enterogastro-oesophageal reflux). Thus, the reduction in the volume of gastric contents achieved with PPI therapy probably has a beneficial effect on both acid and non-acid reflux.[8]

Although *Helicobacter pylori* is a well-established factor in the pathogenesis of peptic ulcer disease the same does not hold true in GORD.[9] The bacterium does not seem to contribute to the motility disturbances, for example in increasing the rate of TLOSRs or in altering gastric emptying (which seems to be delayed in about 40% of patients with GORD). On the contrary, eradication of *Helicobacter pylori* infection can increase the dosage of PPI required to control acid secretion in patients with reflux oesophagitis.[10,11] Finally, on the basis of current knowledge, a recent consensus conference[12] did not recommend systematic research and eradication of the bacterium in GORD and during prolonged antisecretory treatment.

Factors protecting the oesophagus against

Table 1.1   Pharmacological inhibition of TLOSRs in humans.

- NO synthase blockade (L-NMMA)
- CCK_1 – Receptor blockade (e.g. with loxiglumide)
- $5\text{-}HT_3$ – Receptor blockade (e.g. with ondansetron) (granisetron)
- Muscarinic receptor blockade (e.g. with atropine)*
- μ-receptor stimulation (e.g. with morphine)*
- $GABA_b$ – Receptor stimulation (e.g. with baclofen)*

*Presumably through a central effect.
CCK, cholecystokinin; GABA, gamma amino butyric acid.

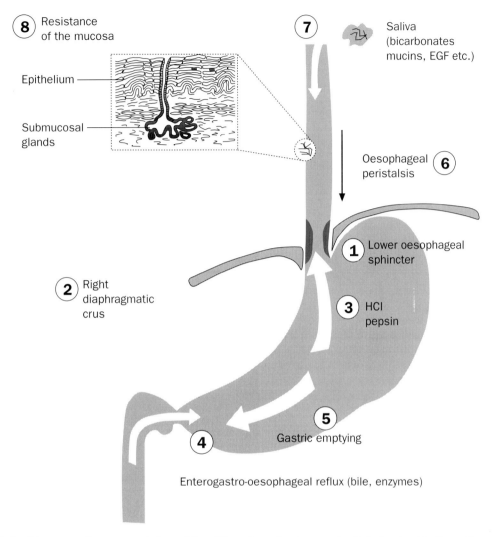

Figure 1.1 Diagrammatic representation of the different mechanisms potentially involved in the pathogenesis of gastro-oesophageal reflux disease (GORD). Anti-reflux barrier consists of (1) the lower oesophageal sphincter (LOS) and the right diaphragmatic crus (2). The components of the refluxate include acid and pepsin (3), and in some instances a non-acid material resulting from enterogastro-oesophageal reflux (4). Delayed gastric emptying is observed in 30 to 40% of GORD patients (5). Oesophageal defence mechanisms rely on oesophageal clearance function and resistance of the oesophageal mucosa. Oesophageal clearance is a two stage phenomenon resulting from the combined action of oesophageal peristaltism (6) and neutralization of acid by swallowed saliva (7). Oesophageal mucosa (8) represents a barrier to ions diffusion and includes several lines of defence. Reproduced with permission from Galmiche JP, Zerbib F (1999).[6]
EGF, epidermal growth factor.

injury by noxious components of the refluxate include:

- Oesophageal clearance, which is frequently abnormal, especially in patients with severe oesophagitis; and
- The resistance of oesophageal mucosa itself (Fig. 1.1).

In addition to peristalsis, saliva plays an important role in oesophageal clearance by neutralizing the minute amounts of acid remaining in the oesophagus after a reflux episode has occurred. Saliva is a complex secretion containing bicarbonates, mucous glycoproteins and epidermal growth factor (EGF), prostaglandin E_2 (PGE$_2$) and transforming growth factor (TGF). The role played by the defence mechanisms of the oesophageal mucosa is probably underestimated. Indeed, symptom relief and healing of reflux oesophagitis require far more potent acid inhibition in GORD than in peptic ulcer disease. Among the mechanisms that may account for reduced resistance to acid of the oesophageal mucosa are:[13]

- A lack of mucus and bicarbonate secretion by surface epithelial cells
- A lack of defensive enhancement by acid-induced prostaglandin release
- Impaired epithelial restitution (which is dependent on cell replication)
- A lack of 'mucous cap' over the injury area

Therefore, oesophageal cells remain readily accessible to luminal acid, while tissue repair requires a neutral pH.

The quality and intensity of oesophageal symptoms are poorly correlated with the severity of lesions seen at endoscopy and the duration of acid exposure measured by pH-metry. For instance, endoscopy-negative patients may experience severe heartburn, with significant impact on quality of life. Interestingly, there is a subset of patients without excess acid reflux but with significant association between symptoms and reflux episodes. Changes in oesophageal sensitivity may be responsible for the intermittent occurrence of symptoms while acid aggression and motor abnormalities persist in the same patient.

AIMS OF TREATMENT AND RATIONALE FOR DIFFERENT THERAPEUTIC APPROACHES

Aims of treatment

The management of GORD requires a consideration of its natural history, which shows great variation between patients.[1] In some patients, usually those referred in tertiary centres, GORD appears as a chronic disease that relapses shortly after discontinuation of treatment, therefore requiring maintenance drug therapy (or surgery) to prevent relapse. On the contrary, in the primary care setting, the disease usually develops in a less severe manner, consisting of intermittent attacks that can easily be treated on an on-demand basis. As already emphasized, most patients are endoscopy-negative or have mild oesophagitis with little (if any) evidence that lesions really worsen with time. In most of them, lesions never develop or, if already present at first assessment, wax and wane without further worsening.[14] Since the severity of oesophagitis is predictive of the therapeutic response and risk of recurrence, endoscopy is usually accepted as a useful assessment, at least once-in-a-life, in patients with GORD of moderate or severe activity.

Finally, there is now a consensus that symptom relief and long-term control of the disease are the primary aims of therapy for most patients. The inclusion of quality-of-life assessments in therapeutic trials is recommended for both drug therapy and anti-reflux surgery. In patients with moderate to severe oesophagitis and/or complications, healing also remains an important therapeutic goal.[12]

Therapeutic strategies

Schematically, there are two therapeutic strategies available for the medical treatment of GORD. The 'step-up' therapeutic approach starts with less active treatments and moves to more active ones only in non-responder patients or in those with very severe disease. This approach is opposed to the 'step-down' strategy, which consists of starting with maximally effective drugs and going towards less powerful treatment after initial remission has been achieved. In fact there is no study evaluating in a direct manner, both completely and reliably, these different management strategies of GORD. Moreover, besides drug therapy, lifestyle and dietary recommendations are a traditional component of the treatment of GORD. Physiological studies have suggested that measures such as raising the head of the bed or elimination of fatty foods may be of benefit because they are able to reduce oesophageal acid exposure. In fact, their therapeutic efficacy has not really been established by well-controlled trials and their relevance is certainly less since the development of very effective drugs for treatment of GORD.

Initial strategy

From a practical standpoint, it is relevant to consider successively the initial therapeutic approach and the long-term management of the disease. An example of an initial strategy recommended by a recent consensus conference[12] (Fig. 1.2) is now described in the list:

1. In the case of intermittent typical symptoms and in the absence of alarming symptoms (e.g. dysphagia or weight loss) an on-demand treatment with antacids, alginates or low-dose H_2-receptor antagonists should be prescribed, these three therapeutic classes having similar symptomatic efficacy (see later).

2. In cases of frequent typical symptoms (once a week or more) without alarming symptoms and in patient aged less than 50 years

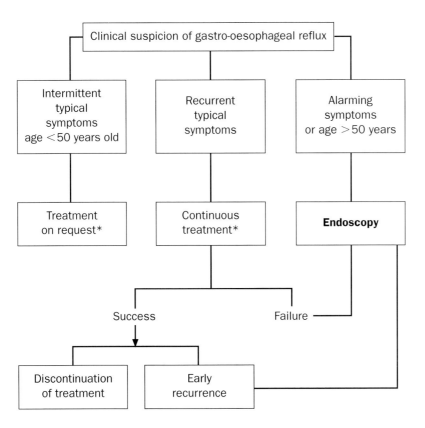

Figure 1.2 Initial management of adult gastro-oesophageal reflux disease according to the recommendations of the French–Belgian Consensus Conference (adapted from reference 12).

*See text for treatment modalities.

old, an empirical treatment can be prescribed for approximately 4 weeks (with PPIs at half dose or standard-dose H_2-receptor antagonists or with cisapride). In cases of symptomatic success, treatment should be discontinued. If the treatment fails to relieve symptoms or in case of early recurrence upper gastrointestinal endoscopy must be performed (if not already performed).

3. In endoscopy-negative patients or in those with only mild or moderate oesophagitis, treatment for 4 weeks with PPIs should be considered. If endoscopic examination is required because of therapeutic failure, full dose PPI should be used. In case of severe oesophagitis or complications, treatment with full dose PPI for 8 weeks should be prescribed at first instance and results assessed by endoscopic examination. In the absence of healing or symptomatic remission, increased doses may be warranted. Extra-digestive manifestations, may justify higher doses or dosing frequency (twice daily instead of once daily).

Long-term management

For the long-term management (Fig. 1.3) the strategy needs to be individualized according to the patient's needs. the following recommendations can be adopted as a general therapeutic guidance:

1. After initial treatment, drug therapy should be discontinued when symptoms have disappeared, except in case of severe or complicated oesophagitis.
2. In common cases of infrequent but recurrent symptoms (without oesophagitis or with non-severe oesophagitis), patients should be treated intermittently according to similar therapeutic modalities that were successful at initial remission.
3. When there are frequent recurrences, when relapses occur early after discontinuation of treatment and there is severely compromised quality of life, maintenance treatment with PPI is indicated.
4. When continuous maintenance treatment is required to control disease activity, anti-

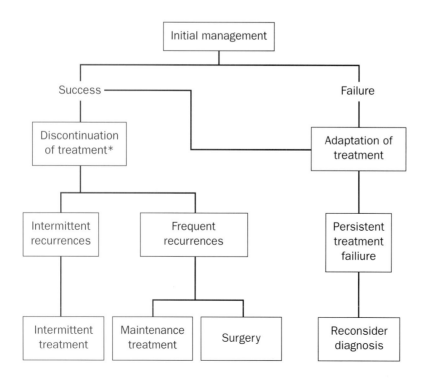

Figure 1.3 Long-term strategy of adult gasto-oesophageal reflux disease according to the recommendations of the French–Belgian Consensus Conference (adapted from reference 12).

reflux surgery should be discussed since it may represent a more cost-effective approach than a lifetime of drug therapy, especially in a young, fit patient.

Management of specific complications
Complications of GORD may require more specific therapeutic approaches.

Peptic stricture is an excellent indication for PPI therapy.[15] In dysphagia, endoscopic dilatation should be associated with medical treatment. In non-healing of oesophagitis, PPI doses should be increased.

The management of oesophageal metaplasia and the prophylaxis of cancer is out of the scope of this chapter but the treatment of symptoms and oesophagitis associated with Barrett's oesophagus relies in general on the same therapeutic principles as in GORD. PPI therapy is efficacious in controlling symptoms and in healing the oesophagitis.[16] Long-term antisecretory treatment, however, does not allow complete regression of Barrett's oesophagus nor prevent the occurrence of dysplasia or cancer.

PRINCIPAL DRUG REGIMENS

The principal drug regimens currently available for the treatment of GORD are summarized in Table 1.2.

PHARMACOLOGY OF RELEVANT DRUGS

Medications available in the treatment of GORD are of several therapeutic classes whose efficacy has been well-documented by controlled-trials, at least for the more recently developed ones.

Topical agents

Antacids, alginates and the association of both yield symptomatic efficacy, which has been documented in some controlled studies.

Epidemiological evidence is probably more convincing with respect to the widespread use of these drugs in primary care as well as for self-medication in patients with mild/intermittent symptoms. Nevertheless, these drugs have no curative or preventive action in oesophagitis.

Antacids
For a review of this class of drugs see reference 17.

Pharmacological aspects
Antacids are preparations that are designed primarily to neutralize gastric acid. Antacids are usually administered either as tablets or suspensions, although there are some granule or gel formulations available. In the liquid formulations, the antacid component can be either soluble in water, and thus in solution (e.g. sodium bicarbonate), or insoluble and present as a finely divided solid (e.g. aluminium hydroxide). Tablets consist of finely divided antacid powder combined with other excipients such as flavourings and binders. Tablets, although more convenient, are considered to be less effective in lowering gastric acidity than liquid preparations.

The effect on gastric pH is of short duration: antacids ingested in the fasting state reduce acidity for only approximately 30 min because of their rapid gastric emptying. When antacids (30 ml) are given 1 and 3 hours after the meal, gastric pH is kept above 2.0 for 3 h. The nocturnal gastric acidity (which normally reaches its peak after midnight) is not adequately controlled by antacids, even when given at bedtime.

Some antacids, especially those containing aluminium, delay gastric emptying of both solids and liquids. This inhibition may be considered a desirable property because rapid gastric emptying of liquid antacids is believed to be the limiting factor in the duration of their neutralizing effect. When a schedule of antacid therapy is ineffective, the *frequency* of administration should be increased rather than the dose. In clinical practice, the control of acidity is

Table 1.2 Principal therapeutic regimens of currently available drugs.

Available drugs	Standard doses (dosing frequency)	Remarks
Antacids and alginates/antacids	One therapeutic unit after meals or on-demand (antacids)	• If ineffective increase dosing frequency rather than daily dose
Cisapride	20–40 mg/day (bid, tid, or qid)	• 20 mg nocte effective for prophylaxis of relapse • Contraindication in patients with cardiac arrhythmia • Caution for drug interferences

H$_2$-receptor antagonists
  Cimetidine
  Ranitidine
  Nizatidine
  Famotidine
	
	800 mg (bid)
	300 mg (bid)
	300 mg (bid)
	20–40 mg (bid)
		• Once-a-day dosing also effective (at dinner rather than bedtime)
		• Low dosages and OTC formulations available for on-demand relief of heartburn

Proton pump inhibitors (PPIs)
  Omeprazole
  Lansoprazole
  Pantoprazole
 	
  Rabeprazole
	
	20 mg (od)
	30 mg (od)
	40 mg (od)
	
	20 mg (od)
		• Half dosages (omeprazole 10 mg or lansoprazole 15 mg) also available for symptomatic treatment and prophylaxis of relapses
		• Higher doses (omeprazole 40–60 mg or lansoprazole 60 mg) for severe or complicated diseases or extraoesophageal manifestations

Combined therapy
  H$_2$-receptor antagonist + cisapride
  PPI + cisapride
	
	Ranitidine 300 mg (bid) + cisapride 40 mg (qid)
	Omeprazole 20 mg (od) + cisapride 30 mg (tid)
		• Less cost-effective than monotherapy with standard-dose PPI
		• More effective than ranitidine + cisapride
		• Not significantly different from monotherapy with omeprazole 20 mg

OTC, over-the-counter.

more easily achieved by the use of an adequate antisecretory drug (i.e. PPIs).

Several studies have suggested that antacids reduce the peptic activity of gastric juice. Aluminium hydroxide has also strong capacity to adsorb bile salts. The binding affinity of bile salts for antacids depend upon the chemical structure of the bile salt and is affected by conjugation.

Clinical efficacy and indications
Although several placebo-controlled trials have failed to establish their efficacy in heartburn, other studies, as well as epidemiological data, suggest that they are likely to be effective in alleviating symptoms. Indeed, most of the controlled trials of antacids in GORD were performed more than 20 years ago and included relatively small numbers of patients, which were not necessarily representative of the population in which antacids are currently administered. There is no evidence that antacids can heal oesophagitis or prevent recurrences. Finally, antacids still represent a useful therapeutic approach in patients with mild or intermittent symptoms, or in the context of self-medication.

Adverse reactions and drug interactions
When large doses of magnesium hydroxide antacids are given, bowel disturbance is often observed. Indeed, there is good correlation between the acid-neutralizing capacity administered and the frequency of diarrhoea. Although in recent formulations an attempt has been made to balance the effects of magnesium by aluminium hydroxide, diarrhoea remains one of the most important limitations to treatment of acid-related diseases with high doses of antacids.

Antacids are usually taken by patients at the time of symptom occurrence. Nevertheless, since antacids may interfere with the absorption of drugs such as antibiotics, patients should be instructed to respect a minimum interval before the next dosing with another drug.

Alginates and alginate/antacids
Mode of action and physicochemical aspects
These pharmaceutical preparations, of which the most widely known is Gaviscon®, contain alginic acid combined with small doses of antacids. Scintigraphic techniques[17,18] have shown that most of the ingested alginic acid is located in the upper half of the stomach where it floats as a raft. Thus, in subjects in whom reflux occurs after treatment with alginic acid, the labelled compound refluxed in preference to the liquid contents of the stomach, such that this viscous foam first contacted the oesophageal mucosa. It is essential that Gaviscon® is taken *after* a meal to ensure gastric floatation. When the alginate/antacid is taken on an empty stomach, the formulation sinks to the base of the greater curvature and 50% is emptied within 20 min of administration. When the formulation is taken 30 min before, the anti-reflux agent does not float on a meal ingested subsequently, instead the food actually displaces the anti-reflux agent from the fundus to the antrum as it is ingested. Once in the antrum, the anti-reflux agent is caught up by the mixing and grinding action of this region. It then becomes diluted with the fluid from the meal and thus it empties ahead of the meal without forming a raft.

Commercial anti-reflux preparations use a wide range of alginate materials. The alginates used in the anti-reflux formulations fall into two groups:

1. The soluble salts (sodium and potassium alginates), which form a gel by reaction with gastric acid; and
2. The insoluble alginates (alginic acid, calcium and magnesium alginate) which primarily form a gel by rehydration.

Often these two types of material may be mixed in a particular formulation. Even in the same formulation the composition varies greatly from country to country. The inclusion of antacids in the formulation increases the neutralization capacity within the raft but decreases the breaking strength and hence the ability of the raft to form a viscous 'plug' in the opening of the oesophagus as a barrier to reflux.

Another component of these anti-reflux formulations that is critical for raft formation is the gas-producing agent. Without it, the formulation would mix and empty with the meal. In contrast, too much gas formation can disrupt and weaken the raft, while gas, which is generated too rapidly or too slowly, will not be trapped in the gel. The rate at which the gas-producing agent can react with the gastric contents will depend on many factors, such as the quantity of particulate antacid present in the formulation and the acid available in the stomach. There will be a competition for free H^+ ions available within the stomach between the gas-producing agent, particulate antacid and food. Generally, the gas-producing agent is sodium bicarbonate. In an attempt to reduce sodium content of some formulations, this has been substituted by the potassium salt; however, these formulations have less buoyancy than those containing sodium bicarbonate.

Pharmacological studies in GORD
In some trials, a significant decrease in the number of reflux episodes and in the percentage time during which the oesophageal pH was in the acidic range has been reported after the administration of eight tablets per day of an alginate-containing preparation (Gaviscon®). Antacid alone (Gaviscon® without alginate) had no effect on oesophageal pH. Other studies, however, failed to show a significant reduction of oesophageal exposure to acid, although doses of Gaviscon® as high as four tablets every 2 h were administered. Usually, Gaviscon® was unable to normalize acid exposure, despite symptomatic improvement.

Clinical trials and indications
The clinical efficacy of Gaviscon® has not been established by large placebo-controlled trials. In the studies in which Gaviscon® appeared to give superior symptomatic improvement compared with placebo, there was no information regarding endoscopic healing. In studies where Gaviscon® was compared with antacids, there

was no statistically significant difference between these drugs in terms of symptom relief and improvement of lesions. In a large open trial of Gaviscon® taken on-demand, however, most patients with mild oesophagitis remained in clinical remission throughout the 6-month study period.[19] On the whole, clinical experience in general practice suggests that alginates or alginate–antacid preparations (Algicon®) are effective in the relief of heartburn but not in the healing of oesophagitis.

Drug interactions and precautions
Although, there is some evidence that the absorption of an H_2-receptor antagonist from a combined formulation of alginate and cimetidine is decreased and slowed, co-administration of cimetidine with liquid Gaviscon® in two separate formulations does not seem to affect the availability of cimetidine. Although alginate/antacids are extremely safe and well-tolerated compounds, patients with cardiac, hepatic or renal failure should be advised that some formulations of Gaviscon® contain substantial amounts of sodium.

Prokinetic compounds

The role of prokinetic drugs in adult GORD is probably less important than in the past, due to the development of potent and safe acid suppressors. Nevertheless, cisapride is still prescribed in infants and children where clinicians are more reluctant to embark in long-term acid suppression. In the future, the development of new compounds (e.g. CCK_1 antagonists or $GABA_b$ agonists) that are capable of inhibiting TLOSRs (Table 1.1) could represent a significant progress in a field of active pharmacological research and competition.[6,20]

Ancillary prokinetics
In the past, several prokinetic agents have been used for the management of GORD. For instance, bethanechol, a cholinergic agent has been shown effective in reducing symptoms and lesions of oesophagitis in both adults and

children. However, it also stimulates gastric acid secretion and is responsible for several side-effects. Similarly, metoclopramide (a $5HT_3$-antagonist), although effective on reflux symptoms at relatively large doses (at least 40 mg/day) is frequently responsible for adverse effects such as drowsiness, bowel disturbance, dizziness or even severe extrapyramidal manifestations. Domperidone is a more recently developed dopamine antagonist related to butyrophenones that has nearly the same pharmacodynamic actions as metoclopramide on œsophageal and gastric motility. Although domperidone does not cross the blood–brain barrier and seldom causes extrapyramidal effects, it may, however, produce symptoms related to hyperprolactinaemia (galactorrhoea, or amenorrhoea). Results similar to those obtained with metoclopramide would be expected in GORD, with domperidone being better tolerated. Although metoclopramide and domperidone are still used in dyspepsia and other gastrointestinal motility-related disorders, they have been virtually abandoned for the treatment of GORD since the development of cisapride.

Cisapride

This compound is a prokinetic drug without an antidopaminergic effect. It is an agonist of 5-HT_4 receptors and releases acetylcholine in the myenteric plexus of the gut. Cisapride increases the amplitude of oesophageal body contractions, increases LOS pressure (especially in reflux patients with a low tone at baseline) and accelerates gastric emptying. Nevertheless, cisapride does not change the rate of TLOSRs. Although cisapride has indirect cholinomimetic effects, it does not affect gastric acid secretion. Cisapride administration (10 or 20 mg, four times a day) enhances salivary secretion in asymptomatic volunteers.[21] This effect may contribute to oesophageal clearance and benefit patients with GORD.

The efficacy of cisapride has been established beyond doubt, both in adults and children. In the short term, cisapride (10 mg four times daily or 20 mg twice daily) is more effective than placebo and equally effective as H_2-receptor antagonists for symptom relief and healing of oesophagitis. Large placebo-controlled trials have shown that maintenance treatment with cisapride (10 or 20 mg twice daily or 20 mg nocte) significantly reduces the 6- and 12-month relapse rate of oesophagitis.[22,23] The therapeutic gain, however, is mainly limited to patients with mild or moderate oesophagitis.

Cisapride is usually well-tolerated, the most frequent side effects being mild diarrhoea, abdominal pain and headache. However, exceptional but lethal cardiac complications (i.e. torsades de pointes) have recently been reported. This adverse effect may reduce the role of cisapride considerably in the treatment of GORD since safe, effective, well-tolerated drugs are now available. The clinician should also be aware of the interaction between cisapride and several other drugs, such as spiramycin and ketoconazole; their concurrent use is absolutely contraindicated. The production licence for cisapride has recently been withdrawn in several countries in Europe and the USA because of life-threatening cardiac side-effects (see also Chapter 7, p. 149).

Combination therapy with antisecretory compounds

Combination therapy of metoclopramide with cimetidine has been investigated in short-term studies. In general, the clinical and endoscopic results obtained by adding this prokinetic compound to cimetidine are not superior to those achieved using cimetidine alone.

The more recent prokinetic agent cisapride has also been used in combination with H_2-receptor antagonists. Cisapride (10 mg twice daily) combined with ranitidine (150 mg twice daily) showed a trend towards improvement over ranitidine alone. Other controlled studies adding cisapride (10 mg four times daily) to either cimetidine or ranitidine resulted in significantly better healing rates than monotherapy with the H_2-receptor antagonist.

In maintenance therapy, adding cisapride (10 mg three times daily) to ranitidine (150 mg twice daily) significantly reduced the relapse rate at 12 months compared with ranitidine alone. The relapse rate observed with ranitidine plus cisapride was not significantly different from that observed with omeprazole alone (20 mg once a day in the morning), but adding cisapride to omeprazole gave better results than those observed with combination therapy using ranitidine.[24] However, for continued relief of heartburn monotherapy with omeprazole alone seems more cost-effective than combined therapy with H_2-receptor antagonists.

Finally, there are few indications for combination therapy using an antisecretory drug and a prokinetic agent. This approach, however, may be reasonable for special patient subgroups such as those whose predominant symptom is regurgitation and those with predominant nocturnal symptoms.[23]

Antisecretory drugs

H_2-receptor antagonists[25,26]
Mode of action and pharmacodynamic studies
Five compounds belonging to this class of drugs, namely cimetidine, ranitidine, nizatidine, famotidine and roxatidine. Although their chemical structure is different, the mechanism of their antisecretory action is identical—a competitive inhibition of H_2-receptors located on the parietal cells, with the consequent reduction of intracellular cyclic AMP concentrations and reduction of acid secretion. The relative potencies of the five H_2-receptor antagonists in inhibiting the secretion of gastric acid vary from 20- to 50-fold, cimetidine and famotidine being the least and the most potent, respectively. Pharmacokinetic parameters are similar among the different compounds, with the exception of oral bioavailability, which is higher for nizatidine and roxatidine. With standard doses, the duration of a serum concentration above the level of 50% inhibition ranges from approximately 6 h for cimetidine to approximately 10 h for the other H_2-receptor antagonists. All the H_2-receptor antagonists suppress acid for about 4–8 h depending on the drug used, cimetidine and nizatidine having a

slightly shorter duration of action than the others. Multiple dosing (i.e. twice-daily administration) is, therefore, the preferred therapeutic regimen for the treatment of GORD.

New formulations of H_2-receptor antagonists
A chewable formulation of cimetidine is now available. The onset of effect of this new formulation proved to be very quick since the medium time for some improvement was less than 20 min and for total pain relief was less than 45 min. A chewable tablet containing cimetidine and alginic acid was also developed and found to be effective for symptom relief in GORD.

Effervescent tablets may also offer a more effective medication for the rapid relief of symptoms. In recent years an effervescent formulation of either cimetidine and ranitidine became available.[27] By combining the immediate effect of a pH buffer with the prolonged systemic effect of an H_2-receptor blockade, these effervescent formulations offer the advantage of a rapid decrease of intragastric acidity.

A new solid dosage form (Pepcid® Rapi-disc (RPD) wafer) of famotidine has recently been introduced in clinical practice. It was designed to disperse, within seconds, on the tongue and to be consumed without water. This convenience and ease of administration should increase compliance, especially in patients with swallowing difficulties. The famotidine wafer, as well as the cimetidine and ranitidine effervescent formulations, will also help to avoid the problems associated with impaired oesophageal transit of conventional dosage forms, since tablets have been shown to lodge in the oesophagus in at least 20% of the subjects.

Clinical efficacy in the short-term treatment of GORD[28,29]
The daily dose of H_2-receptor antagonists given to a patient with GORD initially is usually the conventional one (i.e. cimetidine 800 mg, ranitidine and nizatidine 300 mg, famotidine 40 mg and roxatidine 150 mg). However, as many as 50% of patients fail to respond to such regimens.[29] Some studies have shown that oesophageal exposure to acid was significantly reduced in patients with reflux oesophagitis

who healed after a short course of ranitidine, whereas it was unaffected in patients whose oesophagitis was not healed. As a consequence, in patients with oesophagitis resistant to standard-dose ranitidine, increasing the dose of the drug to 300 mg four times daily is followed by decrease of the total reflux time and improved alleviation of symptoms and healing of oesophagitis. Prolonging the treatment period also improves healing rates but the response rate still remains unsatisfactory when conventional doses are used.

H_2-receptor antagonists for long-term treatment of GORD

In trials of 6–12 months duration with cimetidine (400 mg nocte), ranitidine (150 mg nocte) or famotidine (20 mg or 40 mg nocte), the recurrence rate of erosive oesophagitis has been equivalent to that observed with placebo. However, two large double-blind trials performed with famotidine (20 mg or 40 mg twice daily) showed a significant advantage compared with placebo.[30]

Treatment with standard doses of H_2-receptor antagonists has not been shown conclusively to prevent recurrence of stricture following initial dilatation.

Reasons for limited efficacy of H_2-receptor antagonists in GORD

Although H_2-receptor antagonists are competitive antagonists for the histamine H_2-receptors, acetylcholine or gastrin-stimulated acid secretion is only partially blocked by them. The same holds true for meal-induced acid secretion.

Another important phenomenon, occurring within 2 weeks in patients receiving standard doses of H_2-receptor antagonists, is the development of tolerance, which leads to a reduction in acid inhibition and therefore effectiveness. Tolerance could be caused by up-regulation of either H_2- and gastrin receptors, as well as to increased parietal cell mass following long-term hypergastrinaemia.

Safety of H_2-receptor antagonists

Side-effects are uncommon and reported more frequently with cimetidine. Adverse effects include diarrhoea and other gastrointestinal disturbances, headache, dizziness, rash and tiredness. Rarely bradycardia and atrioventricular block, confusion, hallucinations, seizures, hepatic dysfunction including immune hypersensitivity hepatitis (which is rapidly reversible after drug withdrawal), interstitial nephritis, hypersensitivity reactions (including fever, arthralgia and anaphylaxis) and blood disorders (e.g. thrombocytopenia, neutropenia and pancytopenia) occur. Gynaecomastia and impotence may occur with cimetidine use.

Precautions and contraindications

H_2-receptor antagonists cross the placenta and appear in breast milk. There are no adequate case-control studies to guide use in pregnant or breastfeeding patients. The manufacturer advises avoidance in pregnancy and breastfeeding. The dose of H_2-receptor antagonists should be reduced by 50–75% in renal failure. Cimetidine and nizatidine should be avoided in patients with severe liver disease. Contraindications to H_2-receptor antagonists include known hypersensitivity to the drug.

Drug interactions

Numerous drug interactions have been reported with cimetidine. Clinically important interactions are listed in the following list and cimetidine should be avoided in patients taking these drugs:

- Analgesics, cimetidine increases plasma concentration of opioid analgesics
- Antibacterial agents: cimetidine increases plasma concentration of metronidazole and erythromycin
- Anticoagulants: cimetidine enhances anticoagulant effect of warfarin and nicoumalone
- Antiepileptics: cimetidine increases plasma concentrations of carbamazepine, phenytoin and valproate
- Cardiovascular drugs: cimetidine increases plasma concentrations of amiodarone, flecanide, lignocaine, procainamide, propafenone, quininidine, β-blockers, some calcium-channel blockers

- Other interactions: cimetidine increases plasma concentration of cyclosporin and theophylline

Over-the-counter H_2-receptor antagonists[31]

Since its beginning 20 years ago, the Over-the-Counter (OTC) Review Process has resulted in the switch of many products from prescription to OTC status. This occurrence was attributed to a political initiative to reduce expenditure on pharmaceuticals and physician-based consultation costs. In early 1989, the regulatory authorities in Denmark approved the switch of cimetidine and ranitidine from prescription-only status to OTC availability. Low-dose H_2-receptor antagonists (i.e. 200 mg cimetidine, 75 mg ranitidine and 10 mg famotidine) are effective in preventing and treating heartburn.

In theory, self-medication with H_2-receptor antagonists could mask several disorders and delay interventions for conditions where early detection and treatment could result in improved prognosis. It has been estimated, however, that any change in the interval between symptom occurrence and diagnosis of gastric cancer is likely to be small and have little effect on the overall mortality of gastric cancer in Western communities.

Current role of H_2-receptor antagonists in the management of GORD

H_2-receptor antagonists have been widely used and demonstrated to be safe and efficacious in suppressing acid secretion and in controlling symptoms in mild cases of GORD. They are much less effective in more severe forms of oesophagitis, especially if complicated by stricture or ulcer. Owing to the rapid onset of action, H_2-receptor antagonists seem well-suited for on-demand treatment of reflux symptoms. Effervescent formulations provide more rapid absorption and almost immediate clinical effect.

Proton pump inhibitors (PPIs)

Pharmacodynamics and pharmacokinetics

Omeprazole (20 and 40 mg once daily) was the first PPI evaluated extensively for the treatment of reflux oesophagitis, whereas lansoprazole (30 mg once daily), pantoprazole (40 mg once daily) and rabeprazole (20 mg once daily) have been developed more recently.[32–34] All of these substituted benzimidazoles interact with gastric H^+/K^+-ATPase, the enzyme constituting the final step in the formation of gastric acid. This specific inhibitory action on the 'proton pump' provides a highly selective method of controlling acid secretion. Substituted benzimidazoles are lipophilic weak bases that are absorbed from the small intestine and reach the gastric parietal cells through the bloodstream. Since PPIs are unchanged at physiological pH, they can cross cell membranes; however, in the acidic milieu of the canaliculus of the actively secreting gastric parietal cell, the compounds are exposed to a pH less than 2, cease to be lipophilic, and are trapped and concentrated. PPIs by themselves do not inhibit H^+/K^+-ATPase but at low pH the protonated forms undergo a conversion to a cationic sulfenamide, the active form of the drugs. The sulfenamide reacts with cysteines on the extracellular surface of the proton pump and inactivates the enzyme. This binding is covalent and is irreversible in vivo; acid secretion resumes only with synthesis of new H^+/K^+-ATPase protein. Since in humans the half-life of the proton pump appears to be approximately 18 h, this explains why the antisecretory effect of PPIs is long-lasting.

The pharmacokinetics of the four PPIs currently available is somewhat similar with all of these compounds, exhibiting a short (about 1 h) terminal half-life and a high proportion of protein binding. Lansoprazole and pantoprazole appear to have a better bioavailability, while dose-linearity is found only with pantoprazole and rabeprazole (Table 1.3). While food does not appear to change the bioavailability of PPIs, concomitant administration of antacids delays absorption of omeprazole and lansoprazole. Omeprazole, lansoprazole and to some extent, pantoprazole are metabolized by the cytochrome P_{450} system and the inactive metabolites excreted in the urine. However, dosage adjustments are not usually necessary in hepatic or renal failure.

Table 1.3   Comparative pharmacokinetics of the currently available PPIs.

	Omeprazole (20 mg)	Lansoprazole (30 mg)	Pantoprazole (40 mg)	Rabeprazole (20 mg)
$T_{1/2}$ (h)	0.7	1.3	1.0	1.0
Bioavailability (%)	37–60	80	77	52
Protein binding (%)	95	97	98	96
Dose linearity	No	No	Yes	Yes

Table 1.4   Interaction of the different PPIs with food, antacids and cytochrome P_{450} system.

Drug	Interactions with		
	Food	Antacids	Cytochrome P_{450} system
Omeprazole	No	Yes*	Yes†
Lansoprazole	No	Yes*	Yes†
Pantoprazole	No	No	No
Rabeprazole	No	No	No

*Delayed absorption (little effect on bioavailability).
†Little clinical relevance.

Although of little clinical relevance, the interaction of omeprazole and lansoprazole with the cytochrome P_{450} system should be taken into account when drugs like diazepam are given concomitantly. The more recent PPIs (namely pantoprazole and rabeprazole) appear almost completely free of drug-to-drug interactions (Table 1.4).

The inhibitory effect of PPIs on acid secretion has been established by many studies. However, in contrast to what happens with H_2-receptor antagonists there is frequently a nocturnal breakthrough, that is, a period during which gastric pH remains below pH 4.[35] The addition of ranitidine (150 or 300 mg at night) to ongoing treatment with omeprazole was found to be extremely effective against this nocturnal acid breakthrough phenomenon. Although the relevance of this phenomenon in GORD is presently unknown, it is worthwhile to attempt addition of an H_2-receptor antagonist in Barrett's patients with oesophagitis who respond unsatisfactorily to treatment with a PPI.

Adverse reactions
PPIs as a class have few side-effects. Headache, diarrhoea, nausea and vomiting, constipation, abdominal pain, rashes and dry mouth occur occasionally. Rarely do fever, increase in liver enzymes, hepatitis, hepatic failure, hepatic encephalopathy, toxic epidermal necrolysis, erythema multiforme, urticaria, angio-oedema, taste disturbance, oesophageal candidiasis, alopecia, increased

sweating, depression, agitation, confusion, hallucinations, haematological changes (e.g. leucopenia, agranulocytosis, pancytopenia, thrombocytopenia), interstitial nephritis, gynaecomastia, and impotence occur.

Precautions and contraindications

PPIs appear in breast milk and should be avoided in breastfeeding patients. There are no studies to guide their use in pregnancy and, in general, should be avoided in pregnant patients. Contraindications to PPIs include previous hypersensitivity to the drug.

Short-term efficacy of PPIs in GORD

A meta-analysis of 43 therapeutic trials[36] conducted in patients with moderate to severe oesophagitis has confirmed the clear advantage of PPI over H_2-receptor antagonists, as previously and consistently reported in numerous well-designed individual controlled trials. The proportion of patients successfully treated was nearly double, and the rapidity of healing and symptom relief was approximately twice as fast using PPI, than H_2-receptor antagonists (Table 1.5). The superiority of PPI is obvious, not only in severe cases or in patients refractory to H_2-receptor antagonists but also in patients with mild oesophagitis and in endoscopy-negative patients.[37,38] Quality of life is restored to normal after 4–6 weeks of PPI therapy.[39] Although few studies are available,[40] omeprazole (20 mg or 10 mg daily) clearly provides better results than cisapride (10 mg four times daily).

Efficacy of PPIs in the long-term

Continuous maintenance therapy with PPI is extremely effective when used as a prophylaxis. PPIs are superior to H_2-receptor antagonists, cisapride or a combination of the two.[24] The results of a recent meta-analysis including more than 1200 patients[41] showed that after 6 months of maintenance therapy with 20 mg or 10 mg omeprazole daily, approximately 80% and 70% of patients, respectively, were still in remission. These figures are clearly superior to those obtained with ranitidine or PPI weekend therapy, which is not very effective (Fig. 1.4). Interestingly, as the relief of heartburn during PPI treatment is highly predictive of healing, there is no need for endoscopic monitoring in asymptomatic patients, unless initial endoscopy shows severe oesophagitis or premalignant conditions such as Barrett's oesophagus.[41]

In the primary care setting, intermittent on-demand therapy with omeprazole has also provided excellent results for symptom relief and quality of life. In several countries, PPIs are now available in low dosages for symptomatic treatment of GORD (e.g. omeprazole 10 mg, or lansoprazole 15 mg).

Complications of GORD

In patients with peptic stricture, PPIs are the drug of choice. In a large controlled trial,[15] after endoscopic dilation, more patients were relieved of their dysphagia and returned to a normal diet with a therapeutic regimen of omeprazole

---

Table 1.5 Proportion and speed of healing and symptom relief in moderate to severe esophagitis. Data from a meta-analysis[36] of 7635 patients.

	H_2-receptor antagonist	PPI
Healed (% ± SE)	51.9 ± 17.1	83.6 ± 11.4
Symptom free (% ± SE)	47.6 ± 15.5	77.4 ± 10.4
Rate of healing (%/week ± SE)	5.9 ± 0.2	11.7 ± 0.5
Rate of symptom relief (%/week ± SE)	6.4 ± 0.5	11.5 ± 0.8

SE, standard error of the mean.

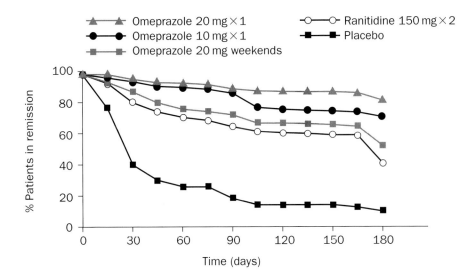

Figure 1.4 Efficacy of long-term treatment for prevention of relapse oesophagitis. Results of a meta-analysis of long-term trials with omeprazole (adapted from Carlsson R et al[41]).

40 mg once daily than with ranitidine 150 mg twice daily. PPIs are also more cost-effective[42] than H$_2$-receptor antagonists and represent the dominant strategy, especially in the older patients.

In patients with Barrett's oesophagus and symptoms of GORD and/or mucosal breaks at endoscopy, PPIs effectively relieve heartburn and heal lesions of oesophagitis.[43] However, even after very prolonged acid suppression with high doses (e.g. lansoprazole 60 mg for 4 years) there is no evidence of complete regression of metaplasia.[16] In some cases, partial regression of intestinal metaplasia and/or replacement by islands of squamous epithelium have been reported. Finally, it is clear that PPI monotherapy is unable to induce clinically relevant regression of metaplasia. Recently, several studies have tested the effects of photo or thermal ablation of Barrett's metaplasia in the anacidic environment provided by high-dose PPI. Although preliminary results are encouraging, further experience is necessary before recommending this approach in routine practice.[16,44]

Safety of PPIs

Although PPIs are extremely well-tolerated

drugs, there is some concern about the risks of potent acid suppression in the long-term.[45]

The occurrence of bacterial intraluminal overgrowth of the small intestine, of infectious diarrhoea or vitamin B$_{12}$ malabsorption is possible during prolonged antisecretory treatment. These disturbances have, in most cases, no significant clinical consequences, and should therefore not be taken into consideration in treatment indications and surveillance.

Hypergastrinemia and hyperplasia of fundic endocrine cells can be induced by powerful and prolonged antisecretory treatments. There have not, however, been any significant clinical consequences during 10 years of clinical use. Surveillance of serum gastrin levels and gastric histology in patients with long-standing PPI treatment is not recommended in clinical practice.

Cost-effectiveness of PPIs

As already emphasized, PPIs definitively represent the most cost-effective drug therapy in patients with severe oesophagitis or complications like peptic stricture. Whether the same holds true in mild moderate disease is, however, more controversial. Should a step-down strategy be applied (i.e. going directly to

PPIs) or a step-up strategy, starting with less effective drugs (e.g. H_2-receptor antagonists or cisapride) and therefore limiting PPI treatment to patients refractory to that initial therapy?

Reports, based on retrospective database analysis and mathematical models, have been conflicting.[46,47] Although the direct cost of PPIs is higher than with other drugs, it is important to remember that indirect costs (e.g. those related to absenteeism) must be considered in a frequently chronic disease like GORD. Finally PPIs seems increasingly more cost-effective as the severity of the disease increases.[48] Once again, 'severity' refers to the whole spectrum of the disease (including endoscopy-negative GORD), not only to the severity of oesophagitis.

CONCLUSIONS AND PERSPECTIVES FOR THE FUTURE

With the development of PPIs, considerable progress has been achieved in the treatment of GORD. Several therapeutic needs are still unmet, however. For example, none of the pro-kinetic drugs currently available are able to correct the underlying motor disorders, especially the rate of TLOSRs. Moreover, even after complete symptom relief and endoscopic healing of oesophagitis with an effective PPI regimen, the disease is not cured, as shown by the frequent relapses observed in many patients. Finally, although the pathogenesis of GORD is now better understood, its aetiology remains unclear. The role of *Helicobacter pylori* is still an area of active research but, so far, there is no evidence that this bacterium plays an important role in the aetiopathogenesis of GORD.

Even if it is reasonable in practice to treat all patients with acid suppression in the first instance, it is crucial to bear in mind the variety of pathophysiological factors that may eventually affect outcome and therapeutic response. Factors such as refluxate composition, mechanisms of mucosal defence, and oesophageal sensitivity may be extremely important, especially for the small subset of patients who fail to respond to an adequate antisecretory regimen.

All of these mechanisms represent potential targets for drug development and future anti-reflux therapy (Table 1.1).

REFERENCES

1. Dent J. Gastro-oesophageal reflux disease. *Digestion* 1998; **59:** 433–445.
2. Locke GR, Talley NJ, Fett SL, Zinsmeister AR, Melton LJ. Prevalence and clinical spectrum of gastroesophageal reflux: a population-based study in Olmsted County, Minnesota. *Gastroenterology* 1997; **112:** 1448–1456.
3. Galmiche JP, Letessier E, Scarpignato C. Treatment of gastro-oesophageal reflux disease in adults. *Brit Med J* 1998; **316:** 1720–1723.
4. Dent J, Brun J, Fendrick M, *et al*. An evidence-based appraisal of reflux disease management—The Genval Workshop Report. *Gut* 1999; **44 (Suppl. 2):** S1–S16.
5. McDougall NI, Johnston BT, Kee F, Collins JSA, McFarland RJ, Love AHG. Natural history of reflux oesophagitis: a 10-year follow-up of its effect on patient symptomatology and quality of life. *Gut* 1996; **38:** 481–486.
6. Galmiche JP, Zerbib F. Mechanisms of gastro-oesophageal reflux disease (GORD) and potential targets for anti-reflux therapy. In: *New Horizons in Gastrointestinal and Liver Disease: Mechanisms and Management*. MJG Farthing, G Bianchi Porro (Eds), John Libbey Eurotext, Paris, 1999, 3–15.
7. Mittal RK, Balaban DH. The esophagogastric junction. *N Engl J Med* 1997; **336:** 924–932.
8. Champion G, Richter JE, Vaezi MF, Singh S, Alexander R. Duodenogastroesophageal reflux: relationship to pH and importance in Barrett's esophagus. *Gastroenterology* 1994; **107:** 747–754.
9. Malfertheiner P, Gerards C. The role of *Helicobacter pylori* in gastroesophageal reflux disease. In: *Gastroenterology and Hepatology. The Next Millenium*. GNJ Tytgat, GJ Krejs (Eds), John Libbey Eurotext, Paris, 1998, 77–87.
10. Labenz J, Tillenburg B, Peitz U, *et al*. *Helicobacter pylori* augments the pH-increasing effect of omeprazole in patients with duodenal ulcer. *Gastroenterology* 1996; **110:** 725–732.
11. Gillen D, Wirz AA, Neithercut WD, Ardill JES, McColl KEL. *Helicobacter pylori* infection potentiates the inhibition of gastric acid secretion by omeprazole. *Gut* 1999; **44:** 468–475.

12. French–Belgian Consensus Conference on Adult Gastro-Oesophageal Reflux Disease 'Diagnosis and Treatment'. *Eur J Gastroenterol Hepatol* 2000; **12:** 129–137.

13. Orlando RC. Why is the high-grade inhibition of gastric acid secretion afforded by proton pump inhibitors often required for healing of reflux esophagitis? An epithelial perspective. *Am J Gastroenterol* 1996; **91:** 1692–1696.

14. Kuster E, Ros E, Toledo-Pimentel V, *et al.* Predictive factors of the long-term outcome in gastro-oesophageal reflux disease: six-year follow-up of 107 patients. *Gut* 1994; **35:** 8–14.

15. Smith PM, Kerr GD, Cockel R, *et al.* A comparison of omeprazole and ranitidine in the prevention of recurrence of benign esophageal stricture. *Gastroenterology* 1994; **107:** 1312–1318.

16. Triadafilopoulos G. Proton pump inhibitors for Barrett's oesophagus. *Gut* 2000; **46:** 144–146.

17. Scarpignato C, Galmiche JP. Antacids and alginates in the treatment of gastroesophageal reflux disease: how do they work and how much are they clinically useful? In: *Advances in Drug Therapy of Gastroesophageal Reflux Disease.* C. Scarpignato (Ed.), Front Gastrointest Research, Karger Basel, 1992; **20:** 153–181.

18. Washington N. *Handbook of Antacids and Anti-reflux agents.* CRC Press, Boca Raton, 1991.

19. Poynard T, and the French Co-operative Study Group. Relapse rate of patients after healing of oesophagitis—a prospective study of alginate as self-care treatment for 6 months. *Aliment Pharmacol Ther* 1993; **7:** 385–392.

20. Zerbib F, Bruley des Varannes S, Scarpignato C, Leray V, D'amato M, Rozé C, Galmiche JP. Endogenous cholecystokinin in postprandial lower esophageal sphincter function and fundic tone in humans. *Am J Physiol* 1998; **275:** G1266–G1273.

21. Goldin GF, Marcinkiewicz M, Zbroch T, Bityutskiy LP, McCallum RW, Sarosiek J. Esophago-protective potential of cisapride. An additional benefit for gastroesophageal reflux disease. *Dig Dis Sci* 1997; **42:** 1362–1369.

22. Blum AL, Adami B, Bouzo MH, Branstatter G, Fumagalli I, Galmiche JP. Effect of cisapride on relapse of esophagitis. A multinational placebo-controlled trial in patients healed with an antisecretory drug. *Dig Dis Sci* 1993; **38:** 551–560.

23. Tytgat GNJ, Janssens J, Reynolds JF, Wienbeck M. Update on the pathophysiology and management of gastro-oesophageal reflux disease: the role of prokinetic therapy. *Eur J Gastroenterol Hepatol* 1996; **8:** 603–611.

24. Vigneri S, Termini R, Leandro G, *et al.* A comparison of five maintenance therapies for reflux esophagitis. *N Engl J Med* 1995; **333:** 1106–1110.

25. Scarpignato C, Galmiche JP. The role of H_2-receptor antagonists in the era of proton pump inhibitors. In: *Guidelines for Management of Symptomatic Gastro-oesophageal Reflux Disease.* L. Lundell (Ed.), Science Press, London, 1998, 55–66.

26. Colin-Jones DG. The role and limitations of H_2-receptor antagonists in the treatment of gastro-oesophageal reflux disease. *Aliment Pharmacol Ther* 1995; **9 (Suppl. 1):** 9–14.

27. Galmiche JP, Shi G, Simon B, Casset-Semanaz F, Slama A. On-demand treatment of gastro-oesophageal reflux symptoms: a study comparing ranitidine 75 mg with placebo and cimetidine 200 mg. *Aliment Pharmacol Ther* 1998; **12:** 909–917.

28. Tytgat GNJ, Nicolai JJ; Reman FC. Efficacy of different doses of cimetidine in the treatment of reflux esophagitis. A review of three large, double-blind, controlled trials. *Gastroenterology* 1990; **99:** 629–634.

29. Koelz HR, Birchler R, Bretholz A, *et al.* Healing and relapse of reflux esophagitis during treatment with ranitidine. *Gastroenterology* 1986; **91:** 1198–1205.

30. Simon TJ, Roberts WG, Berlin RG, Hayden LJ, Berman RS, Reagan JE. Acid suppression by famotidine 20 mg twice daily or 40 mg twice daily in preventing relapse of endoscopic recurrence of erosive esophagitis. *Clin Ther* 1995; **17(6):** 1147–1156.

31. Holt S. Over-the-counter histamine H_2-receptor antagonists. How will they affect the treatment of acid-related diseases? *Drugs* 1994; **47(1):** 1–11.

32. Wilde MI, McTavish D. Omeprazole. An update of its pharmacology and therapeutic use in acid-related disorders. *Drugs* 1994; **48(1):** 91–132.

33. Langtry HD, Wilde MI. Lansoprazole. An update of its pharmacological properties and clinical efficacy in the management of acid-related disorders. *Drugs* 1997; **54(3):** 473–500.

34. Koop H, Schepp W, Dammann HG, Schneider A, Lühmann R, Classen M. Comparative trial of pantoprazole and ranitidine in the treatment of reflux esophagitis. *J Clin Gastroenterol* 1995; **20(3):** 192–195.

35. Peghini PL, Katz PO, Castell DO. Ranitidine controls nocturnal gastric acid breakthrough on

omeprazole: a controlled study in normal subjects. *Gastroenterology* 1998; **115:** 1335–1339.

36. Chiba N, De Cara CJ, Wilkinson JM, Hunt RH. Speed of healing and symptom relief in grade II to IV gastroesophageal reflux disease: a meta-analysis. *Gastroenterology* 1997; **112:** 1798–1810.

37. Bate CM, Griffin SM, Keeling PWN, *et al*. Reflux symptom relief with omeprazole in patients without unequivocal oesophagitis. *Aliment Pharmacol Ther* 1996; **10:** 547–555.

38. Watson RG, Tham TC, Johnston BT, McDougall NI. Double blind cross-over placebo controlled study of omeprazole in the treatment of patients with reflux symptoms and physiological levels of acid reflux—the 'sensitive oesophagus'. *Gut* 1997; **40:** 587–590.

39. Carlsson R, Dent J, Watts R, *et al*. Gastro-oesophageal reflux disease in primary care: an international study of different treatment strategies with omeprazole. *Eur J Gastroenterol Hepatol* 1998; **10:** 119–124.

40. Galmiche JP, Barthélémy P, Hamelin B. Treating the symptoms of gastroesophageal reflux disease: a double-blind comparison of omeprazole and cisapride. *Aliment Pharmacol Ther* 1997; **11:** 765–773.

41. Carlsson R, Galmiche JP, Dent J, Lundell L, Frison L. Prognostic factors influencing relapse of oesophagitis during maintenance therapy with antisecretory drugs: a meta-analysis of long-term omeprazole trials. *Aliment Pharmacol* 1997; **11(3):** 473–482.

42. Marks RD, Richter JE, Rizzo J, *et al*. Omeprazole versus H_2-receptor antagonists in treating patients with peptic stricture and esophagitis. *Gastroenterology* 1994; **106:** 907–915.

43. Sontag DJ, Schnell TG, Chejfec G, Kurucar C, Karpf J, Levine G. Lansoprazole heals erosive reflux oesophagitis inpatients with Barrett oesophagus. *Aliment Pharmacol Ther* 1997; **11:** 147–156.

44. Gossner L, Stolte M, Sroka R, *et al*. Photodynamic ablation of high-grade dysplasia and early cancer in Barrett's esophagus by means of 5-aminolevulinic acid. *Gastroenterology* 1998; **114:** 448–455.

45. Klinkenberg-Knol EC, Festen HPM, Jansen JBMJ, *et al*. Long-term treatment with omeprazole for refractory reflux esophagitis: efficacy and safety. *Ann Intern Med* 1994; **121:** 161–167.

46. Eggleston A, Wigerinck A, Huijghebaert S, Dubois D, Haycox A. Cost-effectiveness of treatment for gastro-oesophageal reflux disease in clinical practice: a clinical database analysis. *Gut* 1998; **42:** 13–16.

47. Heudebert GR, Marks R, Wicox CM, Centor RM. Choice of long-term strategy for the management of patients with severe esophagitis: a cost utility analysis. *Gastroenterology* 1997; **112:** 1078–1086.

48. Harris RA, Kuppermann M, Richter JE. Proton pump inhibitors or histamine-$_2$ receptor antagonists for the prevention of recurrences of erosive reflux esophagitis: a cost-effectiveness analysis. *Am J Gastroenterol* 1997; **92:** 2179–2187.

2

Peptic ulcer disease

Erik AJ Rauws, Guido NJ Tytgat

INTRODUCTION

There are five causes of peptic ulcers:

1. *Helicobacter pylori*-associated peptic ulcer disease (PUD);
2. Non-steroidal anti-inflammatory drug (NSAID)-associated ulcers;
3. Pathological hypersecretory ulcers (e.g. gastrinoma, idiopathic hypersecretory states);
4. Idiopathic PUD; and
5. Miscellaneous causes (Crohn's disease, infection with *H. heilmanii* or viral infections).

In this overview we will focus on the management of *H. pylori*-associated PUD, because the majority of gastroduodenal ulcers in the absence of salicylate or NSAIDs, are related to *H. pylori*. NSAIDs are also a major cause of ulceration. Patients on long-term NSAID treatment have gastric erosions in 20–40%, gastric ulcers in 10–25% and/or duodenal ulcers in 2–5%. However, it is being increasingly recognized that ulcers can occur apparently in the absence of *H. pylori* infection or the use of NSAIDs; these are so-called *idiopathic* ulcers.

H$_2$-receptor antagonists (H$_2$RA) and proton pump inhibitors (PPIs), were shown to be very useful in the treatment of PUD. PPIs are superior to H$_2$RAs both for healing and for maintenance. These drugs are effective because they suppress acid but do not cure the ulcer disease diathesis.[1–3] In duodenal ulcer patients in whom treatment was stopped after 8 weeks, the relapse rate, as determined by endoscopy, was 80% at 1 year and 100% at 2 years.[4] Even patients on maintenance ranitidine (150 mg at night) had a cumulative ulcer relapse after 1 year of 48%.[5] In all patients in whom gastric or duodenal ulcer has been confirmed, the presence of *H. pylori*, and preferably the antimicrobial sensitivity, should be determined, with subsequent short (i.e. 7 days) antimicrobial therapy to cure ulcer disease. PPIs are presently recommended for both the prevention and treatment of gastroduodenal ulcers associated with NSAID use.

PATHOPHYSIOLOGY

Duodenitis and duodenal ulceration

Duodenal ulcer is a multifactorial condition. The aetiology is closely related to enhanced acid secretion, but has been found to be influenced by many other factors, including gender, genetic predisposition, alcohol consumption, drug intake, smoking and, most recently, *H. pylori* infection. The pathogenesis of duodenal ulcer consists of a sequence of several synergistic pathogenetic events. Most duodenal ulcer patients have antral-predominant active chronic gastritis and are colonized by usually virulent (CagA and VacA-positive) *H. pylori* strains.[6–8] Antral *H. pylori* infection impairs the inhibitory feedback control of acid secretion, leading, when combined with increased gastric emptying, to increased duodenal acid load. As a non-specific response to acid injury, gastric metaplasia develops in the duodenum. When *H. pylori* colonizes these foci of gastric metaplasia in the duodenum, active duodenitis develops.[9,10] If duodenitis becomes severe and the inflamed mucosa can no longer maintain its integrity, occasionally and together with other offensive factors (i.e. NSAID), ulcers may develop. The extent of gastric metaplasia is related to the gastric acid output.[10] Duodenitis is resistant to treatment aimed at reducing acidity[11] and healed duodenal ulcers are not accompanied by histologically normal duodenal mucosa. Ulcer healing by itself does not change gastric metaplasia. As in chronic gastritis, the eradication of *H. pylori* leads to resolution of duodenal inflammation.[12] The duodenal ulcer heals, the mucosal defence is restored and in the absence of *H. pylori* infection there is no further ulcer relapse. Acid secretion incompletely returns to normal following cure of the infection, probably the explanation for the regularly observed incomplete resolution of gastric metaplasia.

Gastritis and gastric ulcer

In patients with gastric ulceration, usually a different pattern of gastritis is seen. Gastritis is not confined to the antrum as in duodenal ulcers, but usually extends to the corpus mucosa with varying degrees of atrophy. This impairs the ability of the corpus mucosa to secrete acid. Although inflammation of the antrum stimulates increased gastrin release in these patients, the corpus of the stomach is unable to respond to the gastrin stimulus. Usually, the acid output of gastric ulcer patients is rather low and there-fore excess acid is not the cause of proximal gastric ulcers. It is most likely that the marked *H. pylori*-induced inflammation in the acid-secreting mucosa impairs its resistance to local acid production, even at low levels. Once *H. pylori* has been eradicated, acid secretion improves, sometimes to normal levels.

In Western countries, it is becoming rare to diagnose *H. pylori*-induced gastric ulcer. The majority of today's gastric ulcers, especially complicated ulcers, are drug-induced through the use of aspirin and other non-steroidal anti-flammatory drugs (NSAIDs). Covert or surreptitious intake of these drugs is responsible for a substantial number of *H. pylori*-negative gastric ulcers. NSAID use is associated with reactive gastritis (foveolar hyperplasia, oedema, splaying muscle fibres in the lamina propria, vasodilatation, congestion and paucity of inflammatory cells) in 26–45% of users. Why reactive gastritis develops in some patients when using NSAIDs is unclear but it is not *H. pylori*-associated. The effect of *H. pylori* on NSAID-related gastroduodenal mucosal injury may be established best by evaluating the ulcer recurrence rate after *H. pylori* eradication and subsequent rechallenge with NSAIDs. Whether the pathophysiologic interaction between *H. pylori* and NSAIDs is clinically relevant needs more appropriate clinical trials in patients at risk for ulcers and related complications.[13]

THERAPY OF PEPTIC ULCER THROUGH ACID SUPPRESSION

H$_2$-receptor antagonists

The occupation of H$_2$-receptors by histamine released from mast- and possibly enterochromaffin-like (ECL) cells, activates adenylate cyclase, increasing the intracellular concentrations of cyclic AMP. These increased levels of cyclic AMP activate the proton pump of the parietal cell, to secrete hydrogen ions against a concentration gradient in exchange for potassium ions. H$_2$RAs competitively and selectively inhibit the binding of histamine to the receptor, reducing the intracellular concentrations of cyclic AMP and the secretion of acid by the parietal cells. H_2RAs only partially inhibit the gastrin- or acetylcholine-stimulated acid secretion, probably through a reduction in the potentiation of secretion that occurs in response to simultaneous histamine, gastrin and acetylcholine stimulation.[14]

Proton-pump inhibitors

The proton pump, also called the H^+, K^+-ATPase, is only found on the secretory membrane of the parietal cell. The secretion of hydrochloric acid by the parietal cells finally depends on the proton pump. After activation of the parietal cell, irrespective of the type or route of the stimulus, the H^+, K^+-ATP-ase translocate to the plasma membrane of the secretory canaliculus of the parietal cells. The extracellular aspect of the pump is so exposed to potassium ions and, because of a concomitant increased permeability of the membrane to potassium, the parietal cells are able to secrete acid. PPIs inhibit the activity of H^+, K^+-ATP-ase. PPIs dose-dependently control the gastric acid secretion with a greater antisecretory activity than H_2RA. Meta-analyses have shown a close correlation between reduction of the intragastric acidity and ulcer healing.[15,16] Suppression of nocturnal acidity appears to be of major importance for duodenal ulcer healing.

Acid suppression and ulcer healing

Meta-analyses show that healing occurs in almost all duodenal ulcer patients within 4 weeks if the intragastric milieu is kept above pH 3 for 18 h daily.[15] All available H_2RA (e.g. cimetidine; ranitidine; famotidine; nizatidine and roxatidine), when used in the standard doses, are capable of healing duodenal ulcers to the same degree.[17–21] The rates of complete ulcer healing after 2, 4 and 8 weeks of therapy averages 50%, 80% and 90% respectively. Refractory duodenal ulcers (not healed after 3 months or

more of standard-dose H_2 RA) occur in about 5% of the patients. The cause for refractoriness is rarely found. Acid hypersecretion (Zollinger-Ellison syndrome) is observed only rarely and cannot be responsible for all refractory ulcers. In a few patients inadequate acid suppression has been reported despite high-dose H_2RA. Occasionally, aspirin or NSAIDs, sometimes taken surreptitiously are responsible for refractoriness. Refractory duodenal ulcers usually heal after doubling the dose of H_2RA or, more effectively, after switching to more potent acid inhibition using PPIs.

Compared with duodenal ulcer, healing of *gastric ulcer* is less closely related to acid suppression. All H_2RAs are equally effective in healing gastric ulcers, with healing rates of 60%, 75% and 90% after 4, 6 and 8 weeks, respectively. All gastric ulcers should be biopsied and complete healing should be confirmed since 2–5% of gastric ulcers that appear benign are in fact malignant.[22] Refractory gastric ulcers, if not malignant, often result from the use of aspirin or NSAIDs. However, double-dose H_2RA or PPIs heal these ulcers, although often after more prolonged therapy even if in patients who continue these drugs.

The rates of *duodenal ulcer* healing after 2, 4 and 8 weeks of standard-dose PPI averages 75%, 95% and 100%.[23] Despite the efficacy of PPIs in the treatment of duodenal ulcers, ulcer relapses appear to be similar to those after short-term H_2RA therapy in 30–75% within 6 months.[24] The superiority of PPIs over H_2RAs have been confirmed in many comparative studies. The rates of gastric ulcer healing after 4 and 8 weeks of PPI therapy averages 85% and 98%, respectively. Almost all gastric ulcers heal after standard-dose PPI after 8–12 weeks, even in patients who continue to take NSAIDs. It should be stated that all ulcer-healing data with acid suppressants were obtained mainly in *H. pylori*-infected patients. Whether the efficacy of H_2RAs and PPIs is of the same magnitude in *H. pylori*-negative ulcers is unknown but probably inferior.

Acid suppression and maintenance therapy

Until recently, the management of ulcers consisted of relatively short-term treatment with an acid suppressant drug to heal the ulcer followed by long-term maintenance treatment to prevent ulcer relapses. Ulcer recurrences during maintenance treatment are often painless and may reheal spontaneously during continued therapy. Symptomatic recurrences of duodenal ulcers during maintenance treatment with either 150 mg/day or 300 mg/day ranitidine was 5% at 1 year, 12% at 3 years, 14% at 5 years and 19% at 7 and 9 years.[5,25] PPIs are also superior to H$_2$RAs for ulcer maintenance therapy.[26] In *H. pylori*-positive patients, eradication of *H. pylori* is recommended to prevent ulcer relapses, without the need for any expensive maintenance therapy. However, some patients are *H. pylori* treatment-failures, some continue to experience ulcer relapses despite *H. pylori* eradication, others have co-morbid conditions that increase the risk of recurrences or complications, or are unwilling to complete an anti-*H. pylori* treatment regimen and still need maintenance therapy.

H. PYLORI-NEGATIVE ULCERS

H. pylori-negative duodenal ulcers are rare and should not be confused with false negativity. False-negative testing may occur if inadequate mucosal biopsies are taken or if the patient has or still is taking medication that suppresses *H. pylori*, such as bismuth or PPIs. Some *H. pylori*-negative ulcers may arise as a consequence of false-negative tests, but other factors such as covert or surreptitious intake of over-the-counter aspirin and NSAIDs, acid hypersecretion and idiopathic factors remain important in ulcerogenesis. If all other factors have been eliminated, true *H. pylori*-negative ulcers are rare, and are characterized by a high serum gastrin, high acid-secretory capacity and rapid gastric emptying.[27,28] In these rare cases, ulcer healing and maintenance acid suppressant therapy are indicated.

Interestingly, retrospective data from the USA, reported high proportions of *H. pylori*-negative ulcers.[29] Once NSAID use was excluded, *H. pylori* could not be detected by a variety of diagnostic tests in 39% of duodenal ulcer and 39% of gastric ulcer patients. All adequate explanation for these findings is lacking but may be due to regional variations in *H. pylori* prevalence.

ERADICATION OF *H. PYLORI* AND ULCER HEALING

Until recently, the management of peptic ulcers consisted of short-term acid suppressive therapy for healing followed by long-term maintenance therapy for prevention of ulcer relapse. More than 90% of patients with peptic ulcer are infected with *H. pylori* and it has been shown that successful eradication therapy prevents ulcer relapse and ulcer-associated complications.[30] These observations have radically changed the therapeutic options for peptic ulcer disease from acid suppressive therapy to antimicrobial therapy. All available guidelines recommend eradication of *H. pylori* infection in patients with *H. pylori*-associated peptic ulcer. All *H. pylori*-positive ulcers should be treated, whether the ulcer is active or in remission. This concurs with the European 1996 Maastricht consensus,[31] the 1997 American Digestive Health Foundation International Update Conference[32] and the 1997 Asia Pacific Consensus Conference on the Management of *H. pylori* infection.[33]

There are many randomized controlled trials reporting the efficacy of various combinations of antibiotics and acid-suppressive agents as *H. pylori* eradication regimens.[34,35] The ideal anti-*H. pylori* regimen should be safe, effective, cheap, easy to comply with and well-tolerated. However, none of the drug combinations are able to eradicate *H. pylori* infection in more than 85% of the patients according to intention-to-treat analysis (ITT). The most important factors influencing the efficacy of a therapy are the presence of primary antimicrobial resistance and the level of patient compliance. Treatment regimens are usually classified according to the number of therapeutic agents used. The best of these regimens are PPI, or ranitidine bismuth citrate (RBC)-based triple therapies that provide 85–95% eradication rates in most studies if assessed per-protocol (Table 2.1).

Monotherapy

Monotherapy should never been used to eradicate *H. pylori* because of the unacceptably low efficacy with the available drugs and the frequent emergence of secondary bacterial resistance in those who fail to eradicate the micro-organism. Clarithromycin is currently both in vitro and in vivo the most effective antibiotic against *H. pylori* with eradication rates around 50%, but leads in two out of three failures to clarithromycin resistance.

Dual therapy

Dual therapies comprise use of a PPI or H$_2$RA plus one antibiotic—initially amoxycillin but more recently clarithromycin. Dual therapy gives variable results, usually below 70% and has now been superseded by more effective regimens. Another dual therapy is the combination of ranitidine bismuth citrate (RBC) with clarithromycin given for 14 days. RBC is a salt of ranitidine in which the bismuth and citrate form a complex citrato-bismuth anion, with ranitidine as the cation, which has a high degree of aqueous solubility. It is believed that the greater solubility of RBC especially at lower pH is highly relevant to its superior antipepsin and anti-*H. pylori* effect.[36] The most effective dosing schedule is RBC 400 mg twice daily with clarithromycin 500 mg twice daily for 14 days and reported ITT eradication rates ranging from 76% to 96%. Although effective, 2 weeks of high-dose clarithromycin is expensive and has significant side-effects, which influence compliance negatively.

Triple therapy

Bismuth-based triple therapy comprising a bismuth compound, metronidazole, and tetracycline (or amoxycillin), was used for years as 'the standard' therapy. This regimen is given for 14 days and can achieve eradication rates above 90%. Bismuth (colloidal bismuth subcitrate; bismuth subsalicylate) is usually given four times daily, tetracycline 500 mg four times daily, while metronidazole dosages vary from 200–500 mg three times daily. Patients with metronidazole-resistant strains treated with bismuth-tetracycline-metronidazole for 1 or 2 weeks, showed significantly lower eradication rates than patients with metronidazole-sensitive strains, with a mean decrease in efficacy from 97% to 44%.[37,38] Empiric bismuth-based triple therapy for 7 days can be used safely in areas with a known low prevalence of metronidazole resistance at relatively low cost. In areas with a high prevalence of metronidazole resistance, the course should be extended for 14 days, although better eradication rates can be achieved using alternative regimens without imidazoles or by adding acid suppression (quadruple therapy) to bismuth-based triple therapies. Interestingly, on increasing the dose of metronidazole in bismuth-based triple therapy from 375 mg to 750 mg per day, the *H. pylori* eradication rates increased from 52% to 84% in metronidazole-sensitive strains and in metronidazole-resistant strains from 39% to 64%.[39] Bismuth-based triple therapy has a high rate of side-effects ranging from 7% to 72%,[40] but only 3–3.5% of the patients have to discontinue the therapy as a result of adverse events.[41] The use of bismuth-based triple therapy has declined because of its complexity (4-times daily dosing) and side-effects. Bismuth-based triple therapy is relatively cheap and can be valuable in areas where resources are limited; unfortunately, in these areas metronidazole-resistance is high, leading to poor results.

An alternative can be ranitidine-bismuth-citrate (RBC), which combines the acid-suppressive properties of ranitidine with the antibacterial-cytoprotective properties of

Table 2.1 *H. pylori* eradication rates with certain treatment regimens.

Primary antimicrobial resistance	Advised regimen	*H. pylori* eradication rate (%)
Metronidazole <30% Clarithromycin <15%	Proton pump inhibitor + clarithromycin (500 mg) + amoxycillin Proton pump inhibitor + clarithromycin (250 mg or 500 mg) + metronidazole Ranitidine bismuth citrate or colloidal bismuth citrate (or bismuth subsalicylate) + clarithromycin (500 mg) + metronidazole	85–95
Metronidazole >30% Clarithromycin <15%	Proton pump inhibitor + clarithromycin (500 mg) + amoxycillin Ranitidine bismuth citrate or colloidal bismuth citrate (or bismuth subsalicylate) + clarithromycin (500 mg) + amoxycillin	85–95
Metronidazole >30% Clarithromycin >15%	Proton pump inhibitor + colloidal bismuth citrate (or bismuth subsalicylate) + metronidazole + tetracycline	50–95

bismuth. RBC has proven to be efficacious for the eradication of *H. pylori* when used in combination with two antibiotics (clarithromycin 250 mg daily or tetracycline 500 mg twice daily[42] or amoxycillin 1 g twice daily[43] for 7 days only. The observed ITT eradication rates with the 7-day regimens ranged from 71% to 100%. The *H. pylori* eradication rates for RBC and metronidazole with clarithromycin or tetracycline appear not significantly affected by the sensitivity to metronidazole.[44] RBC-based triple therapy for 7 days containing clarithromycin with either metronidazole or tetracyclin is a simple, effective and well-tolerated regimen for the treatment of *H. pylori* infection. The efficacy of this regimen when there is clarithromycin resistance has not been well-studied, but current data suggest that RBC-clarithromycin with one other antimicrobial, eradicates four out of five clarithromycin-resistant strains.[44]

In one study,[45] 1 week of RBC-based triple therapy appeared to be equally effective as 1 week of PPI-based triple therapy.[45] However, few data are available of head-to-head comparisons in which information on primary resistance is reported.

The most widely used triple therapy today is PPI-based and given for 7 days. PPI triple therapy combines a PPI with any two of the three following antibiotics: nitroimidazole (e.g. metronidazole; tinidazole), clarithromycin and amoxycillin.[46–50] The PPI most extensively investigated is omeprazole, although other PPIs seem to be equally effective. A once-daily standard-dose PPI was used initially, but randomized studies have demonstrated the superiority of twice daily doses or a double-standard dose.[51,52] Lansoprazole, 30 mg twice daily, proved to be superior (83%, ITT) compared with 15 mg twice daily (71%, ITT) in combination with amoxycillin and clarithromycin. Combined with the same antibiotics, pantoprazole, 40 mg twice daily, was more effective (81% per protocol analysis) than 40 mg once daily (59% per protocol analysis). It is clear that addition of an antisecretory agent improves the *H. pylori*-eradication rates, although the precise mechanisms are not completely understood.[53]

In vivo neither H_2RA nor PPIs have any relevant anti-*H. pylori* effect but they enhance the efficacy of acid-sensitive antibiotics. The minimum inhibitory concentration and stability of several antibiotics (amoxycillin) are greater at higher pH.[54,55] Also the pharmacokinetics or tissue distribution of antibiotics might change. PPIs, for example, increase the blood and gastric tissue concentrations of clarithromycin[56] and gastric juice concentrations of amoxycillin.[57] These data, along with the good tissue penetration suggest a favourable profile for eradication of *H. pylori*. Large studies[51,58–60] have evaluated PPI and two antimicrobials in active ulcer patients and those in remission. In the first study, the most successful regimens were omeprazole 20 mg twice daily with clarithromycin 500 mg twice daily and amoxycillin 1 g twice daily (OAC), and omeprazole 20 mg twice daily, with clarithromycin 250 mg twice daily, and metronidazole 400 mg (OCM) twice daily with eradication rates of 95% and 96%, respectively. Similar results have been reported in several other large studies.[61,62] All PPI-triple therapies have their own intrinsic drawbacks, however. If amoxycillin is included, patients who are allergic to penicillin (approximately 10%) will not be able to take it, and perhaps owing to its inclusion there is an increased risk for diarrhoea. If metronidazole is included, the eradication rates are likely to decrease in areas with a high prevalence of imidazole resistance. In a study including *H. pylori*-positive patients with a history of at least one verified duodenal ulcer,[58] the eradication rate was 91% in the OMC group for metronidazole-susceptible *H. pylori* strains versus 76% for the resistant strains. In patients with either active duodenal ulcer or in remission, OAM triple therapy revealed eradication rates in metronidazole-sensitive strains of 85% compared with 60% for metronidazole-resistant strains ($p = <0.001$). If clarithromycin is included, especially when high dosages (500 mg twice daily) are given, side-effects such as taste disturbances and high costs might be a problem. Resistance to clarithromycin is emerging and is expected in the near future to influence eradication rates. In most studies, clarithromycin resistance was uncommon; however, it is thought to have substantial clinical significance by reducing the eradication rate from 95% in sensitive strains to 40% in resistant strains.[63,64] PPI-triple therapy is generally well-tolerated with only mild side-effects (e.g. loose stools, headache, increased liver enzymes). Serious adverse events are very rare and usually result from an allergic reaction.

Quadruple therapy

Addition of a PPI to bismuth-based triple therapy for 7 days improves the efficacy of bismuth-based triple therapy with eradication rates of 93% (ITT) and 95% (PP), respectively.[65-68] In patients with metronidazole-resistant strains there is a trend to lower eradication rates when compared with metronidazole-sensitive strains. Only one study reported a significant decrease in efficacy in metronidazole-resistant versus sensitive strains.[68] Side-effects and dyspeptic complaints are decreased by adding a PPI to bismuth-based triple therapy.[65,69,70] Owing to the complexity of the regimen (four times daily dosing) and the high number of tablets, quadruple therapy, although highly effective, is used mainly as second-line therapy after previous failed therapies.[71]

MANAGEMENT AFTER
H. PYLORI-ERADICATION FAILURE

If the initial therapy fails, second- or even third-line therapies should be employed until H. pylori is eradicated. Although PPI triple, RBC triple and quadruple therapy are effective, a large variation in efficacy exists in treatment studies, with 95% confidence intervals ranging from 80–100%. In routine daily practice, up to 20% of the patients will fail in the eradication of H. pylori owing to non-compliance, bacterial resistance to antimicrobials and treatment-related factors such as number and doses of medications, dosing frequency and treatment duration. In uncomplicated or after the first documented ulcer, routine H. pylori-testing after attempted cure of the infection is not indicated, since in duodenal ulcer disease the resolution of symptoms has proven to be a reliable marker for successful H. pylori eradication.[72]

After healing of a complicated ulcer, or in case of an ulcer relapse, the status of H. pylori and its antimicrobial resistance to metronidazole and clarithromycin should be evaluated, to facilitate the selection for an alternative therapy. The effect of post-treatment resistance has a greater impact on the retreatment efficacy than pretreatment resistance on the initial treatment. Therefore, in general, rescue therapies should not include antibiotics with proven resistance to H. pylori. Usually, after testing for resistance, the choice of the retreatment regimen is easy if there is no evidence of resistance or if resistance has developed to only one drug group (e.g. imidazoles or macrolides). If imidazole-resistance is present, usually replacing the imidazole in PPI-triple therapy with amoxycillin is effective as a second-line treatment.[73,74] If clarithromycin-resistance is present, replacing clarithromycin by an imidazole can be a good second-line PPI-triple regimen. If the resistance pattern is unknown or resistance has been shown for imidazoles as well as macrolides, quadruple therapy is advocated as rescue therapy.[75] In several studies on retreatment with quadruple therapy, secondary imidazole resistance led to an H. pylori-eradication rate of only 50%[76] up to 70–75%.[77]

CLINICAL CONSEQUENCES OF H. PYLORI ERADICATION

Eradication of H. pylori almost completely eliminates ulcer recurrence[30,78] and subsequent complications when compared with traditional ulcer management strategies. After successful H. pylori eradication, no further medical therapy is indicated, which makes this strategy highly cost-effective when compared with maintenance H_2RA or PPI treatment. Several studies[79–86] have shown that eradication of *H. pylori* infection in patients with bleeding ulcers eliminates the risk of recurrent haemorrhage unless NSAIDs are used. In patients who remained *H. pylori* positive, ulcer relapse and rebleeding were common even if acid suppressive therapy was used (Tables 2.2 and 2.3). It is recommended to continue antisecretory therapy after *H. pylori*-eradication therapy until eradication has been confirmed. Maintenance antisecretory therapy should also be continued in the frail and elderly patients or in the presence of serious comorbidity.

Data regarding *H. pylori* in ulcer perforation are scanty. *H. pylori* was detected in 47–80%[87–89] of the patients who presented with perforations. Whether NSAIDs were the cause or false-negative test results and responsible for these lower than expected *H. pylori* detection rates is unclear. Surgical repair of the perforation without further acid-reducing surgery is advised. In *H. pylori*-positive patients, *H. pylori* should be eradicated and eradication confirmed. NSAIDs should be discontinued but, if their use is unavoidable, they should be combined with continued PPI therapy. Quality of life increases after cure of the infection,[90] sick leave decreases and health care expenditure on doctors visits,

Table 2.2 Percentage of patients with rebleeding in *H. pylori*-positive compared with *H. pylori*-negative patients.

			Ulcer rebleeding (%)	
Reference	*n*	Follow up (months)	*H. pylori*-positive	*H. pylori*-negative
Graham *et al*[79]	31	4–26	29	0
Labenz and Borsch[80]	66	6–33	37	0
Jaspersen *et al*[81]	51	12	27	0
Macri *et al*[82]	32	48	82	0
Rokkas *et al*[83]	31	4–14	33	0

Table 2.3 Percentage of patients with rebleeding with microbial therapy compared with H$_2$-receptor antagonist maintenance therapy.

			Ulcer rebleeding (%)	
Reference	*n*	Follow up (months)	Antimicrobial therapy	H$_2$-receptor antagonist maintenance therapy
Santander *et al*[84]	125	12	2.3	12
Riemann *et al*[85]	95	2.5–60	4.2	8.3
Sung *et al*[86]	225	12	0	2

repeat investigations and drugs is reduced. Unfortunately, after *H. pylori*-eradication, many patients experience ulcer- or reflux-related symptoms that require investigation and often long-term treatment with H$_2$RAs or PPIs.

STRESS ULCER BLEEDING

Gastrointestinal bleeding due to stress erosions and ulceration is an important complication in intensive care patients and is associated with high morbidity and up to 50–80% mortality.[91,92] Several factors have been identified that contribute to the development of gastroduodenal mucosal lesions, although the exact pathophysiology is not completely understood. Prophylaxis with acid suppressive, acid neutralizing or cytoprotective agents have been commonly recommended on the basis of the positive outcomes of randomized trials. Routine stress ulcer prophylaxis has been questioned, since recent studies indicate that the current incidence of clinically relevant lesions may be 5% or less, and therefore stress ulcer prophylaxis is only indicated in those at increased risk. The most important prophylactic measure is optimal resuscitation (e.g. from shock, sepsis etc.) aiming to improve oxygenation and haemodynamic status. The risk factors most strongly associated with stress ulcer bleeding are respiratory failure (odds ratio, 15.6) and coagulopathy (odds ratio, 4.3). Cook *et al*[93] reported on 847 patients who had one or both of these risk factors. In 3.7%, clinically important bleeding occurred with a mortality of 48.5%. Without either of these two risk factors, 0.1% had clinically important bleeding, and mortality was only 9.1% ($p < 0.001$). These authors concluded that stress prophylaxis in critically ill patients can be safely withheld unless the patients have coagulopathy or require mechanical ventilation. Cook *et al*[94] also performed a meta-analysis and reported a 50% reduction in relative risk of clinically important bleeding among those patients receiving prophylaxis.

STRESS ULCER PROPHYLAXIS

H$_2$-receptor antagonists

H$_2$RA dose-dependently increase the intragastric pH and reduce pepsin activity. However, even in high dosages the pH is not maintained above pH 4 continuously over 24 h, which is partially explained by the induction of 'tolerance'. Conversely, critically ill patients, especially those with hypotension and requiring mechanical ventilation, have in 40–80% high intragastric pH values without any acid suppression. It is therefore advised to first measure the intragastric pH before considering the use of H$_2$RAs. In patients with hyperacidity, high-dose H$_2$RA (50 mg every 8 h), preferably via continuous infusion is superior to placebo in the prevention of clinically important bleeding. (H$_2$RA are also effective if given orally or via a nasogastric tube.)

Antacids

Antacids dose-dependently neutralize intragastric acid. For optimal results, antacids should be given at 1–2 hourly intervals. Their efficacy decreases if the administration intervals exceeds 3 h. Apart from neutralizing acid and binding of pepsin, aluminium hydroxide-containing antacids stimulate mucosal prostaglandin synthesis, leading to increased mucus and bicarbonate secretion and improved mucosal blood flow. The frequent dosing of antacids, preferably with monitoring of the intragastric pH, is labour-intensive and is often associated with frequent blockages of the nasogastric tube. Side-effects of antacids include hypermagnesaemia, hypophosphataemia, diarrhoea and constipation.

Sucralfate

This is a basic aluminium salt of saccharo-octasulfate with weak antacid properties. Similarly to aluminium-containing antacids, it binds pepsin and also stimulates prostaglandin synthesis, leading to improvement of the mucus layer, mucosal regeneration and mucosal blood flow. Sucralfate (4–6 g/day) is about as effective as antacids in the prevention of stress ulcer bleeding. Administration via nasogastric tube may be associated with technical difficulties.

Prostaglandin analogues

These have not been studied adequately in stress ulcer prophylaxis, as yet there are no data to support their use.

Proton pump inhibitors

These are potent acid suppressive drugs but there are limited data on their use in this setting. As stress ulcers are uncommon if the intragastric pH remains continuously above 4, PPIs may be beneficial in critically ill patients. Levy et al[95] compared intravenous ranitidine 150 mg daily with omeprazole 40 mg daily given orally or by nasogastric tube. Eleven patients (31%) given ranitidine and two patients (6%) given omeprazole developed a clinically important bleeding ($p > 0.05$). The mortality was not different and only related to an increased APACHE II score. The apparent superiority of omeprazole might be the result of its greater potency; however, it is uncertain whether the mean pH is important in the prevention of bleeding stress ulcers. More data are needed before further recommendations can be given.

Cost-effectiveness

Stress ulcer bleeding is reduced by antacids, H_2-receptor antagonists, sucralfate and probably PPIs as well. Since only 5% or less of intensive care (ICU) patients will have clinically relevant bleeding that can be reduced by about 50% with standard prophylaxis, routine prophylaxis is not cost-effective. Also no studies have shown any influence on the mortality compared with placebo or untreated controls. It is advised to give prophylaxis only to patients with coagulopathy and/or who are mechanically ventilated. In patients receiving continuous enteral feeding, usually after the most critical ICU period, stress ulcer prophylaxis may be discontinued.

NSAID-INDUCED GASTROPATHY

Non-aspirin, non-steroidal anti-inflammatory drugs (NSAIDs) are among the most frequently used drugs for musculoskeletal pain and other conditions, including dysmenorrhea. Population-based studies in the USA revealed that 10–20% of persons aged 65 years or older are prescribed NSAIDs, and studies of elderly Medicaid patients showed that 40% received at least one NSAID prescription that covered more that 75% of the year.[96] About one-half of the patients taking NSAID complain of abdominal pain or dyspepsia and a significant number will develop gastrointestinal complications such as bleeding or perforation. The risk for these complications may be increased by a factor 4 to 5, but the risk is strongly dependent on patient risk factors (e.g. previous ulcer disease, age etc.) as well as the kind of NSAID used.[97] Buffered or enteric-coated aspirin and NSAID are often tolerated better but, after rectal administration, are not associated with a reduced incidence of complications. Up to 60% of the patients who take NSAIDs have gastroduodenal lesions such as intramucosal haemorrhage and/or erosions that are of limited clinical significance. The risk in patients taking NSAID therapy of having a gastric or duodenal ulcer is estimated at 10–20% and 2–5%, respectively.[98] Life-threatening complications secondary to NSAID-induced gastrointestinal bleeding can appear without warning symptoms in up to 60% of the patients.[99] The prescribing physician should balance carefully the potential risks of ulcers and their complications against the benefits for the individual patient.

NSAIDs and mechanisms leading to ulceration

NSAIDs, including acetylsalicylic acid, have topical damaging properties that might contribute to their capacity to cause ulceration. Most NSAIDs are weak acids and in an acidic environment non-ionized NSAID diffuses across the cell membrane into epithelial cells. The increased intracellular pH leads to its ionization with subsequent intraepithelial trapping and accumulation.

NSAIDs work by inhibition of cyclo-oxygenase reducing the production of protective prostanoids such as PGE_2 and prostacyclin.[100,101] These prostanoids inhibit acid secretion, stimulate gastric mucus and bicarbonate secretion and cause vasodilatation of the mucosal microcirculation. Cyclo-oxygenase (COX) has two isoforms: the constitutive isoform COX-1, which has several physiologic functions, including maintaining normal function in the GI and renal tracts; and the inducible isoform, COX-2, which is induced and modulated by pro-inflammatory stimuli. Since prostaglandins regulate secretion of mucin and surface active phospholipids, NSAIDs lead to a reduction in mucus barrier function. NSAIDs also inhibit prostaglandin-mediated bicarbonate secretion from gastric and duodenal mucosa and inhibit the mucosal cell proliferation critical to erosion or ulcer formation. NSAIDs may also induce microvascular ischaemia, leading to adherence of cellular elements to the vascular endothelium. The accumulation of activated neutrophils, together with the reduced blood flow might ultimately lead to ischaemic cell damage predisposing to ulceration. In animal models, inhibition of nitric oxide (NO) synthesis promotes NSAID-induced injury, while NO donors reduce NSAID toxicity. Since COX-2 is induced by inflammatory stimuli, it is likely that the anti-inflammatory action of NSAIDs results from the inhibition of COX-2, while the side-effects are largely owing to the inhibition of COX-1. The majority of NSAIDs that are currently available are not completely selective for COX-2 and so adverse reactions from unwanted COX-1 effects are seen often. NSAIDs that have the highest activity against COX-2 and the most favourable COX-2/COX-1 activity ratio will have anti-inflammatory activity with less side-effects than NSAIDs with a less favourable COX-2:COX-1 activity ratio. The discovery of COX-2 has stimulated the development of COX-2 selective NSAIDs. It should be noted, however, that in vitro assays for selectivity, which are considered to indicate safety, do not necessarily correlate with in vivo results.[102,103] In a large 3-month study, nabumetone (1.0–2.0 g daily), naproxen (500–1500 mg daily) and ibuprofen (1200–3200 mg daily) were compared for gastrointestinal complications. Ulcer bleeding and perforation occurred in only 0.03% of patients taking nabumetone compared with 0.5% of the patients on naproxen or ibuprofen ($p = 0.001$). Further studies are awaited, but results to date are promising.[104]

Another approach for developing safer NSAIDs is coupling of a NO-releasing moiety to a NSAID. NO has many of the same properties of prostaglandins in the gastrointestinal tract and is recognized as a mediator of mucosal defence. The NO released will be beneficial by maintaining the mucosal blood flow, will inhibit adherence to the endothelium, inhibit activation of neutrophils and thereby protect the mucosal integrity.[105] These NO-releasing NSAIDs have identical antiinflammatory activity as the native NSAID but have shown to spare the gastroduodenal mucosa when also administered for several weeks.[104,106,107]

Prevention of NSAID-induced gastropathy

Symptoms and mucosal lesions are poorly correlated in NSAID users. Although around 25% of the patients on maintenance NSAIDs suffer abdominal pain, NSAID-associated ulcers are often silent. Symptoms are also poor predictors of NSAID-associated complications. Despite the fact that 10–30% of chronic NSAID users develop peptic ulcers within 3–6 months of usage, the incidence of potentially lethal complications during the same time period is less than 1%.[108] Although there is no strong evidence supporting the advice that patients should take NSAIDs with their meals, many dyspeptic patients benefit from this advice but probably without effect on the ulcer incidence. The most effective preventative measure to NSAID gastropathy is avoiding its use, whenever possible. Several studies of NSAID withdrawal in elderly people show that up to two-thirds using NSAIDs chronically can do just as well without NSAIDs if other analgesics are used (acetaminophen). Reducing the topical damaging effects of NSAIDs, such as enteric coating and producing slow-release formulations have not been effective in reducing the incidence of clinically significant complications such as bleeding or perforation. If NSAIDs are truly indicated, the lowest effective dosage, the shortest duration and the use of a NSAID with a low risk of serious gastrointestinal complications is advocated. Patients at increased risk of serious ulcer complications are older people (above 65–70 years), those with a history of (complicated) ulcer disease, those on higher dosage and more potent NSAIDs or concomitant use of aspirin (for stroke or myocardial ischaemia prevention), as well as patients with other clinical signs of poor general health (e.g. hospitalization, history of renal or heart disease). *H. pylori* infection is not a risk-factor in patients taking NSAIDs for bleeding or perforation. The interaction in mucosal prostaglandin-synthesis between NSAIDs (reduction) and *H. pylori* (stimulation) has been suggested as the mechanism to explain the absence of an additive effect in causing ulceration.[109]

In many studies, differences in faecal blood loss or number of mucosal lesions are compared, while few studies have evaluated well-defined and clinical relevant endpoints such as bleeding, perforation, hospitalization rates and mortality. Since erosions do not lead to complications, they should not be considered when determining the efficacy of any prophylactic agent in long-term clinical studies. Also, the results of any study should be analysed separately for both gastric and duodenal ulcers. The use of ulcer as endpoint in long-term studies is justified by the fact that the major complications such as bleeding and perforation are those associated with peptic ulcer disease. In most studies, the development of acute NSAID-induced damage (usually within 7 days) has been studied in young healthy volunteers, and most of the studies dealing with chronic NSAID-induced injury are retrospective. In clinical practice antacids, H_2RA, PPI, sucralfate or misoprostol, are co-prescribed in many patients, to prevent or treat dyspeptic symptoms and ulcers. Concomitant therapy with either a prostaglandin or acid suppressive agent is only cost-effective in high-risk patients.

Prophylaxis in NSAID gastropathy

NSAIDs threaten mucosal integrity by causing impairment of the mucosal defence and repair mechanisms. Reduction of the aggressiveness of gastric luminal content (acid and pepsin) is probably the most pragmatic approach for prophylaxis of NSAID gastropathy. Universal co-prescription to prevent gastrointestinal side-effects is not indicated; however, high-risk patients should always be protected when NSAIDs are used. The presence of acid appears to be a condition *sine qua non* for NSAID injury to the gastroduodenal mucosa. Animal studies have shown that the degree and the duration of acid-inhibition is a very important factor in the prevention of gastroduodenal mucosal damage.

Prevention of NSAID-related ulcers

Antacid therapy

Aluminium-containing antacids have mainly a gastroprotective effect, independent of their acid buffering capacity, via endogenous prostaglandin release. In short-term studies, antacids at low dose or administered hours before aspirin was given, did not prevent gastroduodenal damage.[110] At high-dose (neutralizing capacity of 1000–1200 mmol of HCl daily) antacids protected adequately when aspirin was taken concomitantly or when taken just before aspirin was ingested.[111] There are no data to support long-term prophylaxis. Apart from practical issues, the results with antacids show that increasing the intragastric pH by antisecretory drugs is more effective in the prevention of NSAID induced injury. In animal as well as in human studies, the relative potency for the prevention of NSAID-induced ulcers is paralleled by their potency in inhibiting histamine-induced acid secretion. The degree and also the duration of their acid inhibitory effect proved to be dominant in the prevention of NSAID-injury.

H_2-receptor antagonist therapy

Several short- and long-term studies have shown that H_2RAs are effective in the prevention of gastroduodenal damage. When given in equivalent acid suppressive dosages, all H_2RAs have a similar effect. At both 4 and 8 weeks, ranitidine (150 mg twice daily) reduced the duodenal ulceration rate from 8% on placebo to 1.5% ($p = 0.024$), but failed to reduce the gastric ulceration rate.[112] In several other placebo-controlled studies, H_2RAs in standard doses only reduce duodenal and not the gastric ulcer rates.[112] H_2RAs might be effective in the prevention of gastric ulcers at high doses. Ranitidine 300 mg twice daily was only effective for the prevention of recurrent (secondary prophylaxis) duodenal ulcers, but not for recurrent gastric ulcer in rheumatoid patients taking NSAIDs.[113] In patients without previous ulcer disease who received long-term (24 weeks) NSAID therapy, the cumulative incidence of gastric ulcer was decreased by high-dose famotidine (40 mg twice daily) from 20% in the placebo to 8% in the famotidine group ($p = 0.003$).[114]

Proton-pump inhibition

The degree and also the duration of acid inhibition appears to be important for the prevention of NSAID-induced injury, suggesting that PPIs should provide superior protection compared with H_2RAs. Several studies (Table 2.4) have shown the efficacy of the PPI omeprazole over placebo,[116–118] H_2RAs[119] and misoprostol[120] in both preventing and healing peptic ulcers associated with NSAID use. Omeprazole (20 mg) appeared to be highly effective in preventing duodenal ulcers when compared with placebo, ranitidine and misoprostol. The rate of duodenal ulceration appeared to be identical with misoprostol and placebo. In the prevention of gastric ulcers, omeprazole and misoprostol were equally effective but misoprostol was less well tolerated mainly owing to a higher incidence of diarrhoea and abdominal pain, as reflected by the higher withdrawal rate from adverse events. So far, no study has reported a reduced complication (e.g. bleeding, perforation) rate in patients using long-term NSAIDs with concomitant PPI compared with placebo.

Misoprostol therapy

NSAIDs strongly inhibit local prostaglandin synthesis leading to decreased mucus and bicarbonate secretion, which are both defensive factors of the mucus barrier against acid back diffusion. Many studies have shown that replacing gastroduodenal mucosal prostaglandins by the use of the PGE analogue misoprostol is effective. In placebo-controlled studies misoprostol reduced the incidence of gastric as well as duodenal ulcers,[112] although the difference did not reach statistical significance in all studies.[113] In a large study of almost 9000 patients with rheumatoid arthritis, patients were randomized to receive either placebo or misoprostol 200 μg four times daily for 6 months.[108] Of the patients on misoprostol, 28% withdrew because of side-effects. Also, 67 serious complications occurred, of which 42 were in patients on placebo. The risk factors for serious complications included age over 75 years, a history of peptic ulcer or bleeding and cardiovascular disease. Patients with all four risk factors would have a 9% risk for a major complication within 6 months. Gastrointestinal bleeding occurred in 56 patients and was not less frequent in patients taking misoprostol. Misoprostol, however, led to fewer perforations (placebo ($n = 7$), misoprostol ($n = 1$)) and gastric outlet obstruction (placebo ($n = 3$),

Table 2.4 Comparative studies on prevention of NSAID-related ulcers.

	Follow-up		Ulcer incidence (*n* (%))			
			Ulcer	Duodenal ulcer	Duodenal + gastric ulcer	Gastric ulcer
Cullen *et al*[115] (PP)	6 months	Omeprazole (20 mg daily)	3 (3.6%)	—		3
		Placebo	14 (16.5%)	6		9
Ekstrom *et al*[117] (SP)	3 months	Omeprazole (20 mg daily)	4 (4.7%)	2		2
		Placebo	15 (16.7%)	9		6
Yeomans *et al*[119] (SP)	6 months	Omeprazole (20 mg daily) *n* = 210	12 (5.7%)	1 (0.5)	0 (0)	11 (5.2%)
		Ranitidine (150 mg twice daily) *n* = 215	42 (19.5%)	7 (3.3)	2 (0.9)	35 (15.3%)
Hawkey *et al*[120] (SP)	6 months	Omeprazole (20 mg daily) *n* = 274	40 (14.6%)	5 (1.8%)	2 (0.7)	33 (12%)
		Misoprostol (200 μg twice daily) *n* = 296	58 (19.6%)	27 (9.1%)	3 (1.0)	28 (9.5%)
		Placebo *n* = 155	66 (42.6%)	16 (10.3%)	3 (1.9)	47 (30.3%)
Bianchi Porro *et al*[118] (PP)	3 weeks	Omeprazole (20 mg daily) *n* = 57		1 (1.7%)		0
		Placebo *n* = 57		1 (1.7%)		7 (12%)

PP, primary ulcer prophylaxis; SP, secondary ulcer prophylaxis.

misoprostol (*n* = 0)). Misoprostol reduced the incidence of upper gastrointestinal complications by 40% over 6 months compared with placebo, but failed to prevent serious adverse events in 60% of the patients and had no effect on mortality. This modest protection and the high incidence of adverse effects has stimulated the use of lower doses of 200 μg twice or three times daily. These lower doses were better tolerated but a significant misoprostol dose–response effect exists in the prevention of gastric (not duodenal) ulcers.[114] When misoprostol 200 μg four times daily was compared with ranitidine 150 mg twice daily for 8 weeks, misoprostol was significantly more effective than ranitidine in the prevention of gastric ulcers (0.56% versus

5.67%, respectively; $p = <0.01$). Misoprostol and ranitidine were equally effective in the prevention of duodenal ulcers (1.1% versus 1.0%, respectively).[116]

Sucralfate therapy

In an acidic environment, the aluminium salt forms a gel with a high affinity for damaged epithelium. It binds bile salts and pepsin, and also increases mucosal defence by the stimulation of bicarbonate and PGE_2 secretion. Only a few long-term prevention studies with sucralfate for NSAID-induced lesions have been performed. In a 6-week placebo-controlled trial, sucralfate 1 g four times daily significantly reduced the severity of symptoms, but failed to influence the incidence of mucosal lesions.[98] In a comparative study during 3 months, sucralfate 1 g four times daily was compared with misoprostol 200 μg four times daily.[121] After 3 months, significantly less gastric ulcers developed in the misoprostol group (1.6%) compared with the sucralfate group (16%).

Healing NSAID-induced ulcers

NSAIDs inhibit cell proliferation in the gastric mucosa at the ulcer margins[122] and thereby delay ulcer healing in patients continuing to take NSAID. In patients on NSAIDs who develop an ulcer, discontinuing the NSAID will usually lead to ulcer healing. If the NSAID cannot been discontinued, H₂RA, PPIs or misoprotol will lead to ulcer healing, although more slowly. Recently two large randomized trials compared ulcer healing with omeprazole 20 or 40 mg daily with misoprostol 200 μg four times daily[120] and ranitidine 150 mg twice daily[119] in patients who continued NSAID therapy. In gastric ulcer patients, at 8 weeks more ulcers had healed with omeprazole 20 mg (83%) and 40 mg (82%), than with ranitidine (64%) ($p = <0.001$ versus omeprazole 20 mg) or misoprostol (74%) ($p = 0.04$ versus omeprazole 20 mg). In duodenal ulcer patients, at 8 weeks, 93% had healed with omeprazole 20 mg, 88% with omeprazole 40 mg, 79% with ranitidine ($p = 0.002$), and 79% with misoprostol ($p < 0.001$). The authors conclude that omeprazole is the treatment of choice for healing NSAID-induced ulcers, based on its efficacy and tolerability, and the optimal dose appears to be 20 mg once daily. There are no published data available for the other PPIs. Omeprazole appears to be more effective than misoprostol in healing NSAID-induced ulcers in *H. pylori*-positive compared with *H. pylori*-negative patients.[123]

In a comparative study of omeprazole 20 mg once daily versus sucralfate 2 g twice daily for 4–8 weeks in ulcer patients and continued NSAID use, omeprazole was significantly superior to sucralfate in gastric ulcer healing both after 4 (87 versus 52%, $p = 0.007$) and 8 weeks (100 versus 82%, $p = 0.04$). No significant differences were observed in duodenal ulcer healing, either at 4 weeks (79 versus 55%) or 8 weeks (95 versus 73%), although a trend was observed in favour of omeprazole.[124] Omeprazole proved statistically superior to sucralfate in gastric and duodenal ulcer healing but only in *H. pylori*-positive patients. The authors stated that it is not always necessary to stop NSAID therapy or to eradicate *H. pylori* in patients who develop gastric or duodenal ulcers.

PHARMACOLOGY OF DRUGS

H₂-receptor antagonists

See Chapter 2 (p. 34).

Proton pump inhibitors

See Chapter 2 (p. 34).

Bismuth

Mode of action

Bismuth inhibits pepsin activity and increases gastric mucosal prostaglandin production and mucus and bicarbonate secretion. It also has antibacterial action against *H. pylori*.

Preparations and indications
Several forms of bismuth are available. Ranitidine bismuth citrate is used in combination with two antibiotics for the eradication of *H. pylori* infection. Colloidal bismuth subcitrate (tripotassium dicitratobismuthate) is used in combination with two antibiotics and a proton pump inhibitor (PPI) for the eradication of *H. pylori* that is resistant to standard treatment.

Adverse reactions
Bismuth preparations may darken the tongue and blacken faeces. Bismuth toxicity leading to encephalopathy and seizures is very rare with short-term administration.

Drug interactions
Reduced absorption of tetracyclines occur with concomitant use with bismuth.

Precautions and contraindications
Bismuth compounds should be avoided in pregnancy and in patients with renal failure.

Misoprostol

Mode of action
Misoprostol is a synthetic prostaglandin E_1 analogue. It replaces protective prostaglandins that are reduced by inhibitors of prostaglandin synthesis, for example NSAIDs.

Indications
Misoprostol is used in the prevention and treatment of NSAID-induced gastric and duodenal ulcers.

Preparations
Misoprostol is available in tablet form.

Dynamics/kinetics
After oral administration there is rapid absorption of misoprostol. It is metabolized to misoprostol acid, with a half-life of 1.5 h.

Elimination is via urine (70% within 24 h) and faeces (15% within 24 h).

Adverse reactions
Diarrhoea and abdominal pain (reduced by taking drug with or after meals) may occur. Less common adverse reactions include nausea and vomiting, flatulence, abnormal vaginal bleeding and dizziness.

Drug interactions
There is an increased risk of central nervous system toxicity with concomitant use with phenylbutazone. Antacids and food diminish absorption, while antacids may enhance diarrhoea.

Precautions and contraindications
Misoprostol is contraindicated in pregnant women or women of childbearing age unless the patient is capable of complying with effective contraceptive measures and has been advised of the risks of taking misoprostol if she became pregnant. It is also contraindicated in breastfeeding patients. Patients with renal impairment should use this drug with caution.

Sucralfate

Sucralfate is a sulphated polysaccharide, sucrose octasulphate, complexed with aluminium hydroxide.

Mode of action
Sucralfate binds to injured gastric mucosa and reduces access to acid and pepsin. It stimulates angiogenesis and the formation of granulation tissue.

Preparations and indications
Tablets and suspension are available for the prevention of stress ulcers.

Dynamics/kinetics
Ulcer adhesion occurs within 1–2 h, and the duration of action of sucralfate is 6 h. the absorption after oral administration is less than 5%.

Adverse reactions

Constipation is the commonest side-effect. Less commonly, diarrhoea, nausea, gastric discomfort, dry mouth, rash, pruritus, headache, vertigo, dizziness and drowsiness occur.

Drug interactions

Sucralfate may reduce the absorption of warfarin, phenytoin, digoxin, ketoconazole, quinolone antibiotics, tetracycline and theophylline. Medications should be taken at least 2 h before sucralfate to minimize these interactions. Sucralfate may increase serum aluminium concentrations when given with aluminium-containing antacids.

Precautions and contraindications

Available evidence suggests that sucralfate is safe during pregnancy and breastfeeding but no definite guidelines are available. Avoid sucralfate in severe renal failure, since aluminium may accumulate.

Clarithromycin

See Chapter 6 (p. 129).

Metronidazole

See Chapter 6 (p. 130).

CONCLUSIONS

In ulcer disease, *H. pylori*-infection should be eradicated obviating need for further long-term acid-suppressive therapy. In complicated ulcer disease (such as bleeding or perforation) eradication should be confirmed before stopping acid-suppressive therapy. In high-risk patients however, prophylaxis should probably be continued irrespective of *H. pylori* status. If *H. pylori* eradication proved unsuccessful, second-line therapy should be employed or life-long acid suppressive therapy is strongly recommended. The use of NSAIDs increases the risk of peptic ulcer complications by 4–5 fold, and it has been calculated that 20–45% of all ulcer complications arise from NSAID use. The prescribing physician should balance carefully the potential risks for ulcers and its complications against the benefits for the individual patient. Based on the patient's risk factors (e.g. previous ulcer disease, age, comorbidity, etc.) universal prophylaxis should be given. PPI therapy proved to be superior to H_2RAs in the prevention of both gastric and duodenal ulcers.

The development of cyclo-oxygenase-2-selective (COX-2) NSAIDs and NO-releasing NSAIDs might provide a highly effective approach to minimize gastroduodenal damage but more data are needed.

REFERENCES

1. Eriksson S, Langstrom G, Rikner L, Carlsson R, Naesdal J. Omeprazole and H_2-receptor antagonists in the acute treatment of duodenal ulcer, gastric ulcer and reflux oesophagitis: a meta-analysis *Eur J Gastroenterol Hepatol* 1995; **7(5):** 467–475.
2. Hunt RH. Peptic ulcer disease: defining the treatment strategies in the era of *Helicobacter pylori*. *Am J Gastroenterol* 1997; **92 (Suppl. 4):** 36S–40S.
3. Howden CW. Optimizing the pharmacology of acid control in acid-related disorders. *Am J Gastroenterol* 1997; **92 (Suppl. 4):** 17S–19S.
4. Bardhan KD, Cole DS, Hawkins BW, Franks CR. Does treatment with cimetidine extended beyond initial healing of duodenal ulcer reduce the subsequent relapse rate? *Br Med J* 1982; **284:** 621–623.
5. Boyd EJ, Penston JG, Johnston DA, Wormsley KG. Does maintenance therapy keep duodenal ulcers healed? *Lancet* 1988; **1:** 1324–1327.
6. Graham DY. *Helicobacter pylori* infection in the pathogenesis of duodenal ulcer and gastric cancer: a model. *Gastroenterology* 1997; **113(6):** 1983–1991.
7. Hamlet A, Thoreson AC, Nilsson O, Svennerholm AM, Olbe L. Duodenal *Helicobacter pylori* infection differs in cagA genotype between asymptomatic subjects and patients with duodenal ulcers. *Gastroenterology* 1999; **116(2):** 259–268.

8. Kuipers EJ. *Helicobacter pylori* and the risk and management of associated diseases: gastritis, ulcer disease, atrophic gastritis and gastric cancer. *Aliment Pharmacol Ther* 1997; **11 (Suppl. 1):** 71–88.

9. Wyatt JI, Rathbone BJ, Dixon MF, Heatley RV. *Campylobacter pyloridis* and acid induced gastric metaplasia in the pathogenesis of duodenitis. *J Clin Pathol* 1987; **40(8):** 841–848.

10. Wyatt JI, Rathbone BJ, Sobala GM, *et al*. Gastric epithelium in the duodenum: its association with *Helicobacter pylori* and inflammation. *J Clin Pathol* 1990; **43(12):** 981–986.

11. Sircus W. Duodenitis: a clinical, endoscopic and histopathologic study. *Quart J Med* 1985; **56(221):** 593–600.

12. Khulusi S, Mendall MA, Badve S, Patel P, Finlayson C, Northfield TC. Effect of *Helicobacter pylori* eradication on gastric metaplasia of the duodenum. *Gut* 1995; **36(2):** 193–197.

13. Hawkey CJ. Personal review: *Helicobacter pylori*, NSAIDs and cognitive dissonance. *Aliment Pharmacol Ther* 1999; **13(6):** 695–702.

14. Freston JW. Overview of medical therapy of peptic ulcer disease. *Gastroenterol Clin North Am* 1990; **19(1):** 121–140.

15. Burget DW, Chiverton SG, Hunt RH. Is there an optimal degree of acid suppression for healing of duodenal ulcers? A model of the relationship between ulcer healing and acid suppression. *Gastroenterology* 1990; **99(2):** 345–351.

16. Bell NJ, Burget D, Howden CW, Wilkinson J, Hunt RH. Appropriate acid suppression for the management of gastro-oesophageal reflux disease. *Digestion* 1992; **51 (Suppl. 1):** 59–67.

17. Gitlin N, McCullough AJ, Smith JL, Mantell G, Berman R. A multicenter, double-blind, randomized, placebo-controlled comparison of nocturnal and twice-a-day famotidine in the treatment of active duodenal ulcer disease. *Gastroenterology* 1987; **92(1):** 48–53.

18. Simon B, Cremer M, Dammann HG, *et al*. 300 mg nizatidine at night versus 300 mg ranitidine at night in patients with duodenal ulcer. A multicentre trial in Europe. *Scand J Gastroenterol Suppl* 1987; **136:** 61–70.

19. Rohner HG, Gugler R. Treatment of active duodenal ulcers with famotidine. A double-blind comparison with ranitidine. *Am J Med* 1986; **81(4B):** 13–16.

20. Soll AH. Duodenal ulcer and drug therapy. In: *Gastrointestinal Disease: Pathophysiology, Diagnosis, Management*. MH Sleisenger, JSE Fordtran (Eds), 4th edn. WB Saunders, Philadelphia, 1989, 879–909.

21. Walt RP, Trotman IF, Frost R, *et al*. Comparison of twice-daily ranitidine with standard cimetidine treatment of duodenal ulcer. *Gut* 1981; **22(4):** 319–322.

22. Feldman M, Burton ME. Histamine$_2$-receptor antagonists. Standard therapy for acid-peptic diseases. 1. *N Engl J Med* 1990; **323(24):** 1672–1680.

23. Wilde MI, McTavish D. Omeprazole. An update of its pharmacology and therapeutic use in acid-related disorders. *Drugs* 1994; **48(1):** 91–132.

24. Graham DY, Colon-Pagan J, Morse RS, *et al*. Ulcer recurrence following duodenal ulcer healing with omeprazole, ranitidine, or placebo: a double-blind, multicenter, 6-month study. The Omeprazole Duodenal Ulcer Study Group. *Gastroenterology* 1992; **102:** 1289–1294.

25. McDougle AM, Lancaster-Smith MJ, Higson DL. Ranitidine maintenance therapy in the prevention of duodenal ulceration; a comparison of 150 mg at night with 300 mg at night. *Aliment Pharmacol Ther* 1995; **9(3):** 287–291.

26. Kovacs TO, Campbell D, Richter J, Haber M, Jennings DE, Rose P. Double-blind comparison of lansoprazole 15 mg, lansoprazole 30 mg and placebo as maintenance therapy in patients with healed duodenal ulcers resistant to H$_2$-receptor antagonists. *Aliment Pharmacol Ther* 1999; **13(7):** 959–967.

27. McColl KE, el Nujumi AM, Chittajallu RS, *et al*. A study of the pathogenesis of *Helicobacter pylori*-negative chronic duodenal ulceration. *Gut* 1993; **34(6):** 762–768.

28. Harris AW, Gummett PA, Phull PS, Jacyna MR, Misiewicz JJ, Baron JH. Recurrence of duodenal ulcer after *Helicobacter pylori* eradication is related to high acid output. *Aliment Pharmacol Ther* 1997; **11(2):** 331–334.

29. Jyotheeswaran S, Shah AN, Jin HO, Potter GD, Ona FV, Chey WY. Prevalence of *Helicobacter pylori* in peptic ulcer patients in greater Rochester, NY: is empirical triple therapy justified? *Am J Gastroenterol* 1998; **93(4):** 574–578.

30. Hopkins RJ, Girardi LS, Turney EA. Relationship between *Helicobacter pylori* eradication and reduced duodenal and gastric ulcer recurrence: a review. *Gastroenterology* 1996; **110(4):** 1244–1252.

31. European *Helicobacter pylori* Study Group. Current European concepts in the management of *Helicobacter pylori* infection. The Maastricht Consensus Report. *Gut* 1997; **41(1):** 8–13.

32. Howden CW. For what conditions is there evidence-based justification for treatment of *Helicobacter pylori* infection? *Gastroenterology* 1997; **113 (Suppl. 6):** S107–S112.

33. Lam SK, Talley NJ. Report of the 1997 Asia Pacific Consensus Conference on the management of *Helicobacter pylori* infection. *J Gastroenterol Hepatol* 1998; **13(1):** 1–12.

34. van der Hulst RW, Keller JJ, Rauws EA, Tytgat GN. Treatment of *Helicobacter pylori* infection: a review of the world literature. *Helicobacter* 1996; **1(1):** 6–19.

35. Pounder RE, Williams MP. The treatment of *Helicobacter pylori* infection. *Aliment Pharmacol Ther* 1997; **11 (Suppl. 1):** 35–41.

36. McColm AA, McLaren A, Klinkert G, *et al.* Ranitidine bismuth citrate: a novel anti-ulcer agent with different physico-chemical characteristics and improved biological activity to a bismuth citrate-ranitidine admixture. *Aliment Pharmacol Ther* 1996; **10(3):** 241–250.

37. de Boer WA, Tytgat GN. How to treat *Helicobacter pylori* infection—should treatment strategies be based on testing bacterial susceptibility? A personal viewpoint. *Eur J Gastroenterol Hepatol* 1996; **8(7):** 709–716.

38. Houben MH, van de Beek D, Hensen EF, de Craen AJ, 't Hoff BW, Tytgat GN. *Helicobacter pylori* eradication therapy in The Netherlands. *Scand J Gastroenterol Suppl* 1999; **230:** 17–22.

39. Roghani HS, Massarrat S, Pahlewanzadeh MR, Dashti M. Effect of two different doses of metronidazole and tetracycline in bismuth triple therapy on eradication of *Helicobacter pylori* and its resistant strains. *Eur J Gastroenterol Hepatol* 1999; **11(7):** 709–712.

40. de Boer WA, Tytgat GN. The best therapy for *Helicobacter pylori* infection: should efficacy or side-effect profile determine our choice? *Scand J Gastroenterol* 1995; **30(5):** 401–407.

41. Chiba N, Hunt RH. Bismuth, metronidazole and tetracycline (BMT)+ acid suppression in *H. pylori* eradication: a meta-analysis [abstract]. *Gut* 1996; **39 (Suppl. 2):** A36–A37.

42. Williams MP, Hamilton MR, Sercombe JC, Pounder RE. Seven-day treatment for *Helicobacter pylori* infection: ranitidine bismuth citrate plus clarithromycin and tetracycline hydrochloride. *Aliment Pharmacol Ther* 1997; **11(4):** 705–710.

43. Savarino V, Mansi C, Mele MR, *et al.* A new 1-week therapy for *Helicobacter pylori* eradication: ranitidine bismuth citrate plus two antibiotics. *Aliment Pharmacol Ther* 1997; **11(4):** 699–703.

44. Sung JJ, Chan FK, Wu JC, *et al.* One-week ranitidine bismuth citrate in combinations with metronidazole, amoxycillin and clarithromycin in the treatment of *Helicobacter pylori* infection: the RBC-MACH study. *Aliment Pharmacol Ther* 1999; **13(8):** 1079–1084.

45. Sung JJ, Leung WK, Ling TK, *et al.* One-week use of ranitidine bismuth citrate, amoxycillin and clarithromycin for the treatment of *Helicobacter pylori*-related duodenal ulcer. *Aliment Pharmacol Ther* 1998; **12(8):** 725–730.

46. Bazzoli F, Zagari M, Fossi S, *et al.* Short-term low-dose triple therapy for the eradication of *Helicobacter pylori*. *Eur J Gastroenterol Hepatol* 1994; **6:** 773–777.

47. Bell GD, Bate CM, Axon AT, *et al.* Addition of metronidazole to omeprazole/amoxycillin dual therapy increases the rate of *Helicobacter pylori* eradication: a double-blind, randomized trial. *Aliment Pharmacol Ther* 1995; **9(5):** 513–520.

48. Labenz J, Stolte M, Peitz U, Tillenburg B, Becker T, Borsch G. One-week triple therapy with omeprazole, amoxycillin and either clarithromycin or metronidazole for cure of *Helicobacter pylori* infection. *Aliment Pharmacol Ther* 1996; **10(2):** 207–210.

49. Misiewicz JJ, Harris AW, Bardhan KD, *et al.* One-week triple therapy for *Helicobacter pylori*: a multicentre comparative study. Lansoprazole Helicobacter Study Group [see comments]. *Gut* 1997; **41(6):** 735–739.

50. Pipkin GA, Williamson R, Wood JR. Review article: one-week clarithromycin triple therapy regimens for eradication of *Helicobacter pylori* [see comments]. *Aliment Pharmacol Ther* 1998; **12(9):** 823–837.

51. Lind T, Veldhuyzen VZ, Unge P, *et al.* Eradication of *Helicobacter pylori* using one-week triple therapies combining omeprazole with two antimicrobials: the MACH I Study. *Helicobacter* 1996; **1(3):** 138–144.

52. Rinaldi V, Zullo A, de Francesco V, *et al.* *Helicobacter pylori* eradication with proton pump inhibitor-based triple therapies and re-treatment with ranitidine bismuth citrate-based triple therapy. *Aliment Pharmacol Ther* 1999; **13(2):** 163–168.

53. Goddard AF. Review article: factors influencing antibiotic transfer across the gastric mucosa. *Aliment Pharmacol Ther* 1998; **12(12):** 1175–1184.

54. Cederbrant G, Kahlmeter G, Schalen C, Kamme C. Additive effect of clarithromycin combined with 14-hydroxy clarithromycin, erythromycin, amoxycillin, metronidazole or omeprazole against *Helicobacter pylori*. *J Antimicrob Chemother* 1994; **34(6):** 1025–1029.

55. Peterson WL. The role of antisecretory drugs in the treatment of *Helicobacter pylori* infection. *Aliment Pharmacol Ther* 1997; **11 (Suppl. 1):** 21–25.

56. Gustavson LE, Kaiser JF, Edmonds AL, Locke CS, DeBartolo ML, Schneck DW. Effect of omeprazole on concentrations of clarithromycin in plasma and gastric tissue at steady state. *Antimicrob Agents Chemother* 1995; **39(9):** 2078–2083.

57. Goddard AF, Jessa MJ, Barrett DA, *et al*. Effect of omeprazole on the distribution of metronidazole, amoxicillin, and clarithromycin in human gastric juice [see comments]. *Gastroenterology* 1996; **111(2):** 358–367.

58. Lind T, Megraud F, Unge P, *et al*. The MACH2 study: role of omeprazole in eradication of *Helicobacter pylori* with 1-week triple therapies [see comments]. *Gastroenterology* 1999; **116(2):** 248–253.

59. Malfertheiner P, Bayerdorffer E, Diete U, *et al*. The GU-MACH study: the effect of 1-week omeprazole triple therapy on *Helicobacter pylori* infection in patients with gastric ulcer. *Aliment Pharmacol Ther* 1999; **13(6):** 703–712.

60. Zanten SJ, Bradette M, Farley A, *et al*. The DU-MACH study: eradication of *Helicobacter pylori* and ulcer healing in patients with acute duodenal ulcer using omeprazole based triple therapy. *Aliment Pharmacol Ther* 1999; **13(3):** 289–295.

61. Moayyedi P, Sahay P, Tompkins DS, Axon AT. Efficacy and optimum dose of omeprazole in a new 1-week triple therapy regimen to eradicate *Helicobacter pylori*. *Eur J Gastroenterol Hepatol* 1995; **7(9):** 835–840.

62. Laine L, Frantz JE, Baker A, Neil GA. A United States multicentre trial of dual and proton pump inhibitor-based triple therapies for *Helicobacter pylori*. *Aliment Pharmacol Ther* 1997; **11(5):** 913–917.

63. Houben MH, Hensen EF, Rauws EA, *et al*. Randomized trial of omeprazole and clarithromycin combined with either metronidazole or amoxicillin in patients with metronidazole-resistant or -susceptible *Helicobacter pylori* strains. *Aliment Pharmacol Ther* 1999; **13(7):** 883–889.

64. van der Wouden EJ, Thijs JC, Zwet AA, Kooy A, Kleibeuker JH. The influence of metronidazole resistance on the efficacy of ranitidine bismuth citrate triple therapy regimens for *Helicobacter pylori* infection. *Aliment Pharmacol Ther* 1999; **13(3):** 297–302.

65. de Boer W, Driessen W, Jansz A, Tytgat G. Effect of acid suppression on efficacy of treatment for *Helicobacter pylori* infection [see comments]. *Lancet* 1995; **345:** 817–820.

66. de Boer WA, Driessen WM, Jansz AR, Tytgat GN. Quadruple therapy compared with dual therapy for eradication of *Helicobacter pylori* in ulcer patients: results of a randomized prospective single-centre study [see comments]. *Eur J Gastroenterol Hepatol* 1995; **7(12):** 1189–1194.

67. de Boer WA, van Etten RJ, Lai JY, Schneeberger PM, van de Wouw BA, Driessen WM. Effectiveness of quadruple therapy using lansoprazole, instead of omeprazole, in curing *Helicobacter pylori* infection. *Helicobacter* 1996; **1(3):** 145–150.

68. van der Hulst RW, van der Ende A, Homan A, Roorda P, Dankert J, Tytgat GN. Influence of metronidazole resistance on efficacy of quadruple therapy for *Helicobacter pylori* eradication [see comments]. *Gut* 1998; **42(2):** 166–169.

69. Hosking SW, Ling TK, Chung SC, *et al*. Duodenal ulcer healing by eradication of *Helicobacter pylori* without anti-acid treatment: randomised controlled trial [see comments]. *Lancet* 1994; **343(8896):** 508–510.

70. Tefera S, Berstad A, Bang CJ, *et al*. Bismuth-based combination therapy for *Helicobacter pylori*-associated peptic ulcer disease (metronidazole for eradication, ranitidine for pain). *Am J Gastroenterol* 1996; **91(5):** 935–941.

71. Lee J, O'Morain C. Consensus or confusion: a review of existing national guidelines on *Helicobacter pylori*-related disease. *Eur J Gastroenterol Hepatol* 1997; **9(5):** 527–531.

72. McColl KE, el Nujumi A, Murray LS, *et al*. Assessment of symptomatic response as predictor of *Helicobacter pylori* status following eradication therapy in patients with ulcer. *Gut* 1998; **42(5):** 618–622.

73. Lerang F, Moum B, Haug JB, *et al*. Highly effect-

ive twice-daily triple therapies for *Helicobacter pylori* infection and peptic ulcer disease: does in vitro metronidazole resistance have any clinical relevance? *Am J Gastroenterol* 1997; **92(2):** 248–253.

74. Gisbert JP, Boixeda D, Moreno L, *et al*. Which therapy should we use when a previous *Helicobacter pylori* eradication therapy fails [abstract]. *Gut* 1997; **41 (Suppl. 1):** A93.

75. Peitz U, Hackelsberger A, Malfertheiner P. A practical approach to patients with refractory *Helicobacter pylori* infection, or who are re-infected after standard therapy. *Drugs* 1999; **57(6):** 905–920.

76. Peitz U, Nush A, Sulliga M, *et al*. Second-line treatment of *Helicobacter pylori* infection [abstract]. *Gut* 1997; **41 (Suppl. 1):** A104.

77. Lee JM, Breslin NP, Hyde DK, Buckley MJ, O'Morain CA. Treatment options for *Helicobacter pylori* infection when proton pump inhibitor-based triple therapy fails in clinical practice. *Aliment Pharmacol Ther* 1999; **13(4):** 489–496.

78. van der Hulst R, Rauws E, Koycu B, *et al*. Prevention of ulcer recurrence after eradication of *Helicobacter pylori*: a prospective long-term follow-up study. *Gastroenterology* 1999; **113:** 1082–1086.

79. Graham DY, Hepps KS, Ramirez FC, Lew GM, Saeed ZA. Treatment of *Helicobacter pylori* reduces the rate of rebleeding in peptic ulcer disease. *Scand J Gastroenterol* 1993; **28(11):** 939–942.

80. Labenz J, Borsch G. Role of *Helicobacter pylori* eradication in the prevention of peptic ulcer bleeding relapse. *Digestion* 1994; **55(1):** 19–23.

81. Jaspersen D, Koerner T, Schorr W, Brennenstuhl M, Raschka C, Hammar CH. *Helicobacter pylori* eradication reduces the rate of rebleeding in ulcer hemorrhage. *Gastrointest Endosc* 1995; **41(1):** 5–7.

82. Macri G, Milani S, Surrenti E, Passaleva MT, Salvadori G, Surrenti C. Eradication of *Helicobacter pylori* reduces the rate of duodenal ulcer rebleeding: a long-term follow-up study. *Am J Gastroenterol* 1998; **93(6):** 925–927.

83. Rokkas T, Karameris A, Mavrogeorgis A, Rallis E, Giannikos N. Eradication of *Helicobacter pylori* reduces the possibility of rebleeding in peptic ulcer disease. *Gastrointest Endosc* 1995; **41(1):** 1–4.

84. Santander C, Gravalos RG, Gomez-Cedenilla A, Cantero J, Pajares JM. Antimicrobial therapy for *Helicobacter pylori* infection versus long-term maintenance antisecretion treatment in the prevention of recurrent hemorrhage from peptic ulcer: prospective nonrandomized trial on 125 patients. *Am J Gastroenterol* 1996; **91(8):** 1549–1552.

85. Riemann JF, Schilling D, Schauwecker P, *et al*. Cure with omeprazole plus amoxicillin versus long-term ranitidine therapy in *Helicobacter pylori*-associated peptic ulcer bleeding. *Gastrointest Endosc* 1997; **46(4):** 299–304.

86. Sung JJ, Leung WK, Suen R, *et al*. One-week antibiotics versus maintenance acid suppression therapy for *Helicobacter pylori*-associated peptic ulcer bleeding. *Dig Dis Sci* 1997; **42(12):** 2524–2528.

87. Reinbach DH, Cruickshank G, McColl KE. Acute perforated duodenal ulcer is not associated with *Helicobacter pylori* infection. *Gut* 1993; **34(10):** 1344–1347.

88. Sebastian M, Chandran VP, Elashaal YI, Sim AJ. *Helicobacter pylori* infection in perforated peptic ulcer disease. *Br J Surg* 1995; **82(3):** 360–362.

89. Chu KM, Kwok KF, Law SY, *et al*. *Helicobacter pylori* status and endoscopy follow-up of patients having a history of perforated duodenal ulcer. *Gastrointest Endosc* 1999; **50(1):** 58–62.

90. Wilhelmsen I. Quality of life and *Helicobacter pylori* eradication. *Scand J Gastroenterol (Suppl)* 1996; **221:** 18–20.

91. Czaja AJ, McAlhany JC, Pruitt BA, Jr. Acute gastroduodenal disease after thermal injury. An endoscopic evaluation of incidence and natural history. *N Engl J Med* 1974; **291(18):** 925–929.

92. Lacroix J, Infante-Rivard C, Jenicek M, Gauthier M. Prophylaxis of upper gastrointestinal bleeding in intensive care units: a meta-analysis [see comments]. *Crit Care Med* 1989; **17(9):** 862–869.

93. Cook DJ, Fuller HD, Guyatt GH, *et al*. Risk factors for gastrointestinal bleeding in critically ill patients. Canadian Critical Care Trials Group. *N Engl J Med* 1994; **330(6):** 377–381.

94. Cook DJ, Witt LG, Cook RJ, Guyatt GH. Stress ulcer prophylaxis in the critically ill: a meta-analysis. *Am J Med* 1991; **91(5):** 519–527.

95. Levy MJ, Seelig CB, Robinson NJ, Ranney JE. Comparison of omeprazole and ranitidine for stress ulcer prophylaxis. *Dig Dis Sci* 1997; **42(6):** 1255–1259.

96. Raskin JB. Gastrointestinal effects of non-steroidal anti-inflammatory therapy. *Am J Med* 1999; **106(5B):** 3S–12S.

97. Garcia Rodriguez LA, Jick H. Risk of upper gastrointestinal bleeding and perforation associated with individual non-steroidal anti-inflammatory drugs. *Lancet* 1994; **343(8900):** 769–772.

98. Caldwell JR, Roth SH, Wu WC, *et al.* Sucralfate treatment of nonsteroidal anti-inflammatory drug-induced gastrointestinal symptoms and mucosal damage. *Am J Med* 1987; **83(3B):** 74–82.

99. Simon B, Dammann HG, Leucht U, Muller P. Ranitidine in the therapy of NSAID-induced gastroduodenal lesions. Results of a randomized, placebo-controlled, double-blind study in patients with rheumatic diseases. *Scand J Gastroenterol (Suppl)* 1988; **23:** 18–21.

100. Vane JR. Inhibition of prostaglandin synthesis as a mechanism of action for aspirin-like drugs. *Nat New Biol* 1971; **231(25):** 232–235.

101. Vane JR, Botting RM. Mechanism of action of nonsteroidal anti-inflammatory drugs. *Am J Med* 1998; **104(3A):** 2S–8S.

102. Laneuville O, Breuer DK, Dewitt DL, Hla T, Funk CD, Smith WL. Differential inhibition of human prostaglandin endoperoxide H synthases-1 and -2 by nonsteroidal anti-inflammatory drugs. *J Pharmacol Exp Ther* 1994; **271(2):** 927–934.

103. Riendeau D, Percival MD, Boyce S, *et al.* Biochemical and pharmacological profile of a tetrasubstituted furanone as a highly selective COX-2 inhibitor. *Br J Pharmacol* 1997; **121(1):** 105–117.

104. Wallace JL. Nonsteroidal anti-inflammatory drugs and gastroenteropathy: the second hundred years. *Gastroenterology* 1997; **112(3):** 1000–1016.

105. Wallace JL, Reuter B, Cicala C, McKnight W, Grisham MB, Cirino G. Novel nonsteroidal anti-inflammatory drug derivatives with markedly reduced ulcerogenic properties in the rat. *Gastroenterology* 1994; **107(1):** 173–179.

106. Cuzzolin L, Conforti A, Adami A, *et al.* Anti-inflammatory potency and gastrointestinal toxicity of a new compound, nitronaproxen. *Pharmacol Res* 1995; **31(1):** 61–65.

107. Davies NM, Roseth AG, Appleyard CB, *et al.* NO-naproxen vs. naproxen: ulcerogenic, analgesic and anti-inflammatory effects. *Aliment Pharmacol Ther* 1997; **11(1):** 69–79.

108. Silverstein FE, Graham DY, Senior JR, *et al.* Misoprostol reduces serious gastrointestinal complications in patients with rheumatoid arthritis receiving nonsteroidal anti-inflammatory drugs. A randomized, double-blind, placebo-controlled trial. *Ann Intern Med* 1995; **123(4):** 241–249.

109. Hudson N, Balsitis M, Filipowicz F, Hawkey CJ. Effect of *Helicobacter pylori* colonisation on gastric mucosal eicosanoid synthesis in patients taking non-steroidal anti-inflammatory drugs. *Gut* 1993; **34(6):** 748–751.

110. Berstad K, Haram EM, Weberg R, Berstad A. Acute damage of gastroduodenal mucosa by acetylsalicylic acid: no prolonged protection by antacids. *Aliment Pharmacol Ther* 1989; **3(6):** 585–590.

111. Domschke W, Hagel J, Ruppin H, Kaduk B. Antacids and gastric mucosal protection. *Scand J Gastroenterol Suppl* 1986; **125:** 144–150.

112. Koch M, Dezi A, Ferrario F, Capurso I. Prevention of nonsteroidal anti-inflammatory drug-induced gastrointestinal mucosal injury. A meta-analysis of randomized controlled clinical trials. *Arch Intern Med* 1996; **156(20):** 2321–2332.

113. Champion GD, Feng PH, Azuma T, *et al.* NSAID-induced gastrointestinal damage. Epidemiology, risk and prevention, with an evaluation of the role of misoprostol. An Asia-Pacific perspective and consensus. *Drugs* 1997; **53(1):** 6–19.

114. Raskin JB, White RH, Jackson JE, *et al.* Misoprostol dosage in the prevention of nonsteroidal anti-inflammatory drug-induced gastric and duodenal ulcers: a comparison of three regimens. *Ann Intern Med* 1995; **123(5):** 344–350.

115. Cullen D, Bardham KD, Eisner M, *et al.* Primary gastroduodenal prophylaxis with omeprazole for non-steroidal anti-inflammatory drug users. *Aliment Pharmacol Ther* 1998; **12:** 135–140.

116. Raskin JB, White RH, Jaszewski R, Korsten MA, Schubert TT, Fort JG. Misoprostol and ranitidine in the prevention of NSAID-induced ulcers: a prospective, double-blind, multicenter study. *Am J Gastroenterol* 1996; **91(2):** 223–227.

117. Ekstrom P, Carling L, Wetterhus S, *et al.* Prevention of peptic ulcer and dyspeptic symptoms with omeprazole in patients receiving continuous non-steroidal anti-inflammatory drug therapy. A Nordic multicentre study [see comments]. *Scand J Gastroenterol* 1996; **31(8):** 753–758.

118. Bianchi Porro G, Lazzaroni M, Petrillo M, Manzionna G, Montrone F, Caruso I.

Prevention of gastroduodenal damage with omeprazole in patients receiving continuous NSAIDs treatment. A double-blind placebo controlled study. *Ital J Gastroenterol Hepatol* 1998; **30(1):** 43–47.

119. Yeomans ND, Tulassay Z, Juhasz L, *et al.* A comparison of omeprazole with ranitidine for ulcers associated with nonsteroidal antiinflammatory drugs. Acid Suppression Trial: Ranitidine versus Omeprazole for NSAID-associated Ulcer Treatment (ASTRONAUT) Study Group [see comments]. *N Engl J Med* 1998; **338(11):** 719–726.

120. Hawkey CJ, Karrasch JA, Szczepanski L, *et al.* Omeprazole compared with misoprostol for ulcers associated with nonsteroidal antiinflammatory drugs. Omeprazole versus Misoprostol for NSAID-induced Ulcer Management (OMNIUM) Study Group. *N Engl J Med* 1998; **338(11):** 727–734.

121. Agrawal NM, Roth S, Graham DY, *et al.* Misoprostol compared with sucralfate in the prevention of nonsteroidal anti-inflammatory drug-induced gastric ulcer. A randomized, controlled trial. *Ann Intern Med* 1991; **115(3):** 195–200.

122. Schmassmann A. Mechanisms of ulcer healing and effects of nonsteroidal anti-inflammatory drugs. *Am J Med* 1998; **104(3A):** 43S–51S.

123. Hawkey CJ, Tulassay Z, Szczepanski L, *et al.* Randomised controlled trial of *Helicobacter pylori* eradication in patients on non-steroidal anti-inflammatory drugs: HELP NSAIDs study. Helicobacter Eradication for Lesion Prevention. *Lancet* 1998; **352(9133):** 1016–1021.

124. Bianchi Porro G, Lazzaroni M, Manzionna G, Petrillo M. Omeprazole and sucralfate in the treatment of NSAID-induced gastric and duodenal ulcer. *Aliment Pharmacol Ther* 1998; **12(4):** 355–360.

3

Emesis

Gareth J Sanger, Paul LR Andrews

INTRODUCTION

The gastrointestinal tract, in common with other epithelialized organs (e.g. skin, respiratory airways), is exposed to the external environment in an interactive and defensive manner. Important protective mechanisms include the mucosal barrier and immune systems. In addition, complex defensive systems operate via the intrinsic and extrinsic nervous systems to provoke behaviours such as intestinal pain, diarrhoea, vomiting, nausea and gastric stasis. These have clear evolutionary advantages for animals that forage for food but they can assume the status of a clinical problem when triggered inappropriately by pathology or drug treatments.[1] Further, severe nausea and vomiting may lead to additional symptoms. For example, negative taste/food aversions are created more readily when a particular food or taste is associated with nausea, than with pain or other sensations.[2] Nausea and vomiting can also be linked to the mechanisms of some forms of anorexia, cachexia[3] and motivational fatigue. In seriously ill patients, the treatment of nausea and dyspnoea has itself been reported to relieve symptoms of pain.[4] It is important, therefore, to realize that the processes of emesis, and its treatment, can have more profound implications than simply the forcible expulsion of gastrointestinal contents.

PATHOPHYSIOLOGY

The mechanisms and mechanics of emesis (nausea, retching and vomiting) have been reviewed extensively.[1,5] In summary, the autonomic (e.g. vagus nerve) and somatic (e.g. phrenic nerve) motor outputs are co-ordinated by brainstem nuclei (especially the parvicellular reticular formation, the Botzinger complex and the nucleus tractus solitarius), which affect gastric, cardiac, respiratory and other functions. The nuclei coordinating emesis have previously been referred to as the 'vomiting centre'. While this is still a useful concept for modelling it is no longer thought to be represented by a single anatomical substrate. Emesis can be evoked or inhibited by drugs, which are assumed to act on pathways projecting to these areas (e.g. via opiate, histamine H_1, cannabinoid receptors), but there are many parallel pathways that lead to these brainstem nuclei and hence, other ways of inducing retching and vomiting. This complexity means that to make a 'universal' anti-emetic drug that blocks emesis whatever the cause is exceedingly difficult. Nevertheless, preclinical studies have identified several potential approaches, including opioid receptor activation,[6] $5HT_{1A}$ receptor antagonism[7] but the most promising of which is NK_1 receptor antagonism.[8,9] The clinical efficacy of this class of agent is currently under investigation but, irrespective of the outcome, the preclinical studies have illustrated that it is possible to make such agents.

To identify which drugs are most effective against different forms of nausea and vomiting, the major causes of emesis have been 'clustered' into groups defined by the predominant emetic pathway (Tables 3.1 and 3.2). The tables also indicate the efficacy of selective 5-hydroxytryptamine$_3$ (5-HT$_3$) receptor antagonists, antiemetic drugs that inhibit the ability of the 5-HT released from the intestinal mucosal enterochromaffin cells to activate and sensitize the vagal nerve afferents terminating in close proximity. This pharmacological selectivity is of enormous value in dissecting the pathways and mechanisms by which drugs and diseases evoke emesis. Figure 3.1 summarizes these pathways, linking them to major classes of antiemetic drug receptor. Included in parenthesis are also those drugs that exert an indirect antiemetic activity because they symptomatically alleviate the cause of the nausea or vomiting (e.g. gastric stasis), rather than interfere with the emetic pathways themselves. Such drugs include the glucocorticoids (e.g. dexamethasone), the partial 5-HT$_4$ receptor agonists (e.g. cisapride, metoclopramide), the somatostatin receptor agonist, octreotide and the benzodiazepines. Finally, the locus at which NK$_1$ receptor antagonists might be expected to exert anti-emetic activity is also indicated but, since these compounds are not generally available for clinical use, no further discussion of their potential use is included in this chapter (see reference 9 for mechanisms of action).

For simplicity, nausea and vomiting can be considered to be generated by five main types of stimulus, and each stimulus may act on more than one pathway.

1. Toxic materials, including drugs, within the lumen of the gut, stimulate predominantly vagal afferents that project to the nucleus tractus solitarius (NTS) and area postrema (AP) in the brainstem and initiate emesis.
2. Absorbed toxic materials including drugs or endogenous agents in the blood, directly stimulate the area postrema (a circumventricular organ where the blood–brain barrier is relatively permeable, located at the caudal extremity of the floor of the fourth ventricle) which, through its outputs, initiates emesis.
3. A pathological situation within the gut (e.g. hypertrophic pyloric stenosis, gastritis) or other visceral organs (e.g. renal failure, myocardial infarct), which directly or indirectly activate the above pathways.
4. A stimulus within the central nervous system (e.g. fear, anticipation, brain trauma, acutely raise intracranial pressure), which evokes the emetic reflex.
5. A disturbance of the vestibular system (e.g. motion sickness, Menière's disease) evokes the emetic reflex. The vestibular system may also modulate the sensitivity of the brainstem emetic pathways, since experimental studies in man have shown that head position changes the sensitivity to the emetic agent apomorphine, which acts on the area postrema.

THERAPEUTIC APPROACHES: RATIONALE

Toxin-, radiation- and drug-induced emesis
(see Table 3.1)

A major site for detecting emetic stimuli lies within the upper gut, which predominantly uses vagal nerve afferents to signal to the NTS within the brainstem and thereby initiate emesis. Stimuli not detected by this mechanism or which are generated elsewhere, or which 'escape' into the systemic circulation, may be detected by hepatic vagal afferents or by the area postrema, via neural links with the NTS.

Cytotoxic, anti-cancer drugs are thought to generate free radicals within the gastrointestinal mucosa, which then stimulate enterochromaffin (EC) cells to release 5-hydroxytryptamine (5-HT). Since the EC cells are in close proximity to the terminals of the vagal nerve afferents, the released 5-HT readily

Table 3.1 Toxin-, radiation- and drug-induced emesis.

Inhibited by 5-HT$_3$ receptor antagonism (sometimes also inhibited by dopamine D$_2$ receptor antagonists)	Inhibited by dopamine D$_2$ receptor antagonists (poorly or unaffected by 5-HT$_3$ receptor antagonism)
Drug/treatment	**Drug/treatment**
· Cytotoxic drugs or radiation (abdominal, whole body) used in anticancer treatment; acute but not delayed emesis, [11,13-15] Interleukin, Interferon [16,17] · Selective serotonin reuptake inhibitors (SSRIs) [18] (also reduced by cisapride) [19] · Protease inhibition in HIV patients · Anti-infective treatments in HIV patients (e.g. high dose co-trimoxazole) [20,21] · Pyrogallol (free-radical scavenger) [22] · Theophylline [23,24] · Acetaminophen intoxication (+N-acetylcysteine treatment) [25,26] · Ipecac [27]	· Apomorphine, Levodopa; unaffected by 5-HT$_3$ receptor antagonists [10] · Systemic/intrathecal morphine; variable inhibition by 5-HT$_3$ receptor antagonists [28-30] · Loperamide; unaffected by 5-HT$_3$ receptor antagonists [12] · PDE IV inhibition (e.g. rolipram); variable effects of 5-HT$_3$ receptor antagonists [31,32] · Anaphylactic shock/histamine; unaffected by 5-HT$_3$ receptor antagonists; AP ablation required [33] · Sodium phosphate; reduced by 5-HT$_3$ receptor antagonists; also reduced by cisapride/metoclopramide [34] · Alcohol: role of dopamine unknown; unaffected by 5-HT$_3$ but prevented by NK$_1$ receptor antagonism [35] · Digitalis; unaffected by 5-HT$_3$ receptor antagonists [36]

Table 3.2 Emesis associated with pregnancy and disease.

Induced via the viscera	Induced predominantly via the CNS	Emesis evoked via multiple central and peripheral causes
Uraemia/chronic renal disease: prevented/ reduced by 5-HT$_3$ receptor antagonists[37]	Anticipation: ongoing anti-cancer treatment; unaffected by 5-HT$_3$ receptor antagonists[42]	Cyclical vomiting syndrome/migraine: unknown effects of 5-HT$_3$ receptor antagonism (cyclical vomiting) or variable (migraine)[48]
Gastrointestinal	Brain damage/trauma:	Postoperative: prevented/reduced by 5-HT$_3$ receptor antagonists[49]
— Acute gastroenteritis; prevented/reduced by 5-HT$_3$ receptor antagonists[38]	— Neurosurgical trauma: prevented/reduced by 5-HT$_3$ receptor antagonists[43]	Pregnancy:
— Distension (e.g. gastric or tube bypassing): reduced by 5-HT$_3$ receptor antagonists[39,40]	— Brainstem lesion (multiple sclerosis and stroke): prevented/reduced by 5-HT$_3$ receptor antagonists[44]	— First trimester: unknown effects of 5-HT$_3$ receptor antagonists
— Bowel obstruction: reduced by 5-HT$_3$ receptor antagonists[41]	— Radiation to brainstem; reduced (moderate radiation[45]) or unaffected (high[46]) by 5-HT$_3$ receptor antagonism	— Hyperemesis gravidarum: reduced by 5-HT$_3$ receptor antagonists[50]
Cardiac:	— Intracranial hypertension; unaffected by 5-HT$_3$ receptor antagonists[47]	Advanced cancer: Carcinoid syndrome VIPoma (dehydration): reduced by 5-HT$_3$ receptor antagonists[51,52]
— Ischaemia: effects of 5-HT$_3$ receptor antagonists are unknown		

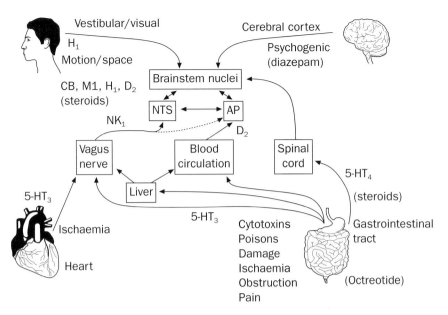

Figure 3.1 The different operative pathways and pharmacologies used by major emetic stimuli. NTS, nucleus tractus solitarius; AP, area postrema; CB, cannabinoid; NK_1, neurokinin-1 receptor; D_2, dopamine; M_1, muscarinic-1 receptor; H_1, histamine.

stimulates 5-HT_3 receptors on these terminals. This process may itself initiate emesis but it is likely that the main role of the 5-HT_3 receptor is to sensitize the vagus nerve to other excitatory substances that are released acutely from the EC cells, such as substance P, or generated by cell death later during the anti-cancer treatment. The result may be the generation of severe and sometimes prolonged forms of nausea and vomiting. During the first 24 h ('acute' phase) emesis can generally be prevented by treatment with 5-HT_3 receptor antagonists; if the emesis is severe and 'delayed' as occurs after high-dose cisplatin, the addition of a corticosteroid is recommended. The mechanisms by which the latter exert anti-emetic activity are unclear but the most obvious possibility is that they reduce oedema at an 'emetic-sensitive site' and remove the generation of emetogenic substances via inhibition of eicosanoid metabolism.[10] However, non-genomic actions of corticosteroids cannot be excluded.

Detailed recommendations for the optimal treatment of nausea and vomiting during anti-cancer therapy have been reviewed by Gralla *et al*.[11] Dopamine D_2 receptor antagonists (selective or non-selective; Table 3.3) for example may also ameliorate mild forms of emesis. Given this activity, albeit often inferior to the efficacy of 5-HT_3 receptor antagonists, it must be concluded that the anti-cancer therapy generates emetogens that operate not only within the gut (via the 5-HT_3 receptor) but which are also liberated into the blood to stimulate D_2 receptors in the area postrema and/or on NTS neurones projecting into the area postrema. A similar process is thought to operate during total body irradiation or during radiation directed to the abdominal areas, in which the evoked emesis is sensitive to inhibition by 5-HT_3 receptor antagonists and, to a lesser extent, by D_2 receptor antagonists.

Several other exogenously administered drugs can evoke emesis. Some are thought to 'irritate' the gastrointestinal tract and, as a result, will release 5-HT from the EC cells to activate the 5-HT_3 receptors on the vagal afferent nerve terminals. This concept is supported by clinical and/or animal data, which show that emesis can be inhibited by selective 5-HT_3 receptor antagonism and sometimes in animals, by abdominal vagotomy. Such drugs include the cytokines interferon or interleukin 2 (emesis also prevented by D_2 receptor antagonism, suggesting that more than one emetic mechanism

Table 3.3 Affinities of common antiemetic drugs for dopamine D_2 and D_3 receptors, α_1-adrenoceptors, histamine H_1, muscarinic (M; subtype not specified) and 5-HT_3 receptors.[a] Data are given as K_i values (nM).

	D_2	D_3	α_1	H_1	M	5-HT_3
Selective/non-selective dopamine D_2 receptor antagonists (multiple of mean D_2 receptor affinity given in parenthesis)						
Thiethylperazine	1.1, 0.5		17 (×21)			
Prochlorperazine	6.8, 7.3, 15, 4.7*	35* (×7)	200 (×21)	100 (×11)	2100 (×225)	1800 (×193)
Chlorpromazine	18, 21, 25, 2.8*	6.1* (×2)	8.8 (×0.4)	28 (×1)	130 (×6)	1900 (×91)
Fluphenazine	3.7, 4.8		8.1 (×2)	60 (×14)	340 (×80)	>10 000
Haloperidol	1.3–1.4, 0.5*, 4.2	9.8 (×4)	14 (×6)	1600 (×696)	>10 000	
Droperidol	1.9–3.0		1.3 (×0.6)	2500 (×1179)	>10 000	4200 (×1953)
Domperidone	0.9, 11, 12, 0.3*	9.5* (×32)	74 (×32)		>10 000	3900 > 10 000
Histamine H_1 receptor antagonists (multiple of mean H_1 receptor affinity given in parenthesis)						
Diphenhydramine	10 000 (×588)			17	120 (×7)	
Promethazine	240 (×83)			2.9	21 (×7)	
Dopamine D_2 and 5-HT_3 receptor antagonist (multiple of mean D_2 receptor affinity given in parenthesis)						
Metoclopramide	34, 160, 240, 270		10 000 (×57)	1100 (×6)	>10 000	120–160 (×1)
Muscarinic receptor antagonist						
Scopolamine	10 000			>10 000	0.8	

[a] Data obtained using native and/or cloned* rat and human receptors.[53-57]

operates), the phosphodiesterase IV enzyme inhibitor—rolipram, certain anti-infective regimens in human immunodeficiency virus (HIV) patients, free-radical generation by pyrogallol and overdoses of theophylline, acetaminophen/diphenhydramine/aspirin combination and colchicine.

The mechanisms of emesis evoked by some other drugs are not yet clear either because the appropriate studies have not yet been carried out or because variable data have been obtained after administration of selective 5-HT$_3$ receptor antagonists (e.g. morphine). In addition, emesis evoked by some drugs (or procedures—see next section) may be inhibited by either 5-HT$_3$ or dopamine D$_2$ receptor antagonism, again suggesting that a circulating drug or toxin has the opportunity to evoke emesis by both releasing 5-HT from the gut and by activating D$_2$ receptors within the area postrema. However, it remains a possibility that, in unusual circumstances, central mechanisms of emesis may also be inhibited by 5-HT$_3$ receptor antagonists, as demonstrated by their ability to inhibit emesis evoked by certain forms of brain trauma.

Finally, some drugs clearly operate directly via the area postrema and/or NTS dendrites and these forms of emesis are not sensitive to inhibition by 5-HT$_3$ receptor antagonism e.g. the dopamine agonist drugs used for Parkinson's disease or loperamide, an opioid receptor agonist that induces emesis and which is unaffected by abdominal vagotomy, by dopamine D$_2$ or 5-HT$_3$ antagonism, but reduced by naloxone and abolished by area postrema ablation.[12]

EMESIS ASSOCIATED WITH DISEASE OR PREGNANCY (see Table 3.2)

Emesis induced via the viscera

Chronic renal disease (uraemia)
Vomiting in this setting may be unaffected by the gastric prokinetic agent and 5-HT$_4$ receptor agonist cisapride,[58] but is reduced or abolished by 5-HT$_3$ receptor antagonism.[37] In addition, improvement in pruritus by 5-HT$_3$ receptor antagonism was also noted in one patient with terminal uraemia[37] and in others with cholestasis.[59] A causal relationship between 5-HT and the symptoms of emesis and pruritis in patients with uraemia has similarities to the 5-HT$_3$ receptor mechanism in the aetiology of emesis in cancer patients receiving cytotoxic therapy, and with the symptoms of pruritis in cholestatic patients. It is suggested[60] that the different combinations of emesis and/or pruritis are partly dependent on the source of 5HT but mostly dependent on the generation of other sensory nerve irritants in a disease-specific manner. Thus, the main action of the 5-HT$_3$ receptors is to sensitize the nerve endings to excitatory actions of other substances.[61] The expression of 5-HT$_3$ receptor function is, therefore, dependent on the accessibility of a particular visceral afferent nerve (within the gut for emesis or skin for pruritis) to pathological amounts of 5-HT and other excitatory substances such as histamine, substance P.

Bowel obstruction
In partial obstruction, particularly when related to a motor disorder or when drug-induced, there is a clear logic to inhibiting the nausea by using drugs that facilitate aboral gastrointestinal propulsion; efficacy, however, is unpredictable.[62] Cisapride or metoclopramide increase gut motility by partially activating the 5-HT$_4$ receptor and facilitating the cholinergic motor pathways within the peristaltic reflex; the affinity and lack of selectivity of these drugs for the 5-HT$_4$ receptor is well-documented[59,63] (see Table 3.3 for metoclopramide). An example of their use is a continuous subcutaneous infusion of metoclopramide to relieve 'narcotic bowel syndrome'.

The selective D$_2$ receptor antagonist domperidone, which poorly penetrates the blood–brain barrier and hence, is generally devoid of the extrapyramidal side-effects of metoclopramide, has no clear intrinsic ability to stimulate gut motility.[64] Instead, its ability to stimulate gut motility is attributed to the removal of an inhibitory, dopamine-mediated influence on the gut. Conditions in which this effect of dopamine becomes apparent must include those in which the gastric stasis is part of the aetiology of nausea. Thus, since domperidone antagonizes at D_2 receptors and thereby exerts anti-emetic activity, it follows that this will also relieve the gastric stasis. Other conditions in which an inappropriate activity of dopamine is exerted on the gut are not so clear but may include dyspepsia or those associated with mental stress.

In total bowel obstruction, the gut may try to initiate propulsive activity against the obstruction, which creates a cycle of distension, secretion, and motor activity, provoking pain, intestinal retropulsion and vomiting; drugs that stimulate gastrointestinal motility are avoided. Treatment includes the use of anti-emetic and analgesic drugs and/or methods of decompression[65,66] although surgical intervention is often the primary intervention in this group of patients. Anti-emetic drugs include the D_2 receptor antagonist haloperidol, an H_1 receptor antagonist such as cyclizine, or the combination of both mechanisms via the use of phenothiazine.[65] High-dose metoclopramide has been used to antagonize at the $5-HT_3$ receptors and inhibit the nausea and vomiting in patients with complete bowel obstruction; morphine was also required to manage the symptoms of colic.[67] Similarly, selective $5-HT_3$ receptor antagonists are reported to control this type of emesis,[41] but without increasing gastrointestinal contractility. These data suggest that 5-HT is involved in the emesis caused by gastrointestinal obstruction.[68] Finally, the emesis may also be relieved by octreotide, a drug with no clear, direct anti-emetic activity. Nevertheless, since octreotide reduces intestinal secretion and facilitates the absorption of water by the intestine, it can remove a cause of the intestinal distension and hence, emesis.[69] For example, immediate termination of intractable, continual vomiting was obtained with octreotide in patients with small bowel obstruction after failure to control with prochlorperazine, metoclopramide, cyclizine or dexamethasone.[70]

Vomiting of cardiac origin

Acute cardiac ischaemia is commonly associated with nausea and vomiting. While this can be inhibited by drugs such as prochlorperazine,[71] the mechanism of emesis may also be linked to activation of the von Bezold-Jarisch, vagovagal reflex.[72] The efferent arm of this reflex evokes transient bradycardia, gastric relaxation and emesis.[73] It can be activated by several different stimuli, including 5-HT at the $5-HT_3$ receptor. It follows, therefore, that emesis evoked during cardiac ischaemia may also be inhibited by $5-HT_3$ receptor antagonists, blocking the action of the 5-HT released from damaged blood platelets at the point of ischaemia.

Emesis evoked predominantly via stimuli in the central nervous system

Anticipatory vomiting

Emesis can be evoked via emotional or anticipatory causes, the latter being especially relevant during repeated courses of anti-cancer chemotherapy. Up to 25% of patients who experience nausea and vomiting in response to anti-cancer treatment may develop anticipatory nausea and vomiting;[42] benzodiazepines have been used to treat this form of emesis.

Brain trauma

The severity of emesis evoked by stereotactic radiosurgery for tumours or for vascular lesions may be correlated directly with the total dose of radiation to the area postrema; treatment is achieved by dopamine D_2 receptor antagonism (droperidol), perhaps in combination with dexamethasone, or by $5-HT_3$ receptor antagonism in combination with corticosteroids (Table 3.2). The latter is one of the few clinical indications in which a central action of $5-HT_3$ receptor antagonism may exert an anti-emetic action. Potentially, a similar involvement of central $5-HT_3$ receptors in the emetic response is also indicated by case reports, which suggests that antagonists at this receptor may control emesis associated with neurosurgical trauma (after failure with promethazine) or the intractable vertigo associated with acute brainstem disorders (Table 3.2).

Emesis evoked via multiple central and peripheral causes

Cyclic vomiting and migraine

This usually occurs in children or adolescents and is characterized by episodes of vomiting of uncertain length or intervals, and an unknown aetiology linked qualitatively to travel sickness and/or migraine or abdominal migraine.[74] The lack of understanding makes treatment difficult; nonetheless, limited success has been achieved by regularizing gut function with prokinetic agents, by the use of mixed D_2 and H_1 receptor antagonists and/or by direct anti-migraine treatment with drugs such as sumatriptan. Similarly, the nausea and vomiting associated with migraine is treated effectively by direct control of the migraine itself. However, when this is not successful, drugs such as prochlorperazine or metoclopramide are effective.[75,76] Selective $5\text{-}HT_3$ receptor antagonists have not been shown to be consistently effective.

Postoperative vomiting

The mechanisms of postoperative emesis may involve factors such as the surgery itself, the effects of the anaesthetics, gastrointestinal distension, inappropriate distribution of blood to emetic-sensitive nerve pathways and the use of opioid analgesics.[8,77] Interestingly, the nausea evoked by intraluminal distension or imitation of the gut may be reduced by $5\text{-}HT_3$ receptor antagonists (Table 3.2), suggesting that such procedures evoke a release of 5-HT from the gut mucosal EC cells. This form of emesis is also inhibited by the various D_2 receptor antagonists and, when the vestibular apparatus is involved, by H_1 or muscarinic receptor antagonists,[77] suggesting that multiple emetic mechanisms must operate.

Vomiting in pregnancy (first trimester) and hyperemesis gravidarum

The mechanisms by which pregnancy can evoke nausea and vomiting are unclear,[78] but a general view is that the central and peripheral emetic pathways are somehow sensitized by the changes in sex steroid hormones.[1] As pregnancy sickness is usually self-limiting it is often managed without the use of drugs. Nevertheless, extensive historical data indicate that the D_2 receptor antagonists metoclopramide and domperidone, the H_1 receptor antagonists promethazine and cyclizine, and the combination of D_2 and H_1 receptor antagonists, chlorpromazine and prochlorperazine, are both effective and not teratogenic.[79] Further, the alleviation of hyperemesis gravidarum by $5\text{-}HT_3$ receptor antagonists (Table 3.1) suggests that 5-HT may also play a role in this severe form of emesis.

Advanced cancer

In the terminally ill patient, the causes of nausea and vomiting may be complex and involve several of the mechanisms discussed previously. In such situations, it is possible to treat rationally, facilitated via an observation of the predominant associated symptoms,[65,80] and by the use of less-selective anti-emetic drugs (e.g. D_2 plus H_1 receptor antagonism). Emesis associated with the carcinoid syndrome[51] or with the dehydration caused by VIPomas[52] may also be inhibited by $5\text{-}HT_3$ receptor antagonism.

Motion sickness

The physiological basis of motion sickness, generated via the vestibular system, is well-established.[81,82] However, the mechanisms by which existing drugs treat motion sickness are unclear and are only assumed to evoke suppressive activity primarily within the brainstem nuclei involved in the motor elements of emesis or within the vestibular nuclei.[81,83] These drugs include antagonists at histamine H_1 receptors (e.g. meclizine), muscarinic receptors (e.g. the M_1–M_5 receptor antagonist scopolamine, possibly acting via M_3 or M_5 receptors[81]) or at any combination of these receptors (e.g. promethazine). Limited anti-nauseant activity can be achieved by simply attempting to overcome the associated gastric stasis;[84] 5-HT$_3$ receptor antagonists in one human study were without anti-emetic activity.[85]

Symptoms associated with emesis

Taste/appetite

Anorexia (loss of appetite, lack of desire for food) often precedes nausea and vomiting;[3] it may be an evolutionary defence mechanism against further ingestion of 'unpleasant' materials. In certain acute clinical conditions when anorexia is drug-induced or associated with a gastric ulcer, it may be treated with metoclopramide or cisapride, especially in the elderly.[86,87] However, conditioned taste aversions associated with emetic stimuli, such as anti-cancer therapies, are difficult to treat and may last for many years. It is not clear whether 5-HT$_3$ receptor antagonists ameliorate reductions in satiety or taste aversion associated with anti-cancer therapies.[88] In rats, reduction in food intake caused by radiation was not prevented by ondansetron,[89] but these data must be treated with caution since rats are incapable of emesis and hence, the mechanisms of satiety and gastric stasis may be different to those of species that can vomit. Similarly, an NK$_1$ receptor antagonist (GR 205171) has been reported to block apomorphine- or amphetamine-induced conditioned taste aversions,[90] suggesting that, if applicable to man, this class of agent may have clinical effects in addition to its action in emesis.

Chronic fatigue

Defined as a perceived (and an actual) decrease in the capacity for physical or mental work, not alleviated by rest.[91] This can be preceded by a 'sickness or illness behaviour' (anorexia, fever, malaise, listlessness, hypersomnia, weakness, depressed activity), evoked by immune and/or inflammatory disorders.[92,93] It may be initiated

via cytokine-induced activation of vagal afferent neurones.[94,95] Thereafter, some form of neuroplasticity must occur to sustain the response after the stimulus has been removed; in cancer patients, the fatigue can persist long after they are free of disease.[53] However, a role of the vagus is supported by a report that the fatigue and emesis associated with acute interferon administration was reduced by the 5-HT$_3$ receptor antagonist granisetron.[17] If confirmed, this is consistent with the ability of the vagus nerve to reflexly suppress skeletal muscle activity[96–98] when activated by, for example, 5-HT[97] and with an increased synthesis of 5-HT by the liver following cytokine treatment.[99]

TREATMENT REGIMENS

Appropriate treatment regimens are dependent on the cause of emesis. Recommendations are found in all standard drug references and in specific working-party articles.[11,100] Treatments may be acute (e.g. as in drug poisoning), preventative (e.g. as for postoperative cases), repetitive (e.g. as for emesis during anticancer chemotherapy) or given on an 'as-need' basis (e.g. hyperemesis gravidarum during pregnancy). If sufficient activity can be achieved, it is usually desirable if the administered drugs have a highly selective action and hence, a minimal side-effect profile (e.g. 5-HT$_3$ receptor antagonists for protection against the emetic effects of radiation during mild-to-moderate anticancer drug-evoked emesis). Sometimes this degree of selectivity cannot be achieved (e.g. extrapyramidal side-effects of D$_2$ receptor antagonists such as haloperidol) or it may be more efficacious and sometimes more desirable to administer 'cocktails' of anti-emetic drugs (e.g. a selective 5-HT$_3$ receptor antagonist plus dexamethasone for the treatment of delayed nausea and vomiting following severe anti-cancer chemotherapy) and/or highly non-selective anti-emetic drugs that have additional, sedating activities, particularly in certain distressful or palliative care situations.

PHARMACOLOGY OF MAJOR DRUGS

The 5-HT$_3$ receptor antagonists are usually considered to be selective in their action, in that low doses have high affinity for the 5-HT$_3$ receptor compared with other receptors.[101] Table 3.3 lists the affinities of other anti-emetic drugs for receptors linked to anti-emetic activities. For the D$_2$ receptor antagonists in particular, matching their affinity for the receptor, versus those of the H$_1$ and muscarinic receptors, provides a guide to the potential of these compounds to exert a relatively wide-spectrum anti-emetic activity and, in addition, a higher incidence of side-effects such as sedation. Adverse events associated with anti-emetic drugs are discussed in detail by Soukop.[102]

Selective and non-selective dopamine D$_2$ receptor antagonists

These comprise:

- Thiethylperazine
- Prochlorperazine
- Chlorpromazine
- Fluphenazine
- Cyclizine
- Haloperidol
- Droperidol
- Domperidone

For nausea and vomiting at established proven doses by antagonism at D$_2$ receptors in the area bostrema.

Extrapyramidal reactions can be the major adverse event, depending on brain penetration and the age of the patient; domperidone poorly crosses the blood–brain barrier and is usually devoid of these reactions. Increased prolactin release means avoidance during pregnancy and breastfeeding. Hypotension and interference with temperature regulation may also occur. Other non-selective activities exert additional anti-emetic therapeutic and/or side-effect activities.

Chlorpromazine

This is used to treat nausea and vomiting of terminal illness, and other indications.

Additional adverse events/contraindications include sedation, agitation in the elderly and antimuscarinic symptoms. It is contraindicated during coma caused by CNS depressants; bone marrow depression; phaeochromocytoma.

Perphenazine

This is used to treat severe nausea, vomiting; and has other indications.

Additional adverse events/contraindications are as for chlorpromazine, but perphenazine is less sedating; extrapyramidal reactions are, however, more frequent.

Prochlorperazine

Used to treat severe nausea, vomiting, and other conditions.

Additional adverse events/contraindications are as for chlorpromazine, but prochlorperazine is less sedating; however, extrapyramidal reactions, especially dystonia are more frequent.

Trifluoperazine

Used in severe nausea, vomiting and in other situations.

Additional adverse events/contraindications are as for chlorpromazine, but there is less sedation, hypotension, hypothermia and antimuscarinic side-effects; extrapyramidal reactions are, however, more frequent—especially dystonia and akathisia.

Domperidone

Used in acute nausea, vomiting; nausea and vomiting following cytotoxic or radiotherapy and functional dyspepsia.

Additional adverse events/contraindications include extrapyramidal side-effects (rare), renal impairment, pregnancy and breastfeeding; domperidone is not recommended for prophylactis of postoperative vomiting or for chronic administration.

Histamine H_1 receptor antagonists

These are:

- Cinnarizine
- Cyclizine
- Dimenhydrinate
- Meclozine
- Promethazine

Histamine H_1 receptor antagonists are used to treat nausea and vomiting using established, proven doses mostly by antagonism at histamine H_1 receptors in vestibular and brainstem nuclei. Other non-selective activities exert additional anti-emetic, therapeutic, side-effect activities. Can cause drowsiness (affects performance of skilled tasks such as driving; enhances effects of alcohol) and antimuscarinic side-effects (dry mouth, blurred vision); cyclizine or cinnarizine are associated with slightly less sedation.

Cyclizine
Used to treat nausea, vomiting, vertigo, motion sickness and labyrinthine disorders.

Additional adverse events/contraindications: may aggravate severe heart failure and counteract haemodynamic benefit of opioids.

Cinnarizine
Cinnarizine is used to treat vestibular disorders, tinnitus, nausea and vomiting in Menière's disease, motion sickness and vascular disease.

Additional adverse events/contraindications are as for cyclizine; allergic skin reactions and fatigue may occur, and caution should be used in hypotension at high doses; rarely, extrapyramidal symptoms occur in the elderly on prolonged therapy. Avoid cinnarizine treatment in porphyria.

Dimenhydrinate
Used in nausea, vomiting, vertigo, motion sickness and labyrinthine disorders.

Additional adverse events/contraindications are as for cyclizine.

Meclozine
Used to treat nausea, vomiting, vertigo, labyrinthine disorders, motion sickness, and other conditions.

Additional adverse events/contraindications are as for cyclizine.

Promethazine
Promethazine is used to treat nausea, vertigo, labyrinthine disorders and motion sickness.

Additional adverse events/contraindications are as for cyclizine but there is more sedation; intramuscular injections may be painful; avoid promethizine in porphyria.

Dopamine D_2 and 5-HT_3 receptor antagonist

Metoclopramide has a mixed pharmacology and is used to treat nausea and vomiting, especially in gastrointestinal disorders and after cytotoxics or radiotherapy, at established conventional doses by antagonism at D_2 receptors in the area postrema and by partially activating gastric enteric 5-HT_4 receptors.

Higher doses antagonize at 5-HT_3 receptors, inhibiting more severe emesis evoked by anti-cancer agents.

Adverse events/contraindications are as for D_2 receptor antagonists; drowsiness also may occur, also diarrhoea, depression, neuroleptic malignant syndrome and cardiac conduction abnormalities following intravenous administration.

Selective 5-HT_3 receptor antagonists

These comprise:

- Granisetron
- Ondansetron
- Tropisetron
- Dolasetron

Selective 5-HT_3 receptor antagonists are used for nausea and vomiting at established, proven doses[64] acting by antagonism at 5-HT_3 receptors, primarily on peripheral vagal afferent nerve terminals. They are associated with mild constipation and with mild headache.

Granisetron

Used to treat nausea and vomiting evoked by cytotoxic chemo- or radiotherapy, also post-operative nausea and vomiting.

Additional adverse events/contraindications include: pregnancy and breastfeeding; rash; transient increases in liver enzymes. Hypersensitivity reactions also reported.

Ondansetron

Used to treat nausea and vomiting evoked by cytotoxic chemo- or radiotherapy; also used to treat postoperative nausea and vomiting.

Additional adverse events/contraindications are: pregnancy and breastfeeding; moderate or severe hepatic impairment; sensation of warmth or flushing; hiccups; occasional alterations in liver enzymes; hypersensitivity reactions; occasional transient visual disturbances and dizziness after intravenous administration; involuntary movements, seizures, chest pain, arrhythmias, hypotension and bradycardia.

Tropisetron

Used to treat nausea and vomiting evoked by cytotoxic chemo- or radiotherapy; postoperative nausea and vomiting.

Additional adverse events/contraindications include: uncontrolled hypertension; pregnancy or breastfeeding; abdominal pain, diarrhoea, dizziness, fatigue, hypersensitivity reactions; collapse; syncope; bradycardia; cardiovascular collapse.

Muscarinic receptor antagonist

Hyoscine or scopolamine are muscarinic receptor antagonists used for premedication and motion sickness at established proven doses by antagonism at muscarinic receptors in the vestibular and brainstem nuclei.

Additional adverse events/contraindications include: drowsiness; dry mouth; dizziness; blurred vision; difficulty with micturition. This type of agent is contraindicated during closed-angle glaucoma.

Cannabinoids

The cannabinoid, nabilone, is used to treat mild-to-moderate nausea and vomiting evoked by cytotoxic chemotherapy that is unresponsive to conventional anti-emetic drugs, at established proven doses. Its mechanism of action is not clear but it is thought to act at cannabinoid receptors within brainstem nuclei co-ordinating the emetic reflex.

Additional adverse events/contraindications include: drowsiness; vertigo; euphoria; dry mouth; ataxia; visual disturbance; concentration difficulties; sleep disturbance; dysphoria; hypotension; headache and nausea; also confusion, disorientation, hallucination, psychosis, depression, decreased co-ordination, tremors, tachycardia, decreased appetite, abdominal pain. Nabilone is contraindicated during severe hepatic impairment, pregnancy and breastfeeding.

REFERENCES

1. Andrews PLR, Davis CJ. The physiology of emesis induced by anti-cancer therapy. In: *Serotonin and the Scientific Basis of Anti-emetic Therapy*. DJM Reynolds, PLR Andrews, CJ Davis (Eds), Oxford Clinical Communications, Oxford, 1995, 25–49.
2. Pelchat ML, Rozin P. The special role of nausea in the acquisition of food dislikes by humans. *Appetite J Intake Res* 1982; **3:** 341–351.
3. Clearfield HR, Roth JLA. Anorexia, nausea and vomiting. In: *Bockus, Gastroenterology*. JE Berk (Ed.), WB Saunders, Philadelphia, 1985, 48–58.
4. Desbiens NA, Mueller-Rizner N, Connors AF, Wenger NS. The relationship of nausea and dyspnea to pain in seriously ill patients. *Pain* 1997; **71:** 149–156.
5. Lang IM. Digestive tract motor correlates of vomiting and nausea. *Can J Physiol Pharmacol*, 1990; **68:** 242–253.
6. Rudd JA, Naylor RJ. Opioid receptor involvement in emesis and anti-emesis. In: *Serotonin*

and the Scientific Basis of Anti-emetic Therapy. DJM Reynolds, PLR Andrews, CJ Davis (Eds), Oxford Clinical Communications, Oxford, 1995, 208–221.

7. Lucot JB. 5HT$_{1A}$ receptor agonists as anti-emetics. In: *Serotonin and the Scientific Basis of Anti-emetic Therapy.* DJM Reynolds, PLR Andrews, CJ Davis (Eds), Oxford Clinical Communications, Oxford, 1995, 222–227.

8. Andrews PLR. Postoperative nausea and vomiting. In: *Problems of the Gastrointestinal Tract in Anesthesia.* MK Herbert, P Holzer, N Roewer (Eds), Springer, Berlin, 1999, 267–288.

9. Fukuda H, Nakamura E, Koga T, Furukawa N, Shiroshita Y. The site of the anti-emetic action of tachykinin NK$_1$ receptor antagonists may exist in the medullary area adjacent to the semi-compact part of the nucleus ambiguus. *Brain Res* 1999; **818:** 439–449.

10. Sanger GJ. The pharmacology of anti-emetic agents. In: *Emesis and Anti-Cancer Therapy: Mechanisms and Treatment.* PLR Andrews, GJ Sanger (Eds), Chapman and Hall, London, 1993, 179–210.

11. Gralla RJ, Osoba D, Kris MG, *et al.* Recommendations for the use of antiemetics: evidence-based, clinical practice guidelines. *J Clin Oncol* 1999; **17:** 2971–2994.

12. Bhandari P, Bingham S, Andrews PLR. The neuropharmacology of loperamide-induced emesis in the ferret: the role of the area postrema, vagus, opiate and 5-HT$_3$ receptors. *Neuropharmacol* 1992; **31:** 735–742.

13. Gandara DR, Roila F, Warr D, *et al.* Consensus proposal for 5-HT$_3$ antagonists in the prevention of acute emesis related to highly emetogenic chemotherapy—dose, schedule and route of administration. *Supportive Care Cancer* 1998; **6:** 237–243.

14. Gregory RE, Ettinger DS. 5-HT$_3$ receptor antagonists for the prevention of chemotherapy-induced nausea and vomiting. A comparison of their pharmacology and clinical efficacy. *Drugs* 1998; **55:** 173–189.

15. Perez EA. A risk–benefit assessment of serotonin 5-HT$_3$ receptor antagonists in antineoplastic therapy-induced emesis. *Drug Safety* 1998; **18:** 43–56.

16. Kim H, Rosenberg SA, Steinberg SM, Cole DJ, Weber J. A randomized double-blinded comparison of the antiemetic efficacy of ondansetron and droperidol in patients receiving high-dose interleukin-2. *J Immunotherapy* 1994; **16:** 60–65.

17. Drapkin R, Barolo JL, Blower PR. Effect of granisetron on performance status during high-dose interferon therapy. *Oncology* 1999; **57:** 303–305.

18. Coupland NJ, Bailey JE, Potokar JP, Nutt DJ. 5-HT$_3$ receptors, nausea, and serotonin reuptake inhibition. *J Clin Psychopharmacol* 1997; **17:** 142–143.

19. Bergeron R, Blier P. Cisapride for the treatment of nausea produced by selective serotonin reuptake inhibitors. *Am J Psychiatry* 1994; **151:** 1084–1086.

20. Gompels M, Mcwilliams S, Ohare M, *et al.* Ondansetron usage in HIV positive patients—a pilot study on the control of nausea and vomiting in patients on high-dose co-trimoxazole for *Pneumocystitis carinii* pneumonia. *Int J STD AIDS* 1993; **4:** 293–296.

21. Arasteh K, Doesche M, Heise W, L'age M. The efficacy of ondansetron for the therapy of metoclopramide (MCP) resistant emesis in the treatment of HIV infection. *AIDS: (2nd Int Congress on Drug Therapy in HIV Infection)*, Scotland, UK, Nov 18–22, 1994, **8 (Suppl. 4)**, S40.

22. Torii Y, Saito H, Matsuki N. Induction of emesis in *Suncus murinus* by pyrogallol a generator of free radicals. *Br J Pharmacol* 1994; **111:** 431–434.

23. Roberts JR, Camey S, Boyle SM, Lee DC. Ondansetron quells drug-resistant emesis in theophylline poisoning. *Am J Emerg Med* 1993; **11:** 609–610.

24. Sage TA, Jones WN, Clark R. Ondansetron in the treatment of intractable nausea associated with theophylline toxicity. *Ann Pharmacother* 1993; **27:** 584–585.

25. Tobias JD, Gregory DF, Deshpande JK. Ondansetron to prevent emesis following N-acetylcysteine for acetaminophen intoxication. *Pediatric Emerg Care* 1992; **8:** 345–346.

26. Reed MD, Marx CM. Ondansetron for treating nausea and vomiting in the poisoned patient. *Ann Pharmacother* 1994; **28:** 331–333.

27. Minton NA. Volunteer models for predicting antiemetic activity of 5-HT$_3$-receptor antagonists. *Br J Clin Pharmacol* 1994; **37:** 525–530.

28. Pitkanen MT, Niemi L, Tuominen MK, Rosenberg PH. Effect of tropisetron, a 5-HT$_3$ receptor antagonist, on analgesia and nausea after intrathecal morphine. *Br J Anaesthesia* 1993; **71:** 681–684.

29. Davies PRF, Warwick P, O'Connor M. Antiemetic efficacy of ondansetron with patient-controlled analgesia. *Anaesthesia* 1996; **51:** 880–882.

30. Koch KL, Bingaman S, Xu L, *et al.* Effect of ondansetron on morphine-induced nausea, gastric myoelectrical activity and plasma vasopressin levels in healthy humans. *Gastroenterol* 1996; **110:** A696.

31. Sheldrick RA, Smith JR, Gale JD. The effect of ondansetron and CP-99,994 on emesis induced by rolipram in conscious ferrets. *Br J Pharmacol* 1995; **116:** 399P.

32. Robichaud A, Tattersall FD, Choudhury I, Rodger IW. Emesis induced by inhibitors of type IV cyclic nucleotide phosphodiesterase (PDE IV) in the ferret. *Neuropharmacol* 1999; **38:** 289–297.

33. Pi WP, Peng MT. Functional development of the central emetic mechanisms in the puppy dog. *Proc Soc Exper Biol Med* 1971; **136:** 802–804.

34. Guller R, Reichlin B, Jost G. Bowel cleansing with sodium phosphate. *Schweizerische Medizinische Wochenschrift* 1996; **126:** 1352–1357.

35. Chen Y, Saito H, Matsuki N. Ethanol-induced emesis in the house musk shrew, suncus murinus. *Life Sci* 1996; **60:** 253–261.

36. Kakimoto S, Saito H, Matsuki N. Involvement of a peripheral mechanism in the emesis induced by cardiac glycosides in suncus murinus. *Biol Pharmaceutical Bull* 1997; **20:** 486–489.

37. Andrews PA, Quan V, Ogg CS. Ondansetron for symptomatic relief in terminal uraemia. *Nephrol Dial Transplant* 1995; **10:** 140.

38. Cubeddu LX, Trujillo LM, Talmaciu I, *et al.* Antiemetic effect of ondansetron in acute gastroenteritis. *Aliment Pharmacol Ther* 1997; **11:** 185–191.

39. Fair R. Ondansetron in nausea. *Pharmaceutical J* 1990; **245:** 514.

40. Kleinerman KB, Deppe SA, Sargent AI. Use of ondansetron for control of projectile vomiting in patients with neurosurgical trauma: two case reports. *Annals Pharmacotherapy* 1993; **27:** 566–568.

41. Baines M, Oliver DJ, Carter RL. Medical management of intestinal obstruction in patients with advanced malignant disease: a clinical and pathological study. *Lancet* 1995; **2:** 990–993.

42. Morrow GR, Roscoe JA, Kirschner JJ, Hynes HE, Rosenbluth RJ. Anticipatory nausea and vomiting in the era of 5-HT$_3$ antiemetics. *Supportive Care Cancer* 1998; **6:** 244–247.

43. Feinle C, Read NW. Ondansetron reduces nausea induced by gastroduodenal stimulation without changing gastric motility. *Am J Physiol* 1996; **271:** G591–G597.

44. Rice GPA, Ebers GC. Ondansetron for intractable vertigo complicating acute brainstem disorders. *Lancet* 1995; **345:** 1182–1183.

45. Bodis S, Alexander E, Kooy H, Loeffler J. The prevention of radiosurgery-induced nausea and vomiting by ondansetron: evidence of a direct effect on the central nervous system chenoreceptor trigger zone. *Surg Neurol* 1994; **42:** 249–252.

46. Alexander E, Siddon RL, Loeffler JS. The acute onset of nausea and vomiting following stereotactic radiosurgery: correlation with total dose to the Area Postrema. *Surg Neurol* 1989; **32:** 40–44.

47. Kacker V, Gupta YK. An experimental model to study intracranial hypertension-induced vomiting in conscious dogs. *Meth Find Exper Clin Pharmacol Res* 1996; **18:** 315–320.

48. Dahlof CGH, Hargreaves RJ. Pathophysiology and pharmacology of migraine. Is there a place for antiemetics in future treatment strategies? *Cephalagia* 1998; **18:** 593–604.

49. Russell D, Kenny GNC. 5-HT$_3$ antagonists in postoperative nausea and vomiting. *Br J Anaesthesia* 1992; **69 (Suppl. 1):** 63S–68S.

50. Tincello DG, Johnstone MJ. Treatment of hyperemesis gravidarum with the 5-HT$_3$ antagonist ondansetron (Zofran). *Postgrad Med J* 1996; **72:** 688–689.

51. Platt AJ, Heddle RM, Rake MO, Smedley H. Ondansetron in carcinoid syndrome, *Lancet* 1993; **339:** 1416.

52. Delahunt JW, Burgess C, Bott V. Ondansetron and VIPoma. *NZ J Med* 1993; **106:** 260.

53. Peroutka SJ, Snyder SH. Antiemetics: neurotransmitter receptor binding predicts therapeutic actions. *Lancet* 1982; **2:** 658–659.

54. Ison PJ, Peroutka SJ. Neurotransmitter receptor binding studies predict antiemetic efficacy and side effects. *Cancer Treat Rep* 1986; **70:** 637–641.

55. Lobbezoo MW, Janszen FHA, Tulp MTM, Zwagemakers JMA. Differential effects of metoclopramide and zetidoline on gastrointestinal motility. *Eur J Pharmacol* 1985; **108:** 105–112.

56. Hamik A, Peroutka SJ. Differential interactions of traditional and novel antiemetics with

dopamine D_2 and 5-hydroxytryptamine$_3$ receptors. *Cancer Chemother Pharmacol* 1989; **24:** 307–310.

57. Sokoloff P, Giros B, Martres MP, Bouthenet M-L, Schwartz J-C. Molecular cloning and characterization of a novel dopamine receptor (D_3) as a target for neuroleptics. *Nature* 1990; **237:** 146–151.

58. Jenkins HR, Verrier-Jones K. Vomiting and chronic renal failure. *Pediatr Nephrol* 1991; **5:** 436.

59. Schworer H, Ramadori G. Cholestatic pruritis—pathophysiology and therapy with special concern on its treatment with 5-hydroxytryptamine subtype-3 receptor antagonists. *Z Gastroenterol* 1995; **33:** 265–274.

60. Sanger GJ, Twycross R. Making sense of emesis, pruritus, 5-HT and 5-HT$_3$ receptor antagonists. *Prog Palliative Care* 1996; **4:** 7–8.

61. Sanger GJ. The involvement of 5-HT$_3$ receptors in visceral function. In: *Central and Peripheral 5-HT$_3$ Receptors*. M Hamon (Ed.), Academic Press, London, 1992, 207–256.

62. Verne GN, Sninsky CA. Chronic intestinal pseudo-obstruction. *Dig Dis* 1995; **13:** 163–181.

63. Sanger GJ. Therapeutic applications of 5-HT$_4$ receptor agonists and antagonists. In: *5-HT$_4$ Receptors in the Brain and Periphery*. RM Eglen (Ed.), Springer, Berlin, 1998, 213–226.

64. Sanger GJ. Effects of metoclopramide and domperidone on cholinergically-mediated contractions of human isolated stomach muscle. *J Pharm Pharmacol* 1985; **37:** 661–664.

65. Regnard C, Comiskey M. Nausea and vomiting in advanced cancer—a flow diagram. *Palliative Med* 1992; **6:** 146–151.

66. Baines MJ. Nausea, vomiting and intestinal obstruction. *Br Med J* 1997; **315:** 1148–1150.

67. Isbister WH, Elder P, Symons L. Non-operative management of malignant intestinal obstruction. *J Roy Coll Surg (Edinb)* 1990; **35:** 369–372.

68. Warner RRP, Feldman MG, Warner GM, Parnes IH, Di Giorgi F. Changes in blood serotonin concentration in mechanical obstruction of the small intestine. II. Findings in patients with intestinal obstruction. *Surgery* 1966; **59:** 758.

69. Riley J, Fallon MT. Octreotide in terminal malignant obstruction of the gastrointestinal tract. *Eur J Palliat Care* 1994; **1:** 23–25.

70. Khoo D, Riley J, Waxman J. Control of emesis in bowel obstruction in terminally ill patients. *Lancet* 1992; **339:** 375–376.

71. Wasserberger J, Ordog GJ, Lau JC, Gilston M, Herman LS. Intravenous prochlorperazine for the rapid control of nausea and vomiting in acute myocardial infarction. *Am J Emerg Med* 1987; **5:** 153–156.

72. Sleight P. Cardiac vomiting. *Br Heart J* 1981; **46:** 5–7.

73. Abrahamsson H, Thoren P. Vomiting and reflex vagal relaxation of the stomach elicited from heart receptors in the cat. *Acta Physiol Scand* 1973; **88:** 433–439.

74. Li BUK, Issenmann RM, Sarna SK (Eds), *2nd International Scientific Symposium on Cyclic Vomiting Syndrome. Dig Dis Sci* 1999; **44:** 1S–120S.

75. Coppola M, Yealy DM. Randomized placebo-controlled evaluation of metoclopramide versus prochlorperazine for the emergency department treatment of migraine. *Ann Emerg Med* 1992; **21:** 1047.

76. Ellis GL, Delaney J, DeHart DA, Owens A. The efficacy of metoclopramide in the treatment of migraine headache. *Annals Emerg Med* 1993; **22:** 191–195.

77. Rose JB, Watcha MF. Postoperative nausea and vomiting in pediatric patients. *Br J Anaesthesia* 1999; **83:** 104–117.

78. Broussard CN, Richter JE. Nausea and vomiting of pregnancy. *Gastroenterol Clin N Am* 1998; **27:** 123–151.

79. Nelson-Piercy C. Treatment of nausea and vomiting in pregnancy. When should it be treated and what can be safely taken? *Drug Safety* 1998; **19:** 155–164.

80. Sykes N. The management of nausea and vomiting. *Practitioner* 1990; **234:** 286–290.

81. Yates BJ, Miller AD, Lucot JB. Physiological basis and pharmacology of motion sickness: an update. *Brain Res Bull* 1998; **47:** 395–406.

82. Jennings RT. Managing space motion sickness. *J Vestibular Res* 1998; **8:** 67–70.

83. Wood CD. Pharmacological countermeasures against motion sickness. In: *Motion and Space Sickness*. GH Crampton (Ed.), CRC Press, Boca Raton, 1990, 343–351.

84. Mitchelson F. No stomach for travel. *Aust J Pharm* 1992; **73:** 627–630.

85. Stott JRR, Barnes GR, Wright RJ, Ruddock CJS. The effect of motion sickness and oculomotor function of GR 38032F, 5-HT$_3$ receptor antagonist with anti-emetic properties. *Br J Clin Pharmacol* 1989; **27:** 1–11.

86. Middleton RSW. The use of metoclopramide in the elderly, *Postgrad Med J* 1973; **49(Suppl.):** 90–93.

87. Morley JE. Anorexia in older persons: epidemiology and optimal treatment. *Drugs Aging* 1996; **8:** 134–155.

88. Rudd JA, Ngan MP, Wai MK. 5-HT$_3$ receptors are not involved in conditioned taste aversions induced by 5-hydroxytryptamine, ipecacuanha or cisplatin. *Eur J Pharmacol* 1998; **352:** 143–149.

89. Winsauer PJ, Verrees JF, O'Halloran KP, Bixler MA, Mele PC. Effects of chlordiazepoxide, 8-OH-DPAT and ondansetron on radiation-induced decreases in food intake in rats. *J Pharm Exper Ther* 1994; **270:** 142–149.

90. McAllister KHM, Pratt JA. GR-205171 blocks apomorphine-induced taste aversion. *Eur J Pharmacol* 1998; **353:** 141–148.

91. Stone P, Richards M, Hardy J. Fatigue in patients with cancer. *Eur J Cancer* 1998; **34:** 1670–1676.

92. Kent S, Bluthe R-M, Kelley KW, Dantzer R. Sickness behavior as a new target for drug development. *Trends Pharmacological Sci* 1992; **13:** 24–28.

93. Andrews PLR. Speculations on the scientific basis of fatigue related to cancer and anti-cancer therapies. *Proc 8th Int Symp Supportive Care in Cancer*, June 19–22, Canada, 1996, 93–95.

94. Watkins LR, Goehler L, Relton JK, *et al.* Blockade of interleukin-1 induced by hyperthermia by subdiaphragmatic vagotomy: evidence for vagal mediation of immune-brain communication. *Neurosci Lett* 1995; **183:** 27–31.

95. Goehler LE, Gaykema RPA, Nguyen KT, *et al.* Interleukin-1-beta in immune cells of the abdominal vagus nerve: a link between the immune and nervous systems? *J Neurosci* 1999; **19:** 2799–2806.

96. Schweitzer A, Wright S. Effects on the knee jerk of stimulation of the central end of the vagus and of various changes in the circulation and respiration. *J Physiol* 1937; **88:** 459–475.

97. Ginzel KH, Muscle relaxation by drugs which stimulate sensory nerve endings. I. The effect of veratrum alkaloids, phenyldiguanide and 5-hydroxytryptamine. *Neuropharmacol* 1973; **12:** 133–148.

98. Pickar JG. The thromboxane A$_2$ mimetic U-46619 inhibits somatomotor activity via a vagal reflex from the lung. *Am J Physiol* 1998; **275:** R706–R712.

99. Fuchs D, Weiss G, Werner-Felmayer G, Wachter H. Cytokine-induced increase in liver serotonin. *Immunol Lett* 1991; **28:** 259.

100. Gora-Harper ML, Balmer C, Castellano FC, *et al.* ASHP: therapeutic guidelines on the pharmacologic management of nausea and vomiting in adult and pediatric patients receiving chemotherapy or radiation surgery or undergoing surgery. *Am J Health Syst Pharm* 1999; **56:** 729–764.

101. Van Wijngaarden I, Tulp MTH, Sondijn W. The concept of selectivity in 5-HT receptor research. *Eur J Pharmacol* 1990; **188:** 301–312.

102. Soukop M. Adverse reactions to antinauseants in common use in the UK. *Adverse Drug React Toxicol Rev* 1998; **17:** 91–113.

4

Gastrointestinal bleeding

Matthew R Banks, Peter D Fairclough

INTRODUCTION

Although there are suggestions that pharmacotherapy may have a beneficial effect in some categories of patients with bleeding peptic ulcer, there is little evidence to support systemic therapy in upper gastrointestinal bleeding. Endoscopic haemostasis using thermal methods or injection therapy has become the mainstay of the treatment of ulcer bleeding.

PATHOPHYSIOLOGY AND THERAPEUTIC RATIONALE

The pathophysiological target for drug therapy is the primary haemostatic plug composed of fibrin and platelets in the eroded vessel in the base of the ulcer or erosion.

Drugs have been used to increase intragastric pH in the hope that the resulting inhibition of fibrin degradation by pepsin and reduced platelet disaggregation at higher pH would stabilize the clot, preventing bleeding and rebleeding after initial haemostasis.[1-3] An alternative, or complementary, approach of inhibiting fibrinolysis by agents such as tranexamic acid has also been little studied. Drugs that reduce splanchnic blood flow, such as somatostatin, have been used to reduce gastrointestinal bleeding. Somatostatin is an endogenous peptide that binds to G-protein-coupled receptors, initiating various functions through a reduction in cytoplasmic cyclic AMP. Its gastrointestinal effects include:

- Inhibition of gastric acid and pepsinogen secretion
- Inhibition of endocrine secretions (e.g. gastrin, cholecystokinin, secretin, vasoactive intestinal peptide (VIP) and motilin)
- Inhibition of intestinal fluid and bicarbonate secretion
- Inhibition of smooth muscle contraction
- Reduction in splanchnic blood flow
- Possibly gastric cytoprotective effects.

All of these may contribute to the effects on gastrointestinal bleeding.

TREATMENT REGIMENS

Anti-secretory therapy

Twenty-seven randomized controlled trials using H_2-receptor antagonists in 2500 patients with upper gastrointestinal bleeding were reviewed by Collins and Langman in 1985.[4] They concluded that the effects of such treatment were modest at most, and that reliable detection of such a modest effect would require a randomized, controlled study of at least 10 000 patients. These early studies were open to criticism because of failure of the drug regimens used to adequately increase intragastric pH, and for inclusion of many patients at low risk of rebleeding, diluting any possible effect.

A subsequent trial of the potent H_2-receptor antagonists, famotidine, addressed these points.[5] In this study, 1005 UK patients with endoscopic stigmata of recent haemorrhage who had not been given endoscopic therapy were allocated randomly to receive intravenous famotidine or placebo. The dosage of famotidine (an initial 10 mg bolus, followed by 3.2 mg/h) had previously been shown to maintain intragastric pH close to 7 in such patients. This study, which was a model of clarity and simplicity, showed no significant effect of the drug therapy on death, rebleeding or surgical intervention.

A similar placebo-controlled study[6] in 1147 patients with upper GI bleeding using the proton pump inhibitor, omeprazole (80 mg i.v. stat, then 40 mg 8-hourly for three doses, followed by 40 mg orally 12-hourly), also showed no overall beneficial effect. This study, however, included patients with a wide variety of pathologies, including ulcers, erosions, varices, Mallory-Weiss tears and gastric cancer, as well as almost 20% of patients in whom no endoscopic diagnosis was made, and endoscopic treatment was allowed.

A later double-blind randomized controlled trial conducted in India[7] enrolled 220 patients exclusively with peptic ulcers with endoscopic stigmata of recent haemorrhage who were not given endoscopic therapy. Oral omeprazole (40 mg 12-hourly for 5 days) was shown to have an effect on continued bleeding and rebleeding (10.9% versus 36.4%, $p < 0.001$), need for surgery (8/110 versus 26/110, $p < 0.001$), and the number of patients requiring transfusion (29.1 versus 70.9%). Mortality was unaffected. Subgroup analysis showed that the benefit was mainly in patients with non-bleeding visible vessels, and not in those with arterial spurting or oozing, as would be expected if the proposed mode of action were in operation.

These and other trials prompted a systematic review of the efficacy of proton pump inhibitors in acute ulcer bleeding.[8] Only four out of 16 randomized controlled trials involving 3154 patients showed a significant reduction in rebleeding rate, four showed a decreased rate of surgical intervention, and none showed a significant reduction in mortality.

The effect of combining endotherapy with acid inhibition has been previously addressed in five studies, enrolling relatively small numbers of patients;[8] only one showed a significant decrease in rebleeding rates. Two studies showed a significant reduction in the need for surgery after initial endotherapy and continuous infusion of omeprazole for 72 h. A more recent trial demonstrated omeprazole given after endotherapy in bleeding peptic ulcers reduced recurrent bleeding and surgery, but not mortality.[9]

The benefits of antisecretory therapy in bleeding peptic ulcer are thus inconclusive. There is possible evidence of modest benefit in some studies but well-designed double-blind randomized studies in large numbers of patients, probably with stratification by stigmata of recent haemorrhage, would be needed to confirm this. Peptic ulcer bleeding has been far better studied than other sources of upper GI bleeding, for which the data are even less strong.

Anti-fibrinolytic therapy

There has been little recent study of the effects of anti-fibrinolytic agents in upper GI bleeding, despite the fact that studies published more than 10 years ago suggested a reduction in mortality.

In a study involving 775 patients treated with cimetidine or tranexamic acid, Barer et al[10] showed that mortality in patients treated with tranexamic acid was 6.3%, compared with 13.5% in controls ($p = 0.0092$). There was, however, no decrease in the rate of rebleeding or surgery. A subsequent meta-analysis of six double-blind placebo controlled trials involving 1267 patients with acute upper GI bleeding treated with tranexamic acid[11] (3–6 g/day intravenously for 2 or 3 days followed by the same dose by mouth for a further 3–5 days in four trials, or 4.5–12 g/day for 2–7 days in two trials), showed a 20–30% reduction in the rate of rebleeding, and a 30–40% reduction in mortality (Table 4.1). Since that time, there have been no substantial trials of the use of anti-fibrinolytic agents in upper gastrointestinal bleeding.

Somatostatin and somatostatin analogues

The plasma half-life of somatostatin itself is too short ($\approx$2 min) for it to be a practical therapeutic agent in anything but acute, short-term situations, although its effect can be prolonged when given by continuous intravenous infusion. The synthetic analogue, octreotide, is equally potent as somatostatin and has a plasma half-life of 90 min; however, it is not yet known whether octreotide has any effects on gastric blood flow, mucus production or pepsin secretion.

Both somatostatin and octreotide have been used in attempts to control non-variceal bleeding in the upper GI tract. The results of trials, however, have been conflicting. Studies showing no benefit of somatostatin over placebo or H_2-antagonists contain low patient numbers and included patients with non-variceal upper GI haemorrhage, of which 80% will cease bleeding spontaneously. In studies excluding low-risk patients and including patients with stigmata prognostic of recurrent bleeding, somatostatin was shown to significantly control bleeding, reduce transfusions requirements, the need for surgery and the time to achieve haemostasis.

Similar results have been achieved in trials comparing somatostatin and placebo or H_2-antagonists for the treatment of bleeding peptic ulcers in high-risk patients. The therapeutic effect of octreotide is far less clear and results of several trials for the treatment of non-variceal upper GI bleeding and peptic ulcer bleeding have not shown any consistent benefit. A recent meta-analysis of 12 placebo-controlled, randomized trials has shown that somatostatin may reduce the risk for continued or recurrent bleeding from acutely bleeding peptic ulcer disease. There was also a reduction in the need for

Table 4.1 Recommended regime for tranexamic acid.

Drug	Dose	Frequency	Route	Duration
Tranexamic acid	3–6 g	Once daily	i.v. initially for: then oral for:	2–3 days 3–5 days

Table 4.2 Recommended regimes for treatment with somatostatin or octreotide.

Drug	Dose	Frequency	Route	Duration
Somatostatin	250 μg	Bolus, then hourly	Intravenous	48–120 h
Octreotide	100 μg	Bolus, then 8-hourly	Subcutaneous or intravenous	72 h

surgery.[12] Somatostatin therapy in acute non-variceal bleeding may be useful as an adjunct before endoscopy or when endoscopy is unsuccessful, contraindicated, or unavailable, but should not be used as an alternative.

Octreotide and somatostatin

Recommended regimes for the use of these drugs are listed in Table 4.2.

Mode of action
These agents decrease intestinal blood flow, increase gastric pH, and enhance gastric mucus secretion.

Kinetics
Octreotide is administered parenterally. It has a half-life of 90 min, and one-third of the dose is extracted by the liver, while one-third is eliminated through the kidneys.

Somatostatin is given parenterally. It has a half-life of 2 min.

Indications
These agents are used as adjunct therapy for acute upper gastrointestinal bleeding.

Adverse reactions
Gastrointestinal disturbance including nausea, vomiting, abdominal pain and bloating, diarrhoea and steatorrhoea, impaired post-prandial glucose tolerance and hepatic disturbance may occur with the use of octreotide and somatostatin.

Drug interactions
These agents reduce the requirements of hypoglycaemic drugs and reduce the plasma levels of cyclosporin.

ANAL FISSURES

Introduction

Anal fissures are breaches in the skin of the distal anal canal, most commonly found in the posterior midline. Drug therapy has recently been revolutionized with the introduction of therapy aimed at reducing anal sphincter pressures, although surgery remains the treatment of choice where pharmacotherapy has failed.

Pathophysiology and therapeutic rationale

The majority of fissures have no underlying cause; however, they may be associated with Crohn's disease, ulcerative colitis or sexually transmitted diseases. There is often spasm of the anal sphincter associated with anal fissures and the maximum resting anal pressure (which relates to internal anal sphincter smooth muscle activity) is often raised.[13] It has been suggested that this spasm perpetuates the ulceration and reduces healing through localized ischaemia and trauma to the lining of the canal.[14] Angiographic studies have demonstrated that the posterior commissure is poorly perfused, and this where most idiopathic fissures occur. Treatments therefore have generally focused on reducing the sphincter pressure through surgical and pharmacological approaches.

Treatment regimens

The current pharmacological regimens favoured include topical application of glycerine trinitrate (GTN) ointment and botulinum toxin A injection of the internal anal sphincter (Table 4.3). Surgery involves a lateral internal anal sphincterotomy, which results in good healing rates (90%); however, incontinence occurs in up to 45% in the early postoperative period and is permanent in 8%.[15] GTN is a donor of nitric oxide (NO), a neurotransmitter that has been shown to be a potent relaxant of vascular and intestinal smooth muscle. Recent trials have shown an 8-week course of 0.2% topical GTN three times daily is effective for over two-thirds of patients with chronic anal fissures.[16] Healing has been shown to be associated with a reduction in the maximum resting anal pressure and higher GTN doses appear to

Table 4.3   Recommended regime for the use of GTN ointment and botulinum toxin A.

Drug	Dose	Frequency	Route	Duration
GTN ointment	0.2% 0.5 ml	Three times per day	Topical peri- and intra-anal	6–8 weeks
Botulinum toxin A	10 U bilaterally in 0.2 ml saline	One set of injections	Internal sphincter injections	

accelerate resolution. The recurrence rate of fissures after GTN treatment, however, is up to one in three, but these can often be treated successfully with repeated courses.

Botulinum toxin A (Botox®) inhibits the release of vesicular acetylcholine from the nerve terminal into the neuromuscular junction, blocking the muscle action potential and subsequent contraction. Botox® injected into the internal anal sphincter improves anal fissure healing and, in a recent study, has been shown to have superior healing rates to GTN (96% after 8 weeks treatment), with fewer recurrent fissures after treatment cessation.[17] For treatment, 10 units of Botox® in 0.2 ml saline are injected into each side of the anterior midline of the internal anal sphincter.

Anal topical GTN
Mode of action
GTN is a nitric oxide donor causing smooth muscle relaxation of the internal anal sphincter, facilitating anal fissure healing.

Indications
Used to treat anal fissures and painful haemorrhoidal disease.

Adverse reactions
Headaches occur in up to 70% of cases; flatulence incontinence and anal burning have been reported in trials; flushing, dizziness, postural hypotension and tachycardia are expected effects of mucosal nitrates.

Drug interactions
Possible interactions of mucosal nitrates are enhanced hypotensive effect of ACE inhibitors, calcium antagonists, α_1 antagonists and other nitrates.

Contraindications
Hypersensitivity to nitrates, hypotensive conditions, hypertrophic obstructive cardiomyopathy, aortic stenosis, closed-angle glaucoma are all contraindications.

Intra-internal anal sphincter Botulinum toxin A injection
Mode of action
This injection causes muscle paralysis through the inhibition of acetylcholine release at the neuromuscular junction.

Indications
It is used to treat anal fissures.

Adverse reactions
None have been reported from recent trials, but faecal incontinence may, in theory, be a possible side-effect.

Contraindications
Generalized disorders of muscle activity, pregnancy and breastfeeding are all contraindications.

Drug interactions
None have been reported.

HAEMORRHOIDS

Introduction

There is little evidence to support the use of pharmacotherapy in the treatment of haemorrhoids and local injection therapy or surgery remains the only effective therapy. However, some drugs aimed at reducing the symptoms of haemorrhoids may be of limited use.

Pathophysiology and therapeutic rationale

Haemorrhoids are probably caused by several factors, the end result of which is congestion and hypertrophy of the internal anal cushions. Anal cushions may become congested because they fail to empty rapidly during the act of defaecation, are abnormally mobile or are trapped by a tight anal sphincter. When the cushions become congested, they are more likely to bleed and become oedematous. This eventually leads to stretching of the muscles and hypertrophy.

During the act of defaecation, the vascular cushions normally rotate outwards; however conditions such as constipation, advancing age and prolonged straining, disturb this normal mechanism and can enhance congestion. Haemorrhoids are more common in pregnancy but this can be considered a normal phenomenon, since they are not more prevalent in non-pregnant multiparous women. It has also been demonstrated that the anal sphincter tone is greater in patients with haemorrhoidal disease, although this is more likely to be a consequence rather than a cause. Common symptoms include bleeding, anal swelling, pain and discomfort, discharge and pruritus. Bleeding may be slight, such as spotting on the toilet paper, or profuse and continuous if the cushions prolapse. Prolapsed cushions have been classified by their extent. First-degree piles do not extend beyond the dentate line, second degree piles extend beyond the dentate line, but spontaneously disappear after straining is complete, third-degree piles can only be digitally reduced after prolapse and fourth-degree piles are permanently outside the anal verge. Complications of haemorrhoidal disease include bleeding, painful thrombosis of the internal and external cushions, and perianal dermatitis.

Treatment regimens

The mainstay of management of haemorrhoids involves local techniques such as sclerosant injections, banding and cryotherapy. For less severe disease, however, topical therapy or suppositories may be considered to treat the pain, discomfort, pruritus and discharge associated with the condition. Bulking agents have been advocated as a treatment to alleviate the discomfort of haemorrhoidal disease but there is little evidence to support this; dietary fibre has proved effective in decreasing symptoms in a few small clinical studies.[18]

Bland topical treatments contain mild astringents such as bismuth subgallate, zinc oxide and hamamelis and may be of symptomatic value. Heparinoids have been suggested to reduce the local oedema associated with congested cushions and to promote resorption of extravasated blood. Local anaesthetics are used to relieve pain and pruritus, although there is little evidence to support their use, which has been associated with local irritation and contact dermatitis.[19] Many preparations contain corticosteroids, which may reduce the local inflammation associated with haemorrhoidal disease. Uncontrolled trials however, have shown little difference between different corticosteroid and non-corticosteroid preparations. There also appears to be little difference between ointments and suppositories.[20,21]

As with fissure-in-ano, internal anal sphincter hypertonia appears to play a role in the pain associated with haemorrhoidal disease. Relaxation of the sphincter with the nitric oxide donor, GTN, may therefore improve symptoms. A small study demonstrated symptomatic improvement after 1 week when 0.5% GTN was applied to the anus in patients with acutely thrombosed external haemorrhoids.[22]

DRUG TREATMENT OF VASCULAR MALFORMATIONS IN THE GASTROINTESTINAL TRACT

Introduction

Vascular anomalies are a common cause of bleeding from the lower gastrointestinal tract, but account for 0–5% of patients presenting with upper GI bleeding. Most vascular ectasias are incidental and do not require treatment and, of the cases responsible for GI bleeding, most can be managed using iron therapy alone. Acute and persistent bleeding is managed primarily by endoscopic therapy or surgery although, for selected patients, sex hormones, octreotide or tranexamic acid may be considered.

Pathophysiology

Vascular ectasias (telangectasias or angiodysplasias) represent an array of pathological identities but can be classified broadly into primary (sporadic) or secondary to conditions such as chronic renal failure, the CREST syndrome, radiotherapy and hereditary haemorrhagic telangectasia (Rendu-Osler-Weber disease). Primary ectasias are the most common and are probably degenerative lesions. Those that are associated with bleeding seem to occur most commonly in the elderly, are often multiple, and are found most commonly in the caecum and ascending colon.[23] The pathogenesis is uncertain; however, injection studies on postmortem samples demonstrate vascular ectasias in most colons from old patients supporting a degenerative role. At colonoscopy, however, primary ectasias are present in up to 3% of patients without any evidence of bleeding and up to 6% of patients with bleeding. The lesions are composed of dilated, distorted, thin-walled vessels in the mucosa and submucosa, and are associated with arteriovenous fistulae and ectatic veins, which probably result from obstruction of vessels piercing the muscular layers. Although cited as a possible association in the past, a recent literature analysis concluded that there was no clear causal relationship between aortic stenosis and colonic angiodysplasia.[24]

The clinical presentation ranges from mild incidental anaemia to massive haemorrhage. The natural history of asymptomatic lesions is benign, and thus they do not require treatment.[25] Ectasias on endoscopy are normally between 0.1 mm–2 cm and are fern-like, composed of multiple vascular fronds originating from a central vessel.

Therapeutic rationale

Once a diagnosis of ectasia has been made, treatments can be instigated acutely during bleeding or to prevent rebleeding. Since little evidence is available for the treatment of specific causes of vascular ectasias, and the pathogenesis remains obscure, drug trials have generally aimed at multiple pathophysiological targets, and thus evidence quoted in this section encompasses ectasias as a heterogeneous group.

Treatment regimens

Acute bleeds can be managed endoscopically with heater probe, bipolar coagulation or laser ablation, all of which have similar efficacy, or by vasopressin infusion into the mesenteric artery or intravenously.[26] If bleeding is severe, surgical resection may be required; however, 90% of acute bleeds resolve spontaneously.

Chronic bleeding is far more common and often requires recurrent blood transfusions. Iron-replacement therapy is the first-line treatment of choice, and may be the only therapy required. Additional treatment may be medical, endoscopic or surgical. Medical therapy mainly includes oestrogens and there have also been small series and case studies suggesting that octreotide, tranexamic acid and danazol may be of benefit.[27–29]

There have been several small trials, series

Table 4.4 Recommended regimens for ethinyloestradiol and norethisterone treatment.

Drug	Dose	Frequency	Route	Duration
Ethinyloestradiol	0.05 mg	Once daily	Oral	6 months
Norethisterone	1 mg	Once daily	Oral	6 months

and case studies with combination oestrogen and progesterone therapy in patients with ectasias. Although there are some negative studies, most suggest that hormone therapy reduces the blood replacement requirements compared with untreated groups or blood requirements before therapy was started (Table 4.4). The patients also represent a selected group, where other forms of treatment have either failed or were inappropriate and where transfusion requirements are high.[30-32]

Therapeutic endoscopy is probably the most effective first-line treatment for chronic bleeding ectasias, although there are no comparative data. If this is either ineffective, technically difficult owing to diffuse or obscure disease, or inappropriate, surgery (for a clear source of bleeding) or hormone therapy should be considered.

Ethinyloestradiol and norethisterone

Mode of action

The mode of action is unknown in the treatment of vascular ectasias.

Indications

Recurrent bleeding due to gastrointestinal ectasia where endoscopic therapy or surgery has failed or is inappropriate is an indication for treatment.

Adverse reactions

These include thrombosis, fluid retention, mood and libido disturbance, hypertension, hepatic impairment; and gynaecomastia and feminization in men.

Drug interactions

Both ethinyloestradiol and norethisterone antagonize the effects of anticoagulants, antidepressants and antihypertensives. They also increase plasma levels of cyclosporin, reduce diuretic effects and increase theopylline plasma levels.

Cautions

Caution should be employed in patients with a family history of thrombosis, obesity, immobilization, hypertension, smoking, diabetes or migraine. The risk of thromboembolism increases with age.

Contraindications

A history of thromboembolism, pregnancy, peripheral vascular disease, ischaemic heart disease, cerebrovascular disease, liver disease, SLE, gallstones, history of cholestatic jaundice are contraindications.

THE PREVENTION OF BLEEDING IN CRITICAL CARE

Introduction

Gastrointestinal bleeding in severely ill patients as a result of stress ulceration is a common problem. The introduction of acid-lowering drugs in these patients has been effective in preventing bleeding in critical care, although the most efficacious drug and regimen remains unclear.

Pathophysiology and therapeutic rationale

Disruption of the mucosa in the upper gastrointestinal tract is common in critically ill patients, and in endoscopic studies, mucosal lesions have been shown to present in 60–100% of cases.[33] Without prophylaxis, the incidence of occult bleeding as a result of stress ulcers is 25% and overt bleeding is 5%, where the mortality associated with overt bleeding is 90%.[34]

The lesions are found typically in the gastric fundus and body and range from submucosal petechiae through to erosions and deep ulcers. More extensive disease can involve the distal oesophagus, gastric antrum and duodenum. The pathophysiology is not well understood but probably involves compromised defensive factors such as mucosal blood flow, mucous production, cell renewal and mucosal permeability and enhanced aggressive factors such as acid and digestive enzymes. Lower gastric pH levels have been demonstrated in critically ill patients.[35] Furthermore, pepsin concentrations are higher in these patients. Decreases in intestinal mucosal blood flow with associated ischaemia and impaired barrier function have been demonstrated in stressed animal models. Animal work has also suggested that stress and starvation leads to a reduction in the hexosamine content of gastric mucus, which may reduce mucosal protection and lead to damage.[36]

There appears to be a relationship between severity of illness and the risk of developing stress ulcers; however, the specific risk factors associated with stress ulcers include sepsis, multiple trauma, severe burns, severe hepatic dysfunction, renal failure and major operations. The probability of stress ulcer bleeding rises as the number of risk factors increases.

Therapeutic rationale

The main thrust in the prevention of stress ulcer bleeding has been to reduce gastric acidity. Early reports demonstrated a reduction in bleeding risk if the gastric pH was maintained above 3.5 by hourly antacid titration.[37] Studies involving ranitidine, cimetidine and antacids demonstrated a reduction in overt and occult bleeding but no individual study has definitely established whether these agents decrease mortality. In a meta-analysis, H_2-receptor antagonists appeared to be superior to antacids both with respect to decreased overt bleeding and also clinically important bleeding.[38] H_2-receptor antagonists are more practical, since antacids generally must be given hourly to attain a satisfactory reduction in gastric acidity. In the same study, sucralfate was shown to be similar to both antacids and H_2-receptor antagonists in reducing clinically significant bleeding but more effective in reducing mortality. Sucralfate was also associated with lower rates of nosocomial pneumonia. Results of a more recent trial, however, comparing ranitidine and sucralfate did not demonstrate any difference between the incidence of nosocomial pneumonia, mortality, or reduction in intensive care unit stay but showed bleeding rates to be significantly lower with ranitidine (1.7% versus 3.8%). Only two trials have demonstrated any advantage of ranitidine over cimetidine in acid reduction, but the side-effect profile of cimetidine is worse than that of ranitidine owing to its P_{450} enzyme binding, enhancing commonly used intensive care drugs such as diazepam, phenytoin labetolol and warfarin. Intravenous cimetidine has also been associated with mental confusion (Table 4.5).

There is little experience with proton pump inhibitors and stress ulcer prophylaxis, probably because intravenous preparations have only recently because widely available. Omeprazole has, however, been shown in numerous studies to reduce gastric pH more effectively than H_2-receptor antagonists beyond 24 h after treatment. Moreover, a recent small study demonstrated that clinically significant bleeding was less in omeprezole- than

Table 4.5 Recommended regimens for treatment with omeprazole, ranitidine, cimetidine and sucralfate.

Drug	Dose	Frequency	Route	Duration
Omeprazole	40 mg	Once daily	NG or oral	Until patient recovery
Ranitidine	50 mg bolus 230 mg	6-hourly Infusion 24 h	Intravenous	Until patient recovery
Cimetidine	300 mg bolus 1200 mg	6-hourly Infusion 24 h	Intravenous	Until patient recovery
Sucralfate	1 g	4-hourly	NG or oral	Until patient recovery

NG, nasogastric.

ranitidine-treated patients, and the incidence of pneumonia was reduced. Also, in a small uncontrolled trial treating high-risk ventilated patients, omeprazole suspension completely prevented overt bleeding (Table 4.5).[39]

REFERENCES

1. Barkham P, Tocantins LM. Action of human gastric juice on human blood clots. *J Appl Physiol* 1953; **6:** 1–7.
2. Hirschowitz BL. Pepsin in the pathogenesis of peptic ulceration. In: *Mechanisms of Peptic Ulcer Healing.* F Halter, A Garner, GNJ Tytgat (Eds), Falk Symposium 59, Dordrecht. The Netherlands, Kluwer, 1991, 183–194.
3. Patchett SE, Enright H, Afdahl N, O'Connell W, O'Donoghue DP. Clot lysis by gastric juice; an in vitro study. *Gut* 1989; **30:** 1704–1707.
4. Collins R, Langman M. Treatment with histamine H_2 antagonists in acute upper gastrointestinal haemorrhage. Implications of randomised trials. *N Engl J Med* 1985; **313:** 660–666.
5. Walt RP, Cottrell J, Mann SG, Freemantle NP, Langman MJ. Continuous intravenous famotidine for haemorrhage from peptic ulcer. *Lancet* 1992; **340:** 1058–1062.
6. Daneshmend TK, Hawkey CJ, Langman MJS,

Logan RFA, Long RG, Walt RP. Omeprazole versus placebo for acute upper gastrointestinal bleeding: randomised double blind controlled trial. *Brit Med J* 1992; **304:** 143–147.
7. Khuroo MS, Yattoo GN, Javid G, *et al.* A comparison of omeprazole and placebo for bleeding peptic ulcer. *N Engl J Med* 1997; **336:** 1054–1058.
8. Bustamente M, Stollman N. The efficacy of proton pump inhibitors in acute ulcer bleeding: a qualitative review. *J Clin Gastroenterol* 2000; **30:** 7–13.
9. Lau JY, Sung JJ, Lee KK, *et al.* Effect of intravenous omeprazole on recurrent bleeding after endoscopic treatment of bleeding peptic ulcers. *N Engl J Med* 2000; **343:** 310–316.
10. Barer D, Ogilvie A, Henry D, *et al.* Cimetidine and tranexamic acid in the treatment of acute upper gastrointestinal tract bleeding. *N Engl J Med* 1983; **308:** 1571–1575.
11. Henry DA, O'Connell DL. Effects of fibrinolytic inhibitors on mortality from upper gastrointestinal haemorrhage. *Brit Med J* 1989; **298:** 1142–1146.
12 Imperiale TF, Birgisson S. Somatostatin or octreotide compared with H_2 antagonists and placebo in the management of acute nonvariceal upper gastrointestinal hemorrhage: a meta-analysis. *Ann Int Med* 1997; **127:** 1062–1071.
13. Arabi Y, Alexander-Williams J, Keighley MR.

Anal pressures in hemorrhoids and anal fissure. *Am J Surg* 1977; **134:** 608–610.

14. Gibbons CP, Read NW. Anal hypertonia in fissures: cause or effect? *Br J Surg* 1986; **73:** 443–445.

15. Nyam DC, Pemberton JH. Long-term results of lateral internal sphincterotomy for chronic anal fissure with particular reference to incidence of fecal incontinence. *Dis Colon Rectum* 1999; **42(10):** 1306–1310.

16. Carpeti EA, Kamm MA, McDonald PJ, Chadwick SJD, Melville D, Phillips RKS. Randomised controlled trial shows that glyceryl trinitrate heals anal fissures, higher doses are not more effective, and there is a high recurrence rate. *Gut* 1999; **44:** 727–730.

17. Brisinda G, Maria G, Bentivoglio AN, Cassetta E, Gui D, Albanese A. A comparison of injections of botulinum toxin and topical nitroglycerin ointment for the treatment of chronic anal fissure. *N Engl J Med* 1999; **341:** 65–69.

18. Klurfeld DM. The role of dietary fibre in gastrointestinal disease. *J Am Diet Assoc* 1987; **87:** 1172–1177.

19. Kawada A, Noguchi H, Hiruma M, Tajima S, Ishibashi A, Marshall J. Fixed drug eruption induced by lidocaine. *Contact Dermatitis* 1996; **35:** 375.

20. Smith RB, Moodie J. Comparative efficacy and tolerability of two ointment and suppository preparations ('Uniroid' and 'Proctosedyl') in the treatment of second-degree haemorrhoids in general practice. *Curr Med Res Opin* 1988; **11:** 32–40.

21. Knoch HG, Klug W, Hubner WD. Ointment treatment of 1st degree hemorrhoids. Comparison of the effectiveness of a phytogenic preparation with two new ointments containing synthetic drugs. *Fortschr Med* 1992; **110:** 135–138.

22. Gorfine SR. Treatment of benign anal disease with topical nitroglycerin. *Dis Colon Rectum* 1995; **38:** 453–456.

23. Boley SJ, Sammartano RJ, Adams A. On the nature and etiology of vascular ectasias of the colon: Degenerative lesions of aging. *Gastroenterology* 1977; **72:** 650.

24. Imperiale TF, Ransohoff DF. Aortic stenosis, idiopathic gastrointestinal bleeding, and angiodysplasia: Is there an association ? *Gastroenterology* 1988; **95:** 1670–1676.

25. Foutch PG, Rex DK, Lieberman DA. Prevalence and natural history of colonic angiodysplasia among healthy asymptomatic people. *Am J Gastroenterol* 1995; **90:** 564–567.

26. Danesh BJ, Spiliadis C, Williams CB. Angiodysplasia, an uncommon cause of colonic bleeding: colonic evaluation of 1050 patients with rectal bleeding and anaemia. *Int J Colon Dis* 1987; **2:** 218.

27. Vujkovac B, Lavre J, Saboviv M. Successful treatment of bleeding from colonic angiodysplasias with tranexamic acid in a hemodialysis patient. *Am J Kidney Dis* 1998; **31:** 536–538.

28. Anderson MR, Aaseby J. Somatostatin in the treatment of gastrointestinal bleeding caused by angiodysplasia. *Scand J Gastroenterol* 1996; **31:** 1037–1039.

29. Rossini FP, Arrigoni A, Pennazio M. Octreotide in the treatment of bleeding due to angiodysplasia of the small intestine. *Am J Gastroenterol* 1993; **88:** 1424–1427.

30. Cutsem E, Rutgeerts P, Vantrappen G. Treatment of bleeding gastrointestinal vascular malformations with oestrogen-progesterone. *Lancet* 1990; **335:** 953–955.

31. Lewis BS, Salomon P, Rivera-MacMurray S, Kornbluth AA, Wenger J, Waye JD. Does hormonal therapy have any benefit for bleeding angiodysplasia. *J Clin Gastroenterol* 1992; **15:** 99–103.

32. Junquera F, Santos J, Saperas E, Armengol JR, Malagelada JR. Estrogen and progesterone treatment in digestive hemorrhage caused by vascular malformations. *Gastroenterol Hepatol* 1995; **18:** 61–65.

33. Czaja AJ, McAlhany JC, Pruitt BA Jr. Acute gastroduodenal disease after thermal injury. An endoscopic evaluation of incidence and natural history. *N Engl J Med* 1974; **291:** 925–929.

34. Schuster DP, Rowley H, Feinstein S, McGue HK, Zuckerman GR. Prospective evaluation of the risk of upper gastrointestinal bleeding after admission to a medical intensive care unit. *Am J Med* 1984; **76:** 623–630.

35. Robbins R, Idjadi F, Stahl WM. Studies of gastric secretion in stressed patients. *Ann Surg* 1972; **175:** 555–562.

36. Robert A, Kauffman GL Jr. Stress ulcers. In: *Gastrointestinal Disease, 3rd edn.* MJ Sleisenger, JS Fordtran (Eds), WB Saunders, Philadelphia, 1984, 612–625.

37. Hastings PR, Skillman JJ, Bushnell LS, Silen W. Antacid titration in the prevention of acute gastrointestinal bleeding. *N Engl J Med* 1978; **298:** 1041–1045.

38. Cook DJ, Reeve BK, Guyatt GH, *et al.* Stress ulcer

prophylaxis in critically ill patients. *J Am Med Assoc* 1996; **275:** 308–314.

39. Lasky MR, Metzler MH, Phillips JO. A prospective study of omeprazole suspension to prevent clinically significant gastrointestinal bleeding from stress ulcers in mechanically ventilated trauma patients. *J Trauma, Injury, Infection, Crit Care* 1998; **44(3):** 527–533.

5

Inflammatory bowel disease

Elizabeth Carty, Anne B Ballinger

INTRODUCTION

Ulcerative colitis (UC) and Crohn's disease (CD) are chronic inflammatory disorders of the gastrointestinal tract. CD is characterized by patchy, transmural granulomatous inflammation of any part of the gastrointestinal tract, although it is most common in the ileocaecal area. UC, in contrast to CD, is limited to the colon, is continuous and involves the mucosa without the formation of granulomas. Both diseases are associated with extraintestinal compli-cations (Table 5.1). The clinical course of some of these complications may parallel that of the underlying bowel disease and thus improve with treatment that is directed primarily against the bowel inflammation.

AETIOPATHOGENESIS OF INFLAMMATORY BOWEL DISEASE

The aetiology of inflammatory bowel disease (IBD) remains unknown, but genetic, immune,

---

Table 5.1   Extraintestinal manifestations of inflammatory bowel disease and their relationship to activity of the bowel disease.

Parallels disease activity in the bowel	Independent of disease activity
Large joint pauciarticular arthropathy	Small joint symmetric polyarthropathy
Episcleritis	Sacroilitis
Erythema nodosum	Ankylosing spondylitis
Pyoderma gangrenosum*	Primary sclerosing cholangitis
Anterior uveitis* (requires topical corticosteroids)	Choledocholithiasis
	Nephrolithiasis
	Amyloidosis (rare)

*Usually related to activity.

infectious and vascular factors all appear to play a role in disease pathogenesis.[1,2] The most popular hypothesis with supporting scientific evidence is that IBD is a heterogeneous group of diseases that result in intestinal inflammation and that genetic and environmental factors are implicated in disease pathogenesis. It is proposed that disruption of the intestinal epithelial integrity may allow bacteria and luminal antigens to trigger an immune response. In the genetically predisposed individual, there is an exaggerated immune response, which may be the result of lack of regulatory or suppressor cell function, or enhanced numbers of effector T cells. In CD, the T-cell immune response is Th1 dominant as manifested by increased production of the pro-inflammatory cytokines, interferon-γ (IFN-γ) and tumour necrosis factor-α (TNF-α) and reduced production of the anti-inflammatory cytokines, interleukin-4 (IL-4) and IL-10. In contrast, in UC there is a Th2 dominant response with increased production of IL-5. Polymorphs, mast cells and eosinophils are also present in enhanced number in the mucosa in Crohn's disease. Increased expression of cell adhesion molecules, such as the intercellular adhesion molecule ICAM1, the vascular cell adhesion molecules VCAM and the selectins, mediate cell recruitment and may be important in the pathogenesis of intestinal inflammation. The functional consequences of enhanced inflammatory cell numbers in the mucosa are increased production of inflammatory mediators such as eicosanoids, proteases, reactive oxygen and nitrogen metabolites, complement and cytokines. As well as ongoing inflammatory processes in the mucosa in CD, there is also defective growth factor production, producing abnormal mucosal repair mechanisms—most notably excessive fibrosis.[2] Evidence from humans with IBD and also from animal models suggests that intestinal bacteria and their products are involved in the initiation and perpetuation of the inflammatory process. However, it is not known whether the antigens that trigger the immune response are the same bacteria responsible for perpetuation of the response.

Cigarette smoking is the most extensively studied environmental factor associated with IBD. Smoking is associated with a two-fold increase in the frequency of CD and increases the risk of disease flares.[3] In contrast to CD, smoking is associated with a reduced frequency of UC and fewer disease flares. The mechanism whereby smoking affects the frequency and course of IBD is not known. All patients with IBD should be advised to stop smoking, in Crohn's disease because of the association with disease activity, and in UC because of the detrimental effects of smoking on cardiorespiratory function.

ULCERATIVE COLITIS

Ulcerative colitis (UC) always begins in the rectum and extends proximally to affect a variable extent of the colon. Mucosal inflammation is in a circumferential and uninterrupted pattern, although patients using topical therapy may have apparent rectal sparing. At the time of diagnosis, disease is confined to the rectum (proctitis) or rectum and sigmoid (proctosigmoiditis) in 27–44% of patients. The frequency of total colonic involvement (pancolitis) varies but is generally present in less than one-third of patients (Fig. 5.1).[4,5] The disease may progress proximally with time in patients who are initially diagnosed as having disease limited to the distal colon. For instance, with disease confined to the rectum or rectosigmoid, extension to the proximal colon occurs in 10–30% of patients after 10 years. Most patients with UC experience a chronic, relapsing, remitting course and will require maintenance treatment in order to reduce the number of relapses.

Therapeutic rationale

The aim of drug therapy is to induce and maintain disease remission. Currently available drugs have anti-inflammatory or immunomodulatory effects and most commonly act by inhibition of pro-inflammatory mediators. The

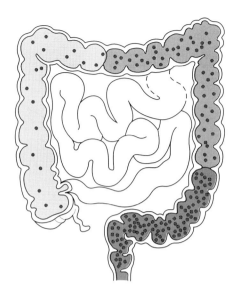

Figure 5.1 Anatomical location of ulcerative colitis. Ulcerative colitis extends proximally from the rectum in a continuous fashion. The extent of proximal spread varies. *Redrawn from The Pentasa slide kit with permission.*

route of drug therapy is dependent on the site and severity (Table 5.2) of disease. Inflammation confined to the rectum or rectosigmoid region (distal colitis) may be amenable to topical therapy whereas more extensive disease will require systemic treatment. Treatment options are summarized in Table 5.3.

Limited disease

Topical treatment is standard therapy for distal disease. The advantages over oral therapy include delivery of higher concentrations of drug to the site of disease, better response rates and fewer side-effects.[7,8] Liquid enemas can deliver drugs as far as the splenic flexure, while foam preparations extend less proximally (to the proximal sigmoid).[9] However, some patients find foam preparations easier to retain, particularly when the disease is active. Suppositories only have effects in the rectum. Aminosalicylates and corticosteroids are both available as enema, foam or suppository. The choice between oral or topical and differing formulations of topical therapy depends on patient preference and site of disease.

Induction of remission
Sulphasalazine 3 g enemas result in a 70% response rate compared with 11% for placebo after 2 weeks' of treatment in patients with proctitis and distal disease.[10] Unlike oral treatment, topical sulphasalazine is well-tolerated, with no adverse effects. Sulphasalazine, however, is a bright orange-yellow in colour by virtue of its azo bond and may produce staining of underwear. Topical mesalazine, the active compound, is therefore the preferred form of treatment. Mesalazine suppositories, 500 mg twice daily, effectively induce remission in proctitis. In patients with distal disease, the efficacy and safety of 4 g 5-aminosalicylic acid (ASA) enemas (one nightly) was assessed over a 6-week study period by Sutherland *et al.*[11] Treatment was well-tolerated and resulted in a response rate of 63% compared with 22% in the placebo group. A later study suggested that 1 g and 2 g enemas were equally effective as 4 g enemas when treating distal disease.[12] Adverse effects of mesalazine enemas were rare and mild in these trials and comprised mainly of anal irritation. A retrospective study has shown an 80% remission rate after 34 weeks' of treatment, suggesting that it is worth persisting in refractory disease.[13]

Table 5.2 Assessment of disease severity* in ulcerative colitis.[6]

	Mild	Severe
Stools per day	≤4	≥6
Rectal bleeding	+/−	+
Fever	None	Mean evening temperature >37.5°C or temperature >37.8°C on 2 days out of 4
Tachycardia	None	>90 beats/min
Anaemia	Not severe	Hb 75% or less of normal
ESR	≤30 mm/h	>30 mm/h

*Moderate, intermediate between severe and mild.

Table 5.3 Summary of therapeutic options in ulcerative colitis.

Mild or moderate proctitis and distal disease	Mild or moderate extensive disease	Severe disease	Severe fulminant acute colitis
Topical 5-ASA* or steroids (may be prescribed alone or in combination)	Oral 5-ASA	Oral corticosteroids	Intravenous corticosteroids
Oral 5-ASA (alone or in combination with topical treatment)			Intravenous cyclosporin
Treat proximal constipation: lactulose, magnesium sulphate			
Refractory disease: oral or intravenous corticosteroids, oral azathioprine, lignocaine or short-chain fatty acid enemas, surgery (proctocolectomy)			

*5-ASA, 5-aminosalicylic acid.

Corticosteroids given as liquid enema, foam or suppository are effective in treating active disease and lead to a clinical response in about 70% of patients with distal UC.[14] Compared with oral preparations, absorption of the topical steroids is only about 40%. However, adrenal suppression and even Cushing's syndrome may occur, especially after prolonged use of topical corticosteroids.[15] Budesonide is a novel steroid, with high local activity, and low systemic activity owing to extensive first-pass metabolism in the liver. As a 2 mg enema, budesonide is effective in acute distal UC. In contrast to prednisolone enemas, adrenal function, as monitored by plasma cortisol levels, is not affected, even with prolonged treatment and may be associated with fewer corticosteroid-related side effects.[16] A meta-analysis in 1997 suggested that mesalazine enemas are more effective than steroid enemas; however, they are more expensive.[17] Some patients may achieve maximum benefit from a combination of oral plus topical mesalazine. Oral corticosteroids are required in a few patients with severe refractory disease. More experimental options include enemas of lignocaine or short-chain fatty acids, and nicotine patches.

Maintenance of remission
Once remission is achieved, therapy can be tapered and administered as maintenance treatment. Mesalazine 0.8–1 g daily effectively maintains remission in UC, both as suppositories for proctitis, and enemas for left-sided colitis.[18,19] In some patients, treatment every second day or three times weekly is sufficient to maintain a remission.[20] Oral mesalazine or azathioprine may be necessary in patients who are not well controlled with topical therapy or prefer oral drug treatment.

Disease extending proximal to the splenic flexure

Induction of remission
Extensive disease cannot be treated adequately using enemas. Mild to moderate disease is treated with mesalazine-containing compounds (Table 5.4) and moderate to severe disease requires oral or intravenous corticosteroids. Oral sulphasalazine 4–6 g/day in four divided doses effectively induces remission in UC[21] but its use can be limited by side-effects. Clinical trials have shown that the newer 5-ASA preparations are equally effective as sulphasalazine for inducing remission and that they are associated with fewer side-effects.[22,23] It is unclear if any of these newer compounds have significant benefits over others in the treatment of acute UC. In one study, balsalazide 2.25 mg three times a day was slightly more effective than

Asacol (800 mg three times daily) in inducing a remission and there appeared to be fewer side-effects with balsalazide.[24] Oral corticosteroids are indicated for moderate to severe UC. Prednisolone 40 mg daily induced remission in about 55% of patients after 3 weeks' of treatment, which was significantly better than the remission rate obtained with a 20 mg daily dosage. There was further benefit with a 60 mg dosage but this associated with a marked increase in adverse effects.[25] Azathioprine or its metabolite, 6-mercaptopurine (6-MP) permits cessation of steroids or a reduction in dose in many patients with persistent symptoms despite prolonged corticosteroid treatment.[26,27] However, onset of action is slow and up to 3–6 months' of treatment may be required to appreciate an optimal effect.

Maintenance of remission
Sulphasalazine and other mesalazine-containing compounds will prevent relapse in quiescent UC. Relapses are about five times more frequent in untreated patients.[28] One study has shown that olsalazine (1.0 g daily) was superior to Asacol (1.2 g daily) in prevention of relapse in UC and may be particularly useful in patients with left-sided UC.[29] Its use has been limited, however, by secretory diarrhoea, which affects up to 10% of patients. Diarrhoea can be minimized by taking the drug with meals and initiating therapy at a low dose and slowly increasing. Whichever therapy is used, it should be continued long-term because the beneficial effects are maintained for many years and the relapse rate is high if drug treatment is stopped.[30] Azathioprine or 6-MP are useful in maintaining a remission in patients who are intolerant, or are not adequately controlled with mesalazine. In one controlled trial, patients who had achieved complete remission while receiving azathioprine were randomized to receive continued azathioprine or placebo. The 1-year rate of relapse was 39% for patients continuing azathioprine and 59% for those taking placebo.[31] Corticosteroids (topical and oral) have not been shown to be of benefit in maintaining remission in UC.

Table 5.4   Oral 5-aminosalicylic acid drugs used in the treatment of inflammatory bowel disease.

Drug	Formulation	Mode of delivery	Site of drug release	Treatment of active disease	Maintenance of remission (daily dose)
Pro-drug					
Sulphasalazine	5-ASA linked to sulphapyridine by azo bond	Azo bond split by bacterial flora to release active drug	Colon	4–6 g in three to four divided doses	1 g three times daily
Balsalazide	5-ASA linked to amino-benzoyl-β-alanine (inert carrier) by azo bond	Azo bond split by bacterial flora to release active drug	Colon	2.25 g three times daily	
Olsalazine	Two molecules of 5-ASA linked by an azo bond	Azo bond split by bacterial flora to release active drug	Colon	1 g three times daily	500 mg twice daily
Coated preparation					
Pentasa	Tablets consist of ethylcellulose-coated microgranules of 5-ASA	5-ASA diffuses through ethylcellulose coating	Jejunum, ileum, colon	2–4 g in two to four divided doses	500 mg three times daily
Asacol	5-ASA tablet core coated with an acrylic-based resin 'Eudragit®-S'	Resin dissolves at pH $\geq$ 7	Distal small bowel, colon	800–1600 mg three times daily	400 mg three times daily
Claversal/mesasal/ salofalk	5-ASA tablet core coated with Eudragit®-L	Dissolves at pH >6	Proximal small bowel onwards		

Acute severe colitis

Acute severe colitis is defined as passage of six or more bloody stools per day with one or more of the following fever of 37.8°C or more, tachycardia >90 beats/min, ESR >30 mm in the first hour and haemoglobin <10.5 g/dl (Table 5.2). Toxic megacolon is defined as colonic dilation, assessed on plain abdominal radiography, of at least 6 cm associated with systemic toxicity. Joint management of the patient between colorectal surgeon and gastroenterologist is mandatory. Treatment is with intravenous hydrocortisone (100 mg 6-hourly) or methylprednisolone (16 mg 6-hourly), which will achieve remission in about 60% of patients.[32,33] When clinically improved, the standard practice is to change treatment to 40 mg oral prednisolone and taper the dose down according to the clinical response.

Intravenous cyclosporin (4 mg/kg/day by continuous infusion) is indicated in selected patients who are refractory to corticosteroids but who do not warrant immediate surgery. In the only published randomized placebo controlled trial of intravenous cyclosporin in severe UC, nine out of the 11 (82%) patients, treated with cyclosporin in addition to ongoing steroid treatment, had a response to treatment, compared with none of the nine patients in the placebo group. The mean length of time to respond in the cyclosporin group was 7 days.[34] In patients who responded, therapy was changed to oral prednisolone and oral cyclosporin (6–8 mg/kg/day) and at 6 months the success rate was 69%.[35] The results of subsequent retrospective studies of cyclosporin treatment in acute UC have been less optimistic and an initial response rate of 56–79% reported. About one-third of these responders subsequently required a colectomy within 18 months.[33,36,37] Data from uncontrolled studies suggest that the subsequent colectomy rate may be reduced by addition of oral azathioprine or 6-mercaptopurine that is initiated during tapering of steroid therapy. A multicentre placebo-controlled trial is underway to evaluate the efficacy of maintenance azathioprine treatment after a severe attack of ulcerative colitis.

In summary, intravenous cyclosporin may be the best option for the patient with new-onset disease who presents with acute severe colitis that is unresponsive to intravenous corticosteroids and who wishes to avoid colectomy. Colectomy may, however, be the preferred option for a patient with chronic and relapsing disease. Mesalazine has no role in the treatment of acute severe colitis and should only be initiated after the acute attack begins to resolve. Total parenteral nutrition has no therapeutic benefit in UC although, in rare cases, may be necessary as a nutritional adjunct.

Summary

Aminosalicylates and steroids remain the important first-line therapies in active UC. Azathioprine is useful to maintain a remission in patients with frequent relapses. Topical treatment with 5-ASA and corticosteroids can be useful in specific patient groups. Novel treatments in particular immunosuppressants continue to be assessed. No single agent is universally successful and drug therapy to cure the disease remains illusive.

EXPERIMENTAL AND NOVEL THERAPIES FOR ULCERATIVE COLITIS

Antibacterial and probiotic therapy

Intestinal luminal flora is thought to be the primary stimulus for inflammation in the gastrointestinal tract of experimental model of colitis and in patients who are genetically susceptible to IBD. Furthermore, experimental work suggests that the onset of inflammation may be associated with an imbalance in the intestinal microflora, with a relative increase in 'harmful' bacteria and reduction in 'beneficial' flora such as lactobacillus and bifidobacteria. The term 'probiotic', refers to living organisms, which, upon ingestion, are beneficial to the host. On the basis of these observations, it has been suggested that manipulation of the intestinal bacterial flora may be beneficial in the treatment of IBD.

Antibiotics

Antibiotics such as tobramycin, ciprofloxacillin and metronidazole have been shown to improve remission rates in steroid-treated patients with active UC.[38] However, antibiotics are usually reserved for patients with acute severe colitis who are ill and febrile, or patients in whom an infective colitis may co-exist. Metronidazole is also useful for patients with pouchitis after ileo pouch-anal anastomosis.

Bismuth

Bismuth inhibits bacterial sulphatases. In a randomized study, bismuth citrate enemas were equally effective as mesalazine enemas and may prove useful in patients refractory to mesalazine.[39]

Probiotics

Treatment with an oral preparation of non-pathogenic *Escherichia coli* is well-tolerated and has similar efficacy to mesalazine (as Asacol, 800 mg three times daily) in maintaining a remission in ulcerative colitis.[40,41] Oral administration of probiotic preparations for 9 months maintained remission in 85% of pouchitis patients compared with none in the placebo group.[42] These preliminary results support the need for further large double-blind randomized trials and additional work to define the mechanism of action.

Immunosuppressants and cytokine therapy

Limited data only are available on the use of anti-tumour necrosis factor (TNF) antibodies in UC. Uncontrolled studies in small numbers of patients have shown a variable response and suggest that the efficacy is certainly less than in patients with CD.[43] A controlled clinical trial of the anti-inflammatory cytokine, IL-10, in patients with mild-to-moderate UC showed a trend in favour of IL-10. However, the number of patients achieving remission was not significantly different from placebo.[44]

There are no controlled data to support long-term use of oral cyclosporin as maintenance therapy in either UC or Crohn's disease, and toxicity limits its usefulness. Cyclosporin enemas are no more effective than placebo in patients with active left-sided ulcerative colitis.[45] In a small open study, the potent immunosuppressive agent tacrolimus, had some benefit in patients with IBD;[46] however, its particular role in the treatment of patients with IBD is not yet clear. The results of methotrexate treatment in patients with UC, unlike Crohn's disease, have been disappointing. At a weekly oral dose of 12.5 mg, methotrexate was not found to be better than placebo in the induction or maintenance of remission in patients with chronic active ulcerative colitis.[47]

Other agents

Heparin

Heparin is an anti-inflammatory agent as well as an anticoagulant and has been promising in case reports and uncontrolled trials of acute UC. In the only randomized controlled trial to date, subcutaneous heparin (10 000 units twice daily) was well-tolerated and superior to placebo in induction of remission in moderate to severe UC (18.2% versus 2.9% at 6 weeks).[48]

Short-chain fatty acids

The use of topical short-chain fatty acids (SCFA) represents a physiological approach to treatment, since butyrate is the key nutrient for the colonocyte and a defect in SCFA metabolism by colonocytes has been postulated to contribute to aetiopathogenesis of UC. Results of randomized controlled trials of SCFA enemas have been disappointing and the largest placebo controlled trial did not demonstrate efficacy in active left-sided UC.[49]

Nicotine

The relative rarity of UC in smokers has led to interest in nicotine as a therapeutic agent.

Nicotine patches were more effective than placebo in active colitis but less effective than prednisolone and with more side-effects.[50] Maintenance therapy with nicotine is ineffective. In an attempt to minimize systemic side-effects, investigators have developed preparations for rectal administration but there are no controlled trials to date.

Local anaesthetics

Neuropeptides can directly modify the immune response. Local anaesthetics have anti-inflammatory properties that are related to inhibition of adrenergic nerves and to anti-inflammatory properties independent of effects on neurones. Uncontrolled studies in patients with distal ulcerative colitis have shown improvement in symptoms, endoscopic appearance and histologic activity after treatment with lignocaine and ropivacaine enemas;[51] however, there are no controlled data to date. Local anaesthetics appear to be well-tolerated and may be worth trying in patients with distal colitis that is resistant to standard medical therapy.

Pouchitis

Pouchitis is a major long-term complication after ileal pouch-anal anastamosis for UC. Only a few treatments have been tested adequately in placebo-controlled trials with adequate numbers of patients. Of these, oral metronidazole is superior to placebo in active chronic pouchitis and oral administration of probiotic bacteria maintains a remission.[42]

CROHN'S DISEASE

Assessment of disease activity in patients with CD is more difficult than in patients with UC because the clinical pattern and disease complications are more heterogeneous. In clinical trials, disease activity is usually assessed on the basis of symptoms, signs and laboratory markers of inflammatory disease; the most widely used index is the Crohn's Disease Activity Index (CDAI). Most of these scoring systems are unsuitable for routine clinical use. The working definitions of the American College of Gastroenterology provide a useful guide for routine clinical practice (Table 5.5). There is a poor correlation between clinical activity and endoscopic findings.

Induction of remission

Mesalazine-containing compounds are useful in patients with mild to moderately active CD. Sulphasalazine is effective only in patients with ileocolonic or colonic disease,[52,53] which is consistent with the release profile of 5-ASA from this preparation in the colon. Pentasa (4 g/day) is superior to placebo in inducing a remission but no significant effect is seen at lower doses.[54] A small study (20 out of 38 patients completing treatment) with Asacol (3.2 g/day) also demonstrated efficacy for mesalazine in patients with mild to moderately active CD.[55] Oral corticosteroids are indicated for patients with moderate to severely active CD. In the American National Co-operative Crohn's Disease Study, patients with active CD were treated with prednisolone at doses of 0.25–0.75 mg/kg/day (depending on the CDAI) or placebo. After 17 weeks, 60% of the prednisolone-treated patients achieved remission compared with 30% of placebo treated (Fig. 5.2).[52] In the European Cooperative Crohn's Disease Study, patients received 48 mg of methylprednisolone (equal to 60 mg prednisolone) tapered to 12 mg over 6 weeks. There was significant benefit in the steroid-treated group irrespective of disease localization.[53] A controlled ileal-release preparation of budesonide (CIR-Entocort, 9 mg once daily) induces remission in 50–70% of patients with mild or moderate disease confined to the distal ileum, ileocaecal region or ascending colon. The CIR capsule is superior to mesalazine and only slightly inferior to 40 mg prednisolone for induction of remission in these patients.[56,57] The incidence of side-effects, such as acne and moon face, is much reduced with budesonide but morning cortisol levels are suppressed,

Table 5.5   Working definition of disease activity in Crohn's disease for clinical practice from the American College of Gastroenterology.

Mild-to-moderate disease	Moderate to severe disease	Severe-fulminant disease	Remission
Outpatients able to tolerate an oral diet without dehydration, toxicity, abdominal tenderness, mass or obstruction	Failed treatment for mild-to-moderate Crohn's disease or patients with prominent symptoms such as fever, weight loss, abdominal pain and tenderness, nausea, vomiting or anaemia	Persisting symptoms with oral steroids, or patients with a high fever, persistent vomiting, obstruction, rebound tenderness, cachexia or abscess	Asymptomatic patients

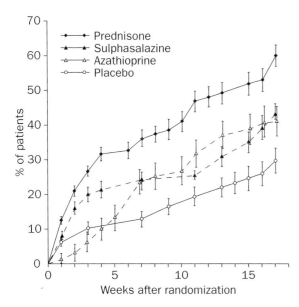

Figure 5.2 Cumulative percent of patients in remission (Crohn's Disease Activity Index) week-by-week.[52] Prednisolone induced remission more rapidly and effectively than placebo. Both sulphasalazine and azathioprine induced remission although neither was as effective as placebo. Reproduced from Summers RW *et al* with permission of Harcourt Health Sciences.[52]

indicating a systemic component in the drug action. The long-term effects of budesonide on bone metabolism are unknown. Treatment with controlled-release budesonide costs much more than prednisolone; nevertheless it might theoretically offer advantages for patients who require frequent course of prednisolone and those at particular risk of adverse effects. Elemental diets (e.g. glucose, amino acids and long-chain triglycerides) were originally used in the treatment of CD because they are devoid of antigens, which are thought to act as important stimuli of the mucosal immune response. The elemental diet is equally effective as corticosteroids for inducing a remission, particularly in small-bowel CD. Recent studies suggest that liquid polymeric diets may have equal efficacy to elemental preparations.[58] Metronidazole, which has both antimicrobial and immunosuppressive properties, has similar efficacy to sulphasalazine but is particularly useful for perianal disease. Patients with severe fulminant disease require hospital admission and treatment with intravenous steroids.

Maintenance of remission

The rate of symptomatic relapse in CD is 40–70% over 2 years.[52] Mesalazine-containing drugs are frequently used as maintenance therapy; however, the results of randomized controlled trials have been conflicting. A meta-analysis in 1997 suggested that, in patients who have their remission induced with medical therapy, the benefit of 5-ASA was small. The number needed to treat with mesalazine to prevent 'one relapse episode' was 16 and when the patients who received mesalazine as postoperative therapy were removed from the analysis, the benefit was not significant. Multivariate analysis in this study suggested that the benefits of mesalazine as maintenance therapy is limited to patients with ileitis, those with prolonged duration of disease and those who have remission induced by surgery.[59] Azathioprine and 6-MP maintain remission in CD and allow a reduction in the dose of corticosteroids in patients whose disease relapses when the dose is reduced.[60,61] Patients who do not tolerate azathioprine owing to minor side-effects such as nausea or abdominal pain may tolerate 6-MP; however, patients who have major side-effects from azathioprine, such as pancreatitis or leucopenia, should not be given 6-MP. The optimum duration of treatment with azathioprine or 6-MP is controversial. A French study has suggested that withdrawal of therapy may be considered in patients who have been in remission for at least 4 years. Owing to the small numbers of patients followed long-term, however, the data must be interpreted with caution and each patient assessed individually.[62] Trials are underway to determine the role of budesonide as maintenance treatment but conventional corticosteroids are not useful (Table 5.6).

Table 5.6   Maintenance of remission in Crohn's disease.

All patients

Stop smoking

   Risk of disease relapse in non-smokers is reduced by about 30% at 5 years

   Smokers have 2-fold increased risk of recurrence compared with non-smokers

   Former smokers have a disease pattern similar to that of non-smokers

Maintenance of remission

   Azathioprine/6-meracaptopurine

   Methotrexate

   Repeated infusions of anti-TNF antibody maintains improvements seen after initial infusions

   Aminosalicyclates ⎫

   Budesonide   ⎬ marginal therapeutic gain

Prevention of postoperative recurrence

   Mesalazine – benefits limited to patients with isolated small bowel disease

   Metronidazole (for 3 months)

   Azathioprine/6-meracaptopurine in high risk patients

Prevention of postoperative recurrence of Crohn's disease

Relapse of intestinal disease after surgical resection is inevitable in CD. Endoscopic recurrence occurs in 29% of patients at 6 months, 56% at 1 year and 85% at 2 years, with symptomatic recurrence in 90% by 3 years.[63] Smoking increases the risk of postoperative recurrence in CD, and all patients who smoke should be advised to stop.[64] Asacol (2.4 g/day), given within 6 weeks of surgery, reduced severe endoscopic recurrence by 55% at 2 years, with an associated reduced symptomatic recurrence rate.[65] Similar results were achieved in a study of Salofalk or Rowasa (3 g/day 5-ASA).[66] A summary of published studies of mesalazine for prevention of postoperative recurrence concluded that the risk reduction for mesalazine-treated patients was 0.04.[67] This means that 25 postoperative patients would have to be treated to prevent one patient having a recurrence after surgery. Based on these results it is difficult to recommend routine mesalazine treatment to all postoperative patients.

In a placebo-controlled trial of 60 patients, metronidazole 20 mg/kg given within 1 week of terminal ileum resection for CD for 3 months, reduced symptomatic recurrence at 1 year to 4% compared with 25% on placebo. However, this difference was not maintained at 2 and 3 years.[68] Long-term use of metronidazole can lead to an irreversible peripheral neuropathy, which may limit its use.[69] Given the possibly higher long-term benefit of mesalazine than metronidazole, selected patients undergoing intestinal resection should be considered for treatment with mesalazine-containing compounds. Budesonide (6 mg/day) reduces postoperative endoscopic recurrence at 1 year for active CD (but not for fibrostenotic disease); however, it does not affect symptomatic recurrence rates.[70]

Symptomatic treatment for Crohn's disease
Codeine phosphate and loperamide may be useful for control of diarrhoea in patients with a previous resection. They should not be used in patients with active colitis. In patients who have had a terminal ileal resection, malabsorption of bile and overflow into the colon induces a secretory diarrhoea. Cholestyramine (4 g/day increased to 4 g three times daily) binds bile salts and may reduce diarrhoea. With extensive ileal resection, however, diarrhoea results from malabsorption of bile and bile acid deficiency, leading to steatorrhoea. This will not be helped by cholestyramine. Some patients with CD, particularly after small-bowel resections, have small-bowel bacterial overgrowth and diarrhoea will respond to antibiotic treatment. NSAIDs should be avoided in patients with UC and CD.

Medical therapy for patients with refractory Crohn's disease

Despite a variety of treatment options, some patients with CD do not adequately respond to conventional therapy or experience side-effects from standard treatment. Recent insights into the immunopathogenic and inflammatory pathways involved in the intestinal inflammatory response have led to the use of novel therapies that target specific aspects of the immune response. Of all the biological therapies that have been tested so far, anti-tumour necrosis factor-alpha (anti-TNF$_\alpha$) antibody treatment appears to be the most effective.

Anti-tumour necrosis factor therapy
Biotechnology agents that have been specifically developed to inhibit TNF-α activity include a murine-human (chimeric) monoclonal anti-TNF antibody (Remicade®, infliximab), a humanized monoclonal anti-TNF antibody (CDP571), and a recombinant TNF receptor fusion protein (etanercept). Of these, infliximab is licensed in Europe and the USA for use in patients with moderate to severe CD that has not responded to conventional therapy, and for patients with enterocuta-

neous fistulae. A single intravenous infusion (5 mg/kg) produced short-term remissions in 13 out of 27 patients compared with only one of 25 placebo controls.[71] After initial treatment, repeat infusions of infliximab at 8-weekly intervals maintained clinical remission in 65% of patients who were followed for up to 44 weeks compared with 37% of controls.[72] For patients with perianal or entero-cutaneous fistulae, three infusions during a 6 week period produced complete fistula closure in 55% of patients compared with 13% of controls. The fistulae stayed closed for approximately 3 months.[73]

Methotrexate
In the only published placebo-controlled trial so far, intramuscular methotrexate, was superior to placebo in induction of remission in patients with chronically active CD. Clinical remission after 16 weeks of intramuscular methotrexate, 25 mg once weekly, was 39.4% in the methotrexate group compared with 19.1% of patients in the placebo group.[74] A significant benefit was seen only in those patients who required 20 mg or more of prednisolone daily in the 2 weeks before randomization. One placebo-controlled trial published in abstract form has shown that low-dose methotrexate is superior to placebo in maintaining a remission in patients who enter a remission on high-dose treatment. After 10 months 65% of methotrexate treated patients (15 mg intramuscular once weekly) remained in remission compared with 39% of those who received placebo. None of the patients who received methotrexate had a severe adverse event. However, the benefits and safety of methotrexate beyond this treatment period are unknown.[75]

Thalidomide
Thalidomide was originally released as a sedative and antiemetic, and discontinued in the 1960s because of teratogenic effects. More recently, thalidomide has been shown to have beneficial anti-inflammatory and immunomodulatory actions; it inhibits production of TNF-α and IL-12, down-regulates integrins, inhibits leucocyte migration and angiogenesis. Two uncontrolled studies have assessed the safety, efficacy and tol-

erance of thalidomide in a total of 34 patients with steroid refractory CD.[76,77] On an intention-to-treat analysis, clinical response was 58% with low-dose therapy (50–100 mg daily) and 55% with high-dose therapy (200–300 mg daily) after 4 weeks of treatment. At Week 12, response rates were 54% with high-dose and 64% with low-dose therapy. Remission rates at 12 weeks were 17–33%. Side-effects included drowsiness requiring a dose reduction in some patients in the high-dose study, pruritus, dermatitis and hypertension. In the high-dose study, two patients had evidence of a sensorimotor neuropathy on electromyography but both had also received long-term treatment with metronidazole. In the low-dose study, some patients reported neuropathic symptoms but there was no objective neurophysiological testing. Teratogenesis with thalidomide remains an important concern. Female patients with child-bearing potential must use two concomitant forms of reliable birth control for 1 month before the first dose and continuing until 1 month after the last dose. Thalidomide may be present in semen and male patients must use condoms. Women must have a pregnancy test within 24 h before beginning treatment and then at intervals during treatment. Despite these strict precautions, there are still concerns regarding the use of thalidomide in patients with CD and it may only be appropriate to use in patients with refractory disease who cannot tolerate other treatments such as infliximab.

Mycophenolate mofetil
Mycophenolate, through its active metabolite mycophenolic acid, inhibits inosine monophosphate dehydrogenase, an enzyme involved in the synthesis of nucleotides containing the purine base guanine. T and B lymphocytes depend primarily on this nucleotide synthesis for their proliferation in response to antigens. It has been used successfully in organ transplantation to reduce graft rejection and is superior to azathioprine in the prevention of acute rejection. A single, controlled clinical trial has suggested that oral mycophenolate (15 mg/kg mycophenolate mofetil for 6 months) is superior to azathioprine in inducing a remission in patients with chronically active CD and a Crohn's Disease Activity Index of greater than 300.[78] The major side-effects are gastrointestinal upset, leucopenia and sepsis; in renal transplant patients, leucopenia and opportunistic infections occur with similar frequency among mycophenolate and azathioprine-treated patients. Further trials are needed, however, to determine the efficacy as maintenance treatment and long-term toxicity compared with azathioprine. Treatment with mycophenolate should be considered in patients with chronically active CD who are allergic or who have not responded to azathioprine/6-MP.[79]

Experimental agents in the treatment of Crohn's disease

New compounds have been developed for the treatment of CD based on a greater understanding of disease pathogenesis. Some of these agents have only been tested so far in animal models of CD, while others have been tested in patients; however, further studies are needed to fully assess the efficacy and safety. These agents are summarized in Table 5.7.

DRUGS IN INFLAMMATORY BOWEL DISEASE DURING PREGNANCY AND BREASTFEEDING

No drugs used in the treatment of IBD are licensed for use during pregnancy or breast-feeding. However, many of the drugs in frequent use for patients with IBD are thought to be safe in pregnancy and, in general, active inflammatory bowel disease is more harmful to the fetus than drug treatment. Patients should be advised to plan conception when the disease is inactive wherever possible, and to continue drugs to prevent relapse if necessary. Mesalazine does not cross the placenta in significant amounts and there are no data to suggest teratogenesis or harm to the fetus at any stage of pregnancy.[80] The newer 5-ASA agents are also probably safe. The risk/benefit ratio should be discussed with the patient and, in

Table 5.7   Potential new therapies for the treatment of Crohn's disease.

Agent	Mode of action
Antisense oligonucleotides	Nucleic acid sequences that bind to RNA or DNA and blocks expression of specific protein
Antisense therapy to block intracellular adhesion molecule-1 (ICAM-1)	
Antisense therapy to nuclear factor kappa B (NFκB)	Inhibits production of transcription factor that activates cytokine genes and mediates pro-inflammatory action of TNF_α
Interleukin-10 and interleukin-11	Increase anti-inflammatory cytokines
Anti-CD4 antibodies	Deplete antigen-activated $CD4^+$ T cells
Anti-integrin 4 antibodies	Inhibit integrin 4 reduces leucocyte migration across vascular endothelium
Fish oil	Eicosapentaenoic acid, the active ingredient, decreases production of pro-inflammatory cytokines, platelet activating factor and reactive oxygen species

situations where the benefit of 5-ASA is limited, such as maintenance of remission in CD, stopping the drug may be advised. Sulphasalazine has the longest history of safe use in pregnancy, however, it is associated with neonatal haemolysis and changing to another 5-ASA agent should be advised if necessary. Steroids should be avoided wherever possible in pregnancy; in patients with CD, nutritional therapy may be an alternative. However, maternal health is important to the fetus and, if necessary in life-threatening disease, such as acute severe colitis, steroids should be used. Immunosuppressants should also be avoided in pregnancy wherever possible; however, some favourable data exist for IBD patients taking azathioprine in pregnancy. In 1990, 16 successful pregnancies in 14 women on the azathioprine were reported.[81] In a case-controlled study of 155 patients, male and female, also demonstrated pregnancy and neonatal problems similar to normal populations in patients on 6-MP.[82] As with steroids, a discussion of the risk/benefit ratio should be discussed with the individual patient.

DRUG INFORMATION FOR THE TREATMENT OF ULCERATIVE COLITIS AND CROHN'S DISEASE

Mesalazine-containing compounds

Mode of action
Mesalazine-containing compounds have a wide variety of anti-inflammatory actions:

- Inhibition of leucocyte migration
- Reduced activation of NFkB
- Reduced synthesis of leucotrienes, thromboxanes, and prostaglandins

But it is not known which of these explains their efficacy in IBD.

Indications
These agents are indicated in the:

- Treatment of mild to moderate UC
- Maintenance of remission in UC

- Maintenance of remission in selected patients with Crohn's disease (CD)

Preparations
The major preparations available are as follows:

- Oral — See Table 5.4
- Topical treatment — Liquid enemas: Pentasa, Salofalk, sulphasalazine
  Foam enemas: Asacol
  Suppositories: Asacol, Pentasa, Salofalk, sulphasalazine

Pharmacokinetics/dynamics
Sulphasalazine, the first aminosalicylate to be used in the treatment of UC, consists of sulphapyridine joined to mesalazine (5-aminosalicylic acid, 5-ASA) by an azo bond (Table 5.4). Sulphasalazine is absorbed from the small intestine, re-excreted in bile and carried to the colon where the azo bond is cleaved by colonic bacteria to release 5-ASA, the active compound for treatment of colitis. The therapeutic activity of sulphasalazine has been attributed to mesalazine, and hypersensitivity and intolerance to sulphapyridine, which is absorbed from the gut. After oral administration, unprotected mesalazine is rapidly and almost completely absorbed from the jejunum, thus limiting its availability in the colon and distal small bowel. Oral preparations have been developed containing 5-ASA without the sulphapyridine carrier but using various modes of drug delivery in order to release active drug at the site of disease (Table 5.4). The therapeutic activity of these compounds is equal to that of sulphasalazine.

Side-effects
Oral sulphasalazine treatment is associated, in about 20% of patients, with side-effects which are attributed to the carrier molecule, sulphapyridine; they include nausea, vomiting, headache, fever, drug rashes, folate deficiency and orange urine. Reversible azoospermia and infertility occur in as many as 80% of men. More serious idiosyncratic side-effects are skin rashes (occasionally associated with photosensitivity),

toxic necrolysis, Stevens-Johnson syndrome, haemolytic anaemia, leucopenia and agranulocytosis. Rarely, neurotoxicity, hepatotoxicity, acute pancreatitis, pulmonary fibrosis, a lupus-like syndrome and haemorrhagic colitis are produced. The incidence of adverse events is less but not negligible with other mesalazine compounds (Table 5.4). After oral administration, they have been shown to cause fever, rash, hepatitis, blood dyscrasias, myocarditis, neuropathy and acute pancreatitis. There are an increasing number of reports of interstitial nephritis and renal failure occurring after treatment with mesalazine. The exact mechanism of induction is unknown and there may only be partial recovery of renal function when the drug is withdrawn, particularly if there is a delay in diagnosis.

Monitoring
A recent article has recommended the following monitoring schedule:

- Serum urea and creatinine measured before treatment commences and then monthly for the first 3 months of treatment
- 3-monthly for the next 9 months
- 6-monthly for the next 5 years and
- Annually thereafter for the duration of treatment[83]

The Committee on Safety of Medicines recommends that patients on any 5-ASA should report immediately any sore throat, fever, malaise or unexplained bleeding.

Contraindications
Serious renal impairment and salicylate hypersensitivity are contraindications to their use. Moreover, sulphasalazine should not be given to patients with sulphonamide sensitivity, porphyria, or glucose-6-phosphate dehydrogenase deficiency.

Corticosteroids

Mode of action
Corticosteroids are lipid-soluble and so enter target cells where they combine with cytoplas-

mic corticosteroid receptors. The steroid/receptor complex then translocates into the nucleus where it binds to promoter regions of several genes, which are then either activated or switched off. Corticosteroids have a wide variety of actions on cellular and humoral immune function, namely:

- Inhibition of leucocyte migration and activation
- Inhibition of cytokine synthesis by suppression of the activation of the nuclear transcription factor NF kappa B (NFκB)
- Reduce a production of pro-inflammatory lipid mediators from arachidonic acid
- Inhibition of phospholipase A_2, cyclo-oxygenase and inducible nitric oxide synthase
- Stimulation of lymphocyte apoptosis in the lamina propria
- Enhancement of sodium and water absorption in the gut

Indications
Treatment of active CD and UC are indications for use. Corticosteroids are, however, ineffective as maintenance therapy.

Preparations
The following preparations are available:

- Oral: Prednisolone, budesonide (CIR-Entocort)
- Intravenous: Hydrocortisone, methyprednisolone
- Topical:
  Enemas—prednisolone sodium phosphate (Predsol), prednisolone metasulphobenzoate (Predfoam), budesonide (Entocort)
  Suppositories—hydrocortisone, prednisolone sodium phosphate (Predsol)

Dynamics/kinetics
Corticosteroids are effective orally since they are protected from first-pass hepatic metabolism by high-affinity binding to plasma proteins. Hydrocortisone and methylprednisolone are used intravenously when a rapid effect is required, such as in acute severe UC. When

intravenous corticosteroids are used they are given 8-hourly to achieve a continuous effect. Equivalent anti-inflammatory doses of steroids used in UC are:

Prednisolone 5 mg = Hydrocortisone 20 mg
= Methylprednisone 4 mg

The novel steroid budesonide is inactivated by first-pass metabolism in the liver giving low systemic absorption, which minimizes hypothalamo-pituitary-adrenal (HPA) suppression, although it may still occur.

Adverse reactions/information for patients
Adverse reactions are as follows:

- Dermatological: acne, moon face, purpura, hirsutes
- Immunological: increased susceptibility to infection, severe chickenpox
- Cardiovascular: hypertension, oedema
- Metabolic: weight gain, diabetes mellitus, hypokalaemia
- Musculoskeletal: osteoporosis (related to dose and duration of treatment), avascular osteonecrosis, proximal myopathy, tendon rupture, growth retardation in children,
- Others: pancreatitis, mood change and psychosis, cataracts

Suppression of the HPA axis is maximal if the drugs are taken in the evening, therefore patients should be advised to take their drugs as a single dose in the morning to minimize side-effects due to HPA suppression.

Patients should be advised not to stop the treatment suddenly, to carry a Steroid Treatment Card, to avoid contact with chicken pox, herpes zoster and measles during treatment and for 3 months after completion of treatment.

Drug interactions
These are as follows:

- Antibiotics: Rifampicin accelerates corticosteroid metabolism (reduces effect)
- Diuretic, hypoglycaemic and hypotensive agents: corticosteroids can antagonize effects
- Anti-epileptic drugs: carbamazepine, phenobarbitone, phenytoin, and primadone accelerate corticosteroid metabolism (which reduces effect)
- Diuretics, Digoxin and B_2-receptor agonists: Corticosteroids can worsen the hypokalaemia associated with these drugs.
- Cyclosporin: At high doses, corticosteroids can increase plasma cyclosporin levels, cyclosporin increases plasma concentrations of corticosteroids

Contraindications
Relative contraindications are diabetes mellitus, some systemic infections and live-virus vaccines and osteoporosis.

Withdrawal of corticosteroids
Gradual withdrawal (over weeks or months) to allow the adrenal gland to recover.

Corticosteroid replacement in the perioperative period
In a patient who takes corticosteroids, the hypothalamo-pituitary-adrenocortical axis (HPA) may be suppressed and the natural stress response to surgery is impaired. Without an adequate cortisol response, the patient is at risk of hypoadrenal crisis. Recent recommendations suggest that patients who have received corticosteroids within 3 months of surgery should be assumed to have some degree of HPA suppression and should receive corticosteroid replacement perioperatively.[84]

For moderate or major surgery
The guidelines are as follows:

1. Morning of surgery: give usual oral corticosteroid dose.
2. At induction: give hydrocortisone bolus, 25 mg intravenously.
3. Subsequently: give hydrocortisone infusion, 100 mg for 24 h stopped after 24 h with moderate surgery or at 48–72 h with major surgery. An alternative regimen is

25–50 mg bolus intravenously every 8 h.
4. Restart usual corticosteroid therapy.

For minor surgery
The following guidelines are used:

1. Morning of surgery: usual oral cortico-steroid dose *or* hydrocortisone bolus (25 mg intravenously) at induction
2. Restart usual corticosteroid therapy post-operatively.

Management of glucocorticoid-induced osteoporosis
Osteopenia (defined as a bone mineral density between 1 and 2.5 standard deviations (SD) below the mean bone density of a sex-matched young adult population) and osteoporosis (bone density below 2.5 SD below the reference population) is common in patients with IBD. The pathogenesis is multifactorial but glucocorticoid therapy is an important contributing factor. Bone densitometry is repeated at yearly intervals to monitor the effects of treatment.[85]

Primary prevention
This should be considered in all patients receiving high doses (15 mg/day or more of pred-nisolone or equivalent) of glucocorticoids for 3 months or more and in patients treated with lower doses (7.5–15 mg/day) who have other strong risk factors for osteoporosis. These include:

- Age over 65 years
- Previous osteoporotic fracture
- Premature menopause (younger than 45 years)
- Premenopausal amenorrhoea and low body weight.

A suitable preventive regimen is at least 1 g of elemental calcium plus 800 IU of vitamin D per day, which is continued until prednisolone or equivalent is lower than 5 mg daily. Hormone replacement therapy should be considered in all postmenopausal women.

Secondary prevention
This should be considered in patients receiving corticosteroids who have reduced bone mineral density and/or a fragility fracture occurs during glucocorticoid treatment. Bone mineral density is measured in the lumbar spine and femoral neck by dual X-ray absorptiometry (DEXA scanning) and reduced bone mineral density defined as a T-score of −1.5 or less (that is 1.5 SD below the reference population). Patients with a T-score above this level who continue to require steroid treatment should be reassessed annually. Patients should be screened for evidence of hypogonadism in men and premenopausal women by measurement of serum testosterone and plasma oestrogen concentrations, respectively. Oestrogen (in women) or testosterone (in men) should be given if hypogonadism is confirmed. If hypogo-nadism is not present or bone loss continues despite replacement, treatment with biphos-phonate should be started. A suitable regimen is 400 mg etidronate daily for 2 weeks, followed by 500 mg calcium for 76 days; this 3-monthly cycle is then repeated.

General measures include weight-bearing exercises, discouraging smoking and excess alcohol and adequate nutrition, including cal-cium and vitamin D supplements in patients with malabsorption. Postmenopausal women should receive hormone replacement therapy. Some patients with Crohn's disease may be suitable for treatment with budesonide, which has reduced systemic absorption compared with prednisolone.

Metronidazole

Mode of action
Metronidazole has antibacterial and anti-inflammatory actions.

Indications
Metronidazole is used for:

- Treating active CD; it has a similar efficacy to sulphasalazine but rarely used
- Treating perianal CD

- Preventing postoperative recurrence of CD
- Treating pouchitis

Preparation

Two preparations of metronidazole are available:

- Oral: 400 mg given three times daily
- Topical: suppository given 500 mg three times daily

Dynamics and kinetics

Metronidazole is absorbed rapidly and most is excreted unchanged in urine.

Adverse reactions

These include:

- Gastrointestinal disturbances: metallic, bitter taste in the mouth, nausea, vomiting
- Neurological symptoms: dizziness, headache, peripheral neuropathy, transient epileptiform seizures
- Disulfiram-like reaction with alcohol—so alcohol should be avoided completely

Monitoring

Monitor patients for clinical evidence of peripheral neuropathy.

Contraindications

Use with caution in severe liver disease, pregnancy and breastfeeding.

Interactions with other drugs

Excretion of metronidazole is reduced by penicillins, aspirin and NSAIDs, with increased risk of toxicity. Disulfiram reacts with alcohol, and the effect of warfarin is increased.

Cyclosporin

Mode of action

Cyclosporin is a potent immunosuppressant and acts primarily by blocking the production of interleukin-2 (IL-2) from T-helper lymphocytes. It also decreases recruitment of cytotoxic T cells and production of IL-3, IL-4, γ-interferon and tumour necrosis factor (TNF)-α.

Indications

Intravenous cyclosporin is useful in selected patients with steroid-refractory acute severe UC.

Preparations

The following preparations are available:

- Intravenous: 4 mg/kg/day
- Oral
  —Sandimmun (6–8 mg/kg/day) with variable absorption
  —Neoral

Dynamics and kinetics

Cyclosporin is strongly hydrophobic and thus must be stabilized with alcohol and polyoxyethylated castor oil (intravenous solution) or alcohol and olive oil (oral solution). It is metabolized by the P_{450} enzyme system.

Adverse reactions

Paresthesias and hypertrichosis are the two most common cyclosporin-induced side-effects. Paresthesiae occur in approximately 30% of patients and typically produce burning and tingling in the hands and feet, which may be associated with a tremor of the hands. These side-effects usually resolve when the dose is reduced. Hypertrichosis is a common side-effect associated with cyclosporin but is a severe cosmetic problem in only a few patients.

Hypertension and/or renal dysfunction occur in about 7% of IBD patients treated with cyclosporin. The exact aetiological mechanisms are unknown but afferent arteriolar vasoconstriction is thought to play an important role. Most patients treated with long-term cyclosporin for autoimmune diseases will show an increase in serum creatinine and a reduction in creatinine clearance, which is dose-dependent and reversible upon dose reduction or discontinuation of therapy. The risk is reduced in these patients by maintaining low serum creatinine levels, not exceeding 30% of baseline. A few patients treated with cyclosporin have been shown to have changes in renal morphology (such as interstitial fibrosis, tubular atrophy and arteriolar changes) which are rarely associated with irreversible loss of renal function.

Other side-effects in IBD patients treated with cyclosporin include:

- Nausea and vomiting (8%)
- Cholestasis (2%)
- Headache (4%)
- Gingival hyperplasia (2%) and
- Anaphylaxis (rarely) with intravenous administration

Grand mal seizures may also complicate cyclosporin therapy; the risk is increased by hypomagnaesemia and hypocholesterolaemia, which both allow easier diffusion of cyclosporin across the blood–brain barrier. A few cases of pneumocystis pneumonia have been reported in UC patients treated with cyclosporin. Prophylactic treatment with low-dose trimethoprim/sulphamethoxazole has been recommended but has not yet been subjected to formal clinical analysis. Cyclosporin is a potent immunosuppressant and there is a theoretical possibility that treatment may increase the risk of cancer; however, to date there has been no increased incidence of malignancy in IBD patients treated with cyclosporin.

Monitoring during cyclosporin treatment
Baseline tests
These include blood pressure, serum urea and electrolytes, magnesium, liver biochemistry, cholesterol, full blood count, and urinalysis.

Monitoring during treatment
Daily blood cyclosporin levels are monitored with intravenous treatment. Monthly trough levels of blood cyclosporin concentrations are monitored in patients receiving oral cyclosporin, although a correlation with clinical response and toxicity has been inconsistent. Cyclosporin concentrations in whole blood should be maintained from 200–800 ng/ml by monoclonal radioimmunoassay or 200–400 ng/ml by high-performance liquid chromatography during intravenous treatment and 150–300 ng/ml (by radioimmunoassay) as the trough level on oral treatment. Blood pressure and serum creatinine should be measured every 2 weeks for the first 3 months of oral treatment and monthly thereafter if the patient is stable. If the serum creatinine rises to more than 30% of baseline levels on two separate occasions, the daily dose of cyclosporin should be reduced.

Contraindications to cyclosporin
Cyclosporin is contraindicated in the following conditions:

- Current malignancy
- Uncontrolled hypertension
- Abnormal renal function
- Uncontrolled infections
- Primary or secondary immunodeficiency
- Hypersensitivity to cyclosporin
- Epilepsy
- Low serum cholesterol or magnesium
- Pregnancy and breastfeeding,
- Co-administration of drugs that interact with cyclosporin (relative contraindication)

Interactions with other drugs
Concomitant administration of certain drugs interact with cyclosporin to:

- Alter blood cyclosporin concentrations (Table 5.8)
- Potentiate renal toxicity: gentamycin, vancomycin, amphotericin B, ketoconazole, NSAIDs
- Reduce clearance of the drug: digoxin

Azathioprine and 6-mercaptopurine

Azathioprine is a derivative of 6-mercaptopurine (6-MP) and can therefore be expected to have similar clinical effects and side-effect profile. However, studies suggest that patients who cannot tolerate azathioprine may be treated with 6-MP without adverse effects.

Indications
Indications for treatment are:

Table 5.8 Drugs and foods that affect blood cyclosporin concentrations.

Drugs that *inhibit* cytochrome P_{450} and *increase* cyclosporin concentrations	Drugs that *induce* cytochrome P_{450} and *decrease* cyclosporin concentrations
Antibiotics	**Antibiotics**
Erythromycin	Rifabutin
Clarithromycin	**Anticonvulsant agents**
Antifungal agents	Carbamazepine
Fluconazole	Phenobarbitone
Itraconazole	Phenytoin
Ketoconazole	**Other agents**
Calcium-channel blockers	Octreotide
Diltiazem	Ticlopidine
Nicardipine	
Verapamil	
Glucocorticoids	
Methylprednisolone	
Other agents	
Allopurinol	
Bromocriptine	
Danazol	
Metoclopramide	
Grapefruit juice	

- Chronically active UC despite corticosteroid treatment
- Maintenance of remission in UC and CD

Preparations
The following preparations are available:

- Azathioprine: 2.0–2.5 mg/kg/day
- 6-MP: 1.0–1.5 mg/kg/day

Mode of action
Azathioprine and 6-MP are metabolized to 6-thioinosinic acid, which is thought to achieve immunosuppression by incorporation into purine nucleotides, disrupting normal purine metabolism and therefore interfering with DNA and RNA synthesis and decreased numbers of B and T lymphocytes. Clinical response may take 3–6 months.

Pharmacokinetics
Azathioprine is metabolized by hepatic xanthine oxidase to 6-MP, which may then enter one of three metabolic pathways:

1. Metabolism to the active end-product, 6-thioinosinic acid, by the enzyme hypoxanthine guanine phosphoribosyl transferase; *or*
2. Conversion to 6-methyl MP by thiopurine methyltransferase; *or*
3. Conversion to the urinary metabolite, 6-thiouric acid, by xanthine oxidase.

A small amount of 6-MP is eliminated unchanged in the urine and metabolites are eventually eliminated in the urine.

Adverse reactions

Allergic
This usually occurs within the first few weeks of starting treatment and is characterized by fever, rash, arthralgia, myalgia, elevation of liver enzymes, hypotension, nausea, vomiting and diarrhoea.

Gastrointestinal
Nausea, vomiting, anorexia and less commonly hepatitis and diarrhoea may occur. Acute pancreatitis occurs in 3–15% of patients, usually within the first few weeks of starting treatment, is often benign and resolves on drug withdrawal.

Myelosuppression
In 739 IBD patients treated with azathioprine for a median period of 12 months, 37 (5%) patients developed asymptomatic leucopaenia, which required a dose reduction. Nine (1%) patients developed severe leucopaenia of whom two died of sepsis.[86] Myelotoxicity may occur at any time during treatment. 1 in 300 individuals have very low levels of methyltransferase, resulting in reduced metabolism of azathioprine and 6-MP, and increased risk of toxicity. Heterozygotes (11% of the population) are also at increased risk of toxicity. Some centres now measure the levels of red cell thiopurine methyltransferase before starting azathioprine or 6-MP. Patients with very low red cell methyltransferase levels are highly likely to develop severe myelosuppression and should not be given azathioprine or 6-MP.

Malignancy
Chronic immunosuppression may potentially increase the risk of neoplasia particular lymphoma. However, in two large studies evaluating more than 1000 IBD patients treated with long-term azathioprine or 6-MP, there was no overall excess of cancer.[87,88]

Drug interactions
Allopurinol increases toxicity of azathioprine and 6-MP by inhibiting xanthine oxidase. The two drugs should not be used together if at all possible. However, if necessary, the dose of azathioprine or 6-MP must be reduced to one-quarter or of one-third of normal.

Dose adjustment in renal impairment
Within creatinine clearance of 10–50 ml/min, administer 75% of the normal dose. With a creatinine clearance less than 10 ml/min, administer 50% of the normal dose.

Monitoring during treatment
Weekly full blood counts for the first 4 weeks of treatment should be undertaken, and 4–6 weekly thereafter.

Contraindications
Contraindications to treatment are as follows:

- Previous pancreatitis associated with azathioprine use
- Concomitant allopurinol treatment (relative)
- Patients with very low red cell thiopurine methyltransferase levels (see under adverse reactions)

Infliximab

Mode of action
Anti-TNF antibody binds to and inhibits the action of soluble TNF. Antibodies also bind to TNF-α on the surface of immune cells and initiate complement or effector cell-mediated lysis, thus depleting this cell population.

Indications
Infliximab is used to treat:

- Moderate to severe active refractory CD
- Fistulizing CD that is unresponsive to conventional treatment

Dose
A dose of 5 mg/kg body weight by intravenous infusion administered over a 2-hour period. For

fistulizing disease, two further infusions at 2 and 6 weeks after the initial infusion are given.

Pharmacokinetics
Infliximab has a serum half-life of approximately 10 days.

Adverse reactions
Adverse reactions are as follows:

- Acute infusion reactions occurring during, or in the 2 hours following infusion: fever and chills (4%), pruritus and urticaria (1%), chest pain, hypotension, hypertension and dyspnoea (1%). If occurs slow infusion rate, or stop temporarily until symptoms subside. Discontinue infusion if severe symptoms. Medication for treatment of hypersensitivity reactions should be available for immediate use.
- Delayed hypersensitivity reactions (e.g. myalgia, rash, fever, arthralgia, pruritus, urticaria) up to 2 weeks after infusion. More common in patients treated with infliximab over 12 weeks previously.
- Autoimmunity: development of anti-double-stranded (ds) DNA antibodies, rarely lupus-like syndrome. Resolution of symptoms and disappearance of anti-ds DNA after discontinuation of infliximab.
- Human anti-chimeric antibody development may diminish therapeutic effect and increase likelihood of developing infusion reactions.
- Chronic exposure to immunosuppressants may increase susceptibility to malignancy and lymphoma. Effect of infliximab on these phenomena is unknown.
- Infections, serious in less than 3%.

Information for patients
Patients should be warned of side-effects. Female patients should avoid pregnancy or breastfeeding for 6 months after treatment.

Drug interactions
There are no interactions with drugs commonly used in the treatment of CD.

Contraindications
These include:

- Active infections and/or abscesses
- History of hypersensitivity to infliximab or murine proteins
- After a drug (infliximab)-free interval of over 14 weeks, since hypersensitivity reactions more common (relative contraindication).
- No experience of infliximab in pregnancy.

Monitoring during treatment
Blood pressure and pulse half-hourly during, and for 2 hours after infusion.

Methotrexate

Indications
Methotrexate is used to treat chronically active, steroid-dependent CD in which other therapies have failed.

Dose
The dosage is 25 mg intramuscularly for 16 weeks to induce remission; maintenance treatment is 7.5–15 mg i.m. or orally weekly.

Mode of action
Methotrexate is a competitive dihydrofolate reductase inhibitor, resulting in impaired DNA synthesis. Its additional anti-inflammatory effects result from inhibition of IL-1 and induction of apoptosis of selected T-cell populations.

Pharmacokinetics/dynamics
Oral methotrexate up to 0.1 mg/kg is completely absorbed, at doses above this absorption may not be complete. Peak serum concentrations occur 0.5–2 h after intramuscular injection. Methotrexate is 50% protein bound in the circulation. It is actively transported across cell membranes and so is widely distributed. Methotrexate is retained for several weeks in the kidney and for months in the liver. There is little, if any, metabolism of the drug; most is excreted by the kidneys, while small amounts are excreted in the faeces via bile.

Adverse reactions/information for patients

Serious adverse reactions include:

- Myelosuppression
- Teratogenesis
- Hypersensitivity pneumonitis
- Hepatic fibrosis

Minor adverse reactions include:

- Gastrointestinal upset
- Stomatitis or soreness of the mouth
- Alopecia
- Macrocytosis
- Skin rashes
- Malaise/fatigue
- Headache

Folic acid supplementation (1 mg/day) may decrease gastrointestinal side-effects without affecting drug efficacy.

Patients should be cautioned against pregnancy and breastfeeding. Discontinue in men and women 3 months before conception. Patients are advised to avoid alcohol, even in moderation, which may increase the risk of liver toxicity.

Drug interactions

Profound leukopenia may occur with drugs with anti-folate properties (e.g. co-trimoxazole) and azathioprine or 6-mercaptopurine. Concomitant use of any other renal- or hepato-toxic drugs (including alcohol) should be avoided. Toxicity may be increased by drugs that compete for protein binding, such as salicylates, diuretics, hypoglycaemic agents, sulphonamides, phenytoin, chloramphenicol and other antibiotics.

Monitoring during treatment

- Before starting treatment: full blood count, liver biochemistry, urea and electrolytes, chest radiography and urinalysis.
- During treatment: liver biochemistry and full blood count every 2 weeks, and then at 2-monthly intervals during maintenance treatment.

In IBD patients with normal liver function tests there is no need for liver biopsy before treatment commences. It is suggested that a liver biopsy should be performed after 2 g total dose (irrespective of liver biochemistry) but the role of routine liver biopsy in IBD patients taking methotrexate remains to be determined

Contraindications

Pre-existing renal, haematological, hepatic or pulmonary disease, pregnancy and breastfeeding are all contraindications to treatment.

COLLAGENOUS AND LYMPHOCYTIC COLITIS (MICROSCOPIC COLITIS)

Introduction

There are two main types of microscopic colitis:

1. Lymphocytic colitis (which is characterized by a subepithelial lymphocytic infiltrate in the colonic mucosa); and
2. Collagenous colitis (which is characterized by a thickened subepithelial collagen band).

Some patients have a mixed form with both thickening of the collagenous plate and an increased number of intraepithelial lymphocytes.[89] Microscopic colitis is characterized by non-bloody chronic watery diarrhoea. Diarrhoea is the result of decreased absorption of water and electrolytes, which is thought to occur secondary to the inflammatory cell infiltrate. The colon appears normal on barium enema examination and, at colonoscopy, and the diagnosis is made by histological examination of colonic biopsies. The aetiology of collagenous and lymphocytic colitis is unknown and the two conditions may represent two distinct disease entities. Collagenous colitis has been reported after long-term NSAID use and diarrhoea may improve with drug cessation.

Therapeutic rationale

There are few well-controlled trials to guide the treatment of patients with microscopic colitis.

Most treatments are based on reports of small numbers of patients.[90] Some patients run a relapsing/remitting course and require intermittent treatment only. Loperamide is frequently recommended as the initial treatment and is used for symptomatic control of diarrhoea. Loperamide may have to be given at high dosage (4 mg three times daily or more) to be effective. Orally administered 5-aminosalicylic acid (5-ASA) drugs, such as sulphasalazine and mesalazine, have been used in dosages similar to those used in IBD patients, with response rates of 25–75%. A retrospective study of treatment in patients with collagenous colitis recommended that cholestyramine is used in patients who do not respond to loperamide or 5-ASA drugs.[90] Cholestyramine (4 g four times daily) has been used on the basis that the inflammatory cell infiltrate and collagen deposition results from bacterial toxins (which bind to cholestyramine) and mucosal injury.[91] The efficacy of cholestyramine may also be related to bile-acid malabsorption, which is common in patients with collagenous colitis. Preliminary studies suggest that bismuth subsalicylate (three 262 mg tablets three times daily for 8 weeks), which has antimicrobial properties, may reduce diarrhoea and benefits may persist for some months after stopping treatment. In resistant cases, oral prednisolone, oral budesonide[92] (3 mg three times daily) and subcutaneous octreotide[93] have been used. Oral prednisolone is a very effective treatment in these patients; however, relapse often occurs after drug withdrawal, and the dose required to maintain remission is often unacceptably high, at more than 20 mg daily.[90] Unlike ulcerative colitis and Crohn's disease, microscopic colitis rarely requires surgery. Nevertheless, ileostomy is required rarely for severe symptoms that are refractory to medical therapy.

PHARMACOLOGY OF DRUGS USED TO TREAT COLLAGENOUS AND LYMPHOCYTIC COLITIS

Loperamide

Mode of action
Loperamide acts directly on the intestinal musculature to inhibit peristalsis and prolong transit time enhancing fluid and electrolyte absorption through the intestinal mucosa.

Dynamics/kinetics
Its onset of action is 0.5–1 h. Over 50% is converted on first-pass hepatic metabolism to inactive metabolites, faecal and urinary excretion of metabolites and unchanged drug (40%).

Adverse reactions
Drowsiness, abdominal cramps and bloating, paralytic ileus, constipation, skin rashes including urticaria.

Drug interactions
Phenothiazines and tricyclic antidepressants may potentiate the adverse effects of loperamide.

Contraindications/precautions
Loperamide is contraindicated where inhibition of peristalsis should be avoided, such as acute severe colitis, some cases of infectious diarrhoea and pseudomembranous colitis. It should be used with caution in patients with liver disease (large first-pass hepatic metabolism).

Bismuth subsalicylate

In addition, bismuth subsalicylate has aspirin-like side-effects and is contraindicated in patients with a coagulopathy. There is increased toxicity of aspirin, warfarin and hypoglycaemics with bismuth subsalicylate.

5-aminosalicylate

See p. 89.

Prednisolone

See p. 91.

Budesonide

See p. 84.

Octreotide

See Chapter 13 (p. 304).

Cholestyramine

See Chapter 12 (p. 262).

EOSINOPHILIC GASTROENTERITIS

Eosinophilic gastroenteritis is a rare disorder characterized by eosinophilic infiltration of the bowel wall, peripheral eosinophilia in most cases and a variety of gastrointestinal symptoms, which may be diagnosed initially as irritable bowel syndrome. The aetiopathogenesis of eosinophilic gastroenteritis is poorly understood. An allergic component has been proposed in some patients but avoidance of specific foods does not usually result in clinical benefit.

The signs and symptoms are related to the layer(s) and extent of bowel involvement with eosinophilic infiltration. The stomach and proximal small bowel are most commonly affected, although any part of the gastrointestinal tract, including the bile ducts, may be involved. Mucosal disease, muscle layer disease and subserosal disease may exist. The most common symptoms associated with mucosal disease are abdominal pain, diarrhoea, nausea and vomiting. Eosinophilic infiltration of the muscle layer of the gastrointestinal tract results in obstructive-type symptoms, such as vomiting and abdominal distension. Subserosal disease may present with any of the above symptoms and ascites.

There are no randomized controlled trials to guide the clinician in the treatment of patients with eosinophilic gastroenteritis. The response to dietary modification and food withdrawal is usually poor. Diarrhoea is treated symptomatically with loperamide. Patients with severe symptoms of malabsorption may respond to oral prednisolone (p. 91).

REFERENCES

1. Fiocchi C. Inflammatory bowel disease: etiology and pathogenesis. *Gastroenterology* 1998; **115:** 182–205.
2. Di Mola FF, Friess H, Scheuren A, *et al.* Transforming growth factor-betas and their signalling receptors are co-expressed in Crohn's disease. *Ann Surg* 1999; **229:** 67–75.
3. Sutherland LR, Ramcharan S, Bryant H, Fick G. Effect of cigarette smoking on recurrence of Crohn's disease. *Gastroenterology* 1990; **98:** 1123–1128.
4. Haug K, Schrumpt E, Barstad S, Fluge G. Epidemiology of ulcerative colitis in western Norway. *Scand J Gastroenterol* 1988; **23:** 517–522.
5. Langholz E, Munkholm P, Davidsen M, Binder V. Course of ulcerative colitis: analysis of changes in disease activity over years. *Gastroenterology* 1994; **107:** 3–11.
6. Truelove SC and Witts LJ. Cortisone in ulcerative colitis: preliminary report on a therapeutic trial. *Brit Med J* 1954; **2:** 375–378.
7. Kam L, Cohen H, Dooley C, *et al.* A comparison of mesalamine suspension enema and oral sulphasalazine for treatment of active distal ulcerative colitis in adults. *Am J Gastroenterol* 1996; **91:** 1338–1342.
8. Campieri M, Gionchetti P, Rizzello F, *et al.* A controlled randomized trial comparing oral versus rectal mesalazine in the treatment of ulcerative proctitis. *Gastroenterology* 1996; **110:** A876.
9. Farthing MJ, Rutland MD, Clark ML. Retrograde spread of hydrocortisone containing foam given

intrarectally in ulcerative colitis. *Br Med J* 1979; **2:** 822–824.

10. Palmer KR, Goepel JR, Holdsworth CD. Sulphasalazine retention enemas in ulcerative colitis: a double-blind trial. *Br Med J* 1981; **282:** 1571–1573.

11. Sutherland LR, Martin F, Greer S, *et al.* 5-ASA enema in the treatment of distal ulcerative colitis, proctosigmoiditis and proctitis. *Gastroenterology* 1987; **92:** 1894–1898.

12. Campieri TM, Gionchetti P, Belluzzi A, *et al.* Optimum dosage of 5-ASA as rectal enemas in patients with active ulcerative colitis. *Gut* 1991; **32:** 929–931.

13. Biddle WL, Miner PB. Long-term use of mesalazine enemas to induce remission in ulcerative colitis. *Gastroenterology* 1990; **99:** 113–118.

14. Somerville KW, Langman MJ, Kane SP, MacGilchrist AJ, Watkinson G, Salmon P. Effect of treatment on symptoms and quality of life in patients with ulcerative colitis: comparative trial of hydrocortisone acetate foam and prednisolone 21-phosphate enemas. *Brit Med J Clin Res Ed* 1985; **291:** 866.

15. Tsuruoka S, Sugimoto K, Fujimura A. Drug-induced Cushings syndrome in a patient with ulcerative colitis after betamethasone enema: evaluation of plasma drug concentration. *Ther Drug Monit* 1998; **20:** 387–389.

16. Danielsson A, Lofberg R, Persson T, *et al.* A steroid enema, budesonide, lacking systemic effects for the treatment of distal ulcerative colitis or proctitis. *Scand J Gastroenterol* 1992; **27:** 9–12.

17. Marshall JK, Irvine EJ. Rectal corticosteroids versus alternative treatments in ulcerative colitis: a meta-analysis. *Gut* 1997; **40:** 775–781.

18. D'Arienzo A, Panarese A, D'Armiento FP, *et al.* 5-Aminosalicylic acid suppositories in the maintenance of remission in idiopathic proctitis or proctosigmoiditis: a double-blind placebo-controlled clinical trial. *Am J Gastroenterol* 1990; **85:** 1079–1082.

19. Biddle WL, Greenberger NJ, Swan JT, *et al.* 5-Aminosalicyclic acid enemas: effective agent in maintaining remission in left-sided ulcerative colitis. *Gastroenterology* 1988; **94:** 1075–1079.

20. Marteau P, Crand J, Foucault M, Rambaud J-C. use of mesalazine slow-release suppositories 1 g three times per week to maintain remission of ulcerative proctitis: a randomised double blind placebo controlled multicentre study. *Gut* 1998; **42:** 195–199.

21. Dick AP, Grayson MJ, Carpenter RG, *et al.* Controlled trial of sulphasalazine in the treatment of ulcerative colitis. *Gut* 1964; **5:** 437–442.

22. Sninsky GA, Corr DH, Shanahan F, *et al.* Oral mesalazine (Asacol) for mildly to moderately active ulcerative colitis: a multicentre study. *Ann Intern Med* 1991; **115:** 350–355.

23. Sutherland BR, May GR, Shaffer LA. Sulphasalazine revisited: a meta-analysis of 5-aminosalicylic acid in the treatment of ulcerative colitis. *Ann Intern Med* 1993; **118:** 540–549.

24. Green JR, Lobo AJ, Holdsworth CD, *et al.* Balsalazide is more effective and better tolerated than mesalamine in the treatment of acute ulcerative colitis. The Abacus Investigator Group. *Gastroenterology* 1998; **114:** 15–22,

25. Baron JH, Connell AM, Kanaghinis TG, Lennard-Jones JE, Jones FA. Outpatients treatment of ulcerative colitis: comparison between three doses of oral prednisolone. *Br Med J* 1962; **2:** 441–442.

26. Rosenberg JL, Wall AJ, Levin B, *et al.* A controlled trial of azathioprine in the management of chronic ulcerative colitis. *Gastroenterology* 1975; **69:** 96–99.

27. Kirk AP, Lennard-Jones JE. Controlled trial of azathioprine in chronic ulcerative colitis. *Brit Med J* 1982; **284:** 1291–1292.

28. Dissanayake AS, Truelove SC. A controlled therapeutic trial of long-term maintenance treatment of ulcerative colitis with sulphasalazine. *Gut* 1973; **14:** 923.

29. Courtney MG, Nunes DP, Bergin CF, *et al.* Randomised comparison of olsalazine and mesalazine in prevention of relapses in ulcerative colitis. *Lancet* 1992; **339:** 1279–1281.

30. Stein RB, Hanauer SB. Medical therapy for inflammatory bowel disease. *Gastroenterol Clin N Am* 1999; **28:** 297–321.

31. Hawthorne AB, Logan RFA, Hawkey CJ, *et al.* Randomised controlled trial of azathioprine withdrawal in ulcerative colitis. *Brit Med J* 1992; **305:** 20–22.

32. Jarnerot G, Rolny P, Sandberg-Gertzen H. Intensive intravenous treatment of ulcerative colitis. *Gastroenterology* 1985; **89:** 1005–1013.

33. Hyde GM, Thillainayagam AV, Jewell DP. Intravenous cyclosporin as rescue therapy in severe ulcerative colitis; time for a reappraisal. *Eur J Gastroenterol Hepatol* 1998; **10:** 411–413.

34. Lichtiger S, Present DG, Kornbluth A, *et al.* Cyclosporin in severe ulcerative colitis refractory

to steroid therapy. *New Engl J Med* 1994; **330:** 1841–1845.

35. Kronbluth A, Lichtiger S, Present D, *et al*. Long-term results of oral cyclosporin in patients with severe ulcerative colitis: a double-blind randomized, multi-center trial. *Gastroenterology* 1994; **106:** A714.

36. Cohen RD, Stein R, Hanauer SB. Intravenous cyclosporin in ulcerative colitis: a five-year experience. *Am J Gastrol* 1999; **94:** 1587–1592.

37. Wenzl HH, Petritsch W, Aichbichler BW, Hinterleitner TA, Fleischmann G, Krejs GJ. Short-term efficacy and long-term outcome of cyclosporine treatment in patients with severe ulcerative colitis. *Z Gastroenterol* 1998; **36:** 287–293.

38. Present DH. Ciprofloxacin as a treatment for ulcerative colitis—not yet. *Gastroenterology* 1998; **15:** 1289–1291.

39. Pullan RD, Ganesh S, Mani V, *et al*. Comparison of bismuth citrate and 5-aminosalicylic acid enemas in distal ulcerative colitis: a controlled trial. *Gut* 1993; **34:** 676.

40. Kruis W, Schütz E, Eric P, Fixa B, Judmaier G, Stolte M. Double-blind comparison of an oral *Escherichia coli* preparation and mesalazine in maintaining remission of ulcerative colitis. *Aliment Pharmacol Ther* 1997; **11:** 853–858.

41. Rembacken BJ, Snelling AM, Hawkey PM, Chalmers DM, Axon ATR. Non-pathogenic *Escherichia coli* versus mesalazine for the treatment of ulcerative colitis: a randomised trial. *Lancet* 1999; **354:** 635–639.

42. Gionchetti P, Rizzello F, Venturi A, *et al*. Maintenance treatment of chronic pouchitis: a randomised placebo-controlled, double-blind trial with a new probiotic preparation. *Gastroenterology* 1998; **114:** G4037 [Abstract].

43. Evans RC, Clarke L, Heath P, Stephens S, Morris AI, Rhodes JM. Treatment of ulcerative colitis with an engineered human anti-TNF$_{alpha}$ antibody CDP571. *Aliment Pharmacol Ther* 1997; **11:** 1031–1035.

44. Schreiber S, Fedorak RN, Wild G, *et al*. Safety and tolerance of rHuIL-10 treatment in patients with mild/moderate active ulcerative colitis. *Gastroenterology* 1998; **114:** A1080.

45. Sandborn WJ, Tremaine WJ, Schroeder KW, *et al*. A placebo-controlled trial of cyclosporine enemas for mildly to moderately active left-sided ulcerative colitis. *Gastroenterology* 1994; **106:** 1429–1435.

46. Fellermann K, Ludwig D, Stahl M, David-Walek T, Stange EF. Steroid-unresponsive acute attacks of inflammatory bowel disease: immunomodulation by tacrolimus (FK506). *Am J Gastroenterol* 1998; **3:** 1860–1866.

47. Oren R, Arber N, Odes S, *et al*. Methotrexate in chronic active ulcerative colitis: a double-blind, randomized, Israeli multicenter trial. *Gastroenterology* 1996; **110:** 1416–1421.

48. Korzenik JR, Robert ME, Bitton A, *et al*. A multicenter, randomised controlled trial of heparin for the treatment of ulcerative colitis. *Gastroenterology* 1999; **116:** A752.

49. Scheppach W, Sommer H, Kirchner T, *et al*. Effect of butyrate enemas on the colonic mucosa in distal ulcerative colitis. *Gastroenterology* 1992; **103:** 51–57.

50. Thomas GA, Rhodes J, Ragunath K, *et al*. Transdermal nicotine compared with oral prednisolone therapy for active ulcerative colitis. *Eur J Gastroenterol Hepatol* 1996; **8:** 769–776.

51. Arlander E, Ost A, Stahlberg D, Lofberg R. Ropivacaine gel in active distal ulcerative colitis and proctitis—a pharmacokinetic and exploratory clinical study. *Aliment Pharmacol Ther* 1996; **10:** 73–81.

52. Summers RW, Switz DM, Sessions JT Jr, *et al*. National Cooperative Crohn's Disease Study (NCCDS): results of drug treatment. *Gastroenterology* 1979; **77:** 847–869.

53. Malchow H, Ewe K, Brandes JW, *et al*. European Crohn's Disease Study (ECCDS): results of drug treatment. *Gastroenterology* 1984; **86:** 249–266.

54. Singleton JW, Hanauer HB, Gitnick GL, *et al*. and the Pentasa Crohn's Disease Study Group. Mesalamine capsules for the treatment of active Crohn's disease; results of a 16-week trial. *Gastroenterology* 1993; **104:** 1293–1301.

55. Tremain WJ, Schroeder KW, Harrison JM, *et al*. A randomised double-blind, placebo-controlled trial of the oral mesalamine (5-ASA) preparation. Asacol, in the treatment of symptomatic Crohn's colitis and ileocolitis. *J Clin Gastroenterol* 1994; **19:** 278–282.

56. Thomsen OO, Cortot A, Jewell D, *et al*. Budesonide led to a greater remission rate and fewer severe adverse events than did mesalamine in Crohn's disease. *N Engl J Med* 1998; **339:** 370–374.

57. Rutgeerts P, Lofberg R, Malchow H, *et al*. A comparison of budesonide and prednisolone for active Crohn's disease. *N Engl J Med* 1994; **331:** 842–845.

58. Klein S, Kinney J, Khursheed J, *et al*. Nutrition support in clinical practice: review of published data and recommendations for future research directions. *J Parenter Enteral Nutr* 1997; **21**: 133.

59. Camma C, Giunta M, Rosselli M, *et al*. Mesalamine in the maintenance treatment of Crohn's disease: a meta-analysis adjusted for confounding variables. *Gastroenterology* 1997; **113**: 1465–1473.

60. Pearson DC, May GR, Fick GH, *et al*. Azathioprine and 6-mercaptopurine in Crohn's disease: a meta-analysis. *Ann Int Med* 1995; **122**: 132–142.

61. O'Donaghue DP, Dawson AM, Powell-Tuck J, *et al*. Double-blind withdrawal trial of azathioprine as maintenance treatment for Crohn's disease. *Lancet* 1978; **2**: 955–957.

62. Bouchnik Y, Lemann M, Mary JY, *et al*. Long-term follow-up of patients with Crohn's disease treated with azathioprine or 6-mercaptopurine. *Lancet* 1996; **347**: 215–219.

63. Rutgeerts P, Heboes K, Vantrappen G, *et al*. Predictability of the post-operative course of Crohn's disease. *Gastroenterology* 1990; **99**: 956–963.

64. Breuer-Katschinski BD, Hollander N, Goebell H. Effect of cigarette smoking on the course of Crohn's disease. *Eur J Gastroenterol Hepatol* 1996; **8**: 225–228.

65. Caprilli R, Andreoli A, Capurso L, *et al*. Oral mesalasine (5-aminosalicylic acid; Asacol) for the prevention of post-operative recurrence of Crohn's disease. *Aliment Pharmacol Ther* 1994; **8**: 35–43.

66. McCleod RS, Wolff BG, Steinhert AH, *et al*. Prophylactic mesalamine treatment decreases postoperative recurrence of Crohn's disease. *Gastroenterology* 1995; **109**: 404–413.

67. Sutherland LR. Mesalamine for the prevention of postoperative recurrence: is nearly there the same as being there. *Gastroenterology* 2000; **118**: 436–438.

68. Rutgeerts P, Hiele M, Heboes K, *et al*. Controlled trial of metronidazole treatment for prevention of Crohn's recurrence after ileal resection. *Gastroenterology* 1995; **108**: 1617–1621.

69. Duffy LF, Daum F, Fisher SE, *et al*. Peripheral neuropathy in Crohn's disease patients treated with metronidazole. *Gastroenterology* 1985; **88**: 681–684.

70. Hellers G, Cortot A, Jewell DP, *et al*. Oral Budesonide for prevention of post-surgical recurrence Crohn's disease. *Gastroenterology* 1999; **116**: 294–300.

71. Targan SR, Hanauer SB, Van Deventer SJ, *et al*. A short-term study of chimeric monoclonal antibody to cA2 to tumour necrosis factor alpha for Crohn's disease. *N Engl J Med* 1997; **337**: 1029–1035.

72. Rutgeerts P, D'Haens G, van Deventer S, *et al*. Retreatment with anti-TNF-α chimeric antibody (cA2) effectively maintains cA2-induced remission in Crohn's disease. *Gastroenterology* 1997; **112**: A1078.

73. Present D, Rutgeerts P, Targan S, *et al*. Infliximab for the treatment of fistulas in patients with Crohn's disease. *N Engl J Med* 1999; **340**: 1398–1405.

74. Feagan BG, Rochon J, Fedorak RN, *et al*. Methotrexate for the treatment of Crohn's disease. *N Engl J Med* 1995; **332**: 292–297.

75. Feagan BG, Fedorak RN, Irvine EJ, *et al*. A comparison of methotrexate with placebo for the maintenance of remission of Crohn's disease. North American Crohn's Study Group. *New Engl J Med* 2000; **342**: 1627–1632.

76. Ehrenpreis ED, Kane SV, Cohen LB, Cohen RD, Hanauer SB. Thalidomide therapy for patients with refractory Crohn's disease: an open-label trial. *Gastroenterology* 1999; **117**: 1271–1277.

77. Vasiliauskas EA, Kam LY, Abreu-Martin MT, *et al*. An open-label pilot study of low-dose thalidomide in chronically active steroid-dependent Crohn's disease. *Gastroenterology* 1999; **117**: 1278–1287.

78. Neurath MF, Wanitschke R, Peters M, Krummenauer F, Meyer zum Buschenfelde K-H, Schlaak JF. Randomised trial of mycophenolate mofetil versus azathioprine for treatment of chronic active Crohn's disease. *Gut* 1999; **44**: 625–628.

79. Present DH. Is mycophenolate mofetil a new alternative in the treatment of inflammatory bowel disease? *Gut* 1999; **44**: 592–593.

80. Trallori G, D'Albasio G, Bardizzi G, *et al*. 5-Aminosalicylic acid in pregnancy: clinical report. *Ital J Gastroenterol* 1994; **26**: 75–78.

81. Alstead EM, Ritchie JK, Lennard-Jones LE, *et al*. Safety of azathioprine in pregnancy in inflammatory bowel disease. *Gastroenterology* 1990; **99**: 443–446.

82. Francella A, Dayan A, Rubin P, *et al*. 6-Mercaptopurine is safe therapy for child bearing patients with inflammatory bowel disease: a case-controlled study. *Gastroenterology* 1996; **110**: A909.

83. Corrigan G, Stevens PE. Interstitial nephritis associated with the use of mesalazine in inflammatory bowel disease. *Aliment Pharmacol Ther* 2000; **14:** 1–6.

84. Anonymous. Drugs in the peri-operative period: 2—Corticosteroids and therapy for diabetes mellitus. *Drugs Ther Bull* 1999; **37(9):** 68–70.

85. Compston JE. Management of bone disease in patients on long-term glucocorticoid therapy. *Gut* 1999; **44:** 770–772.

86. Connell WR, Kamm MA, Lennard-Jones JE, Ritchie JK. Bone marrow toxicity from azathioprine: twenty-seven year experience in inflammatory bowel disease. *Gut* 1993; **34:** 1081–1085.

87. Connell WR, Kamm MA, Dickson M, *et al*. Long-term neoplasia risk after azathioprine treatment in inflammatory bowel disease. *Lancet* 1994; **343:** 1249–1252.

88. Present DH, Meltzer SJ, Krumholz MP, *et al*. 6-mercaptopurine in the management of inflammatory bowel disease: short and long-term toxicity. *Ann Intern Med* 1989; **111:** 641–649.

89. Tremaine WJ. Collagenous colitis and lymphocytic colitis. *J Clin Gastroenterol* 2000; **30:** 245–249.

90. Bohr J, Tysk C, Eriksson S, Abrahamsson H, Jarnerot G. Collagenous colitis: a retrospective study of clinical presentation and treatment in 163 patients. *Gut* 1996; **39:** 846–851.

91. Ung KA, Gillberg R, Kilander A, Abrahamsson H. Role of bile acids and bile acid binding agents in patients with collagenous colitis. *Gut* 2000; **46:** 170–175.

92. Tromm A, Griga T, Mollmann HW, May B, Muller KM, Fisseler-Eckhoff A. Budesonide for the treatment of collagenous colitis: first results of a pilot trial. *Am J Gastroenterol* 1999; **94:** 1871–1875.

93. Fisher NC, Tutt A, Sim E, Scarpello JH, Green JR. Collagenous colitis responsive to octreotide therapy. *J Clin Gastroenterol* 1996; **23:** 300–301.

6

Gastrointestinal and liver infections

Michael JG Farthing

INTRODUCTION

Infections of the gastrointestinal tract and liver are the most common disorders of the alimentary tract in both the industrialized and in the resource-poor countries of the world. In the developing world, microbial enteropathogens are highly prevalent, with the major reservoirs being water, food, animals and humans. Infectious diarrhoea is responsible for the death of up to four million pre-school children each year. In some African countries, children may suffer up to seven attacks of acute diarrhoea annually, each of which contributes to the infection–malnutrition cycle, which, in many, ultimately results in impaired growth and development.

Despite major public health interventions to ensure water quality and sewage disposal, intestinal infections are increasing in many industrialized countries. These include food-borne infections, such as *Salmonella* spp., *Campylobacter jejuni* and *Enterohaemorrhagic Escherichia coli*, and waterborne infections such as *Giardia intestinalis* and *Cryptosporidium parvum*. Other factors contributing to this increase in infectious diarrhoea include the widespread use of broad-spectrum antibiotics, impaired host immunity owing to HIV infection and cancer chemotherapy, and the increase in foreign travel. A recent survey in general practice in the UK has revealed a high incidence of infectious diarrhoea[1] and reports to the Public Health Laboratory Service continue to increase for several micro-organisms particularly *Campylobacter jejuni* (Fig. 6.1). *Salmonella* spp. infections have also been rising steadily during the past decade but, for the first time in 1999, have shown a decline, which can probably be attributed to the introduction of vaccination of chicken flocks against *Salmonella* spp.

Although diarrhoea is the most common manifestation of gastrointestinal infection, there are several other important clinical syndromes, including oesophagitis (from candidiasis, cytomegalovirus infection), gastritis (from anisakiasis), intestinal obstruction (from tuberculosis, schistosomiasis) and proctitis and perianal disease (from chlamydia infections, herpes simplex virus infection and gonorrhoea). Some infections may be carried by the host without symptoms.

Bacterial and parasitic infections of the liver and biliary tract are also a major cause of morbidity and mortality worldwide, producing liver abscess, cholangitis and biliary obstruction and chronic liver disease with portal hypertension.

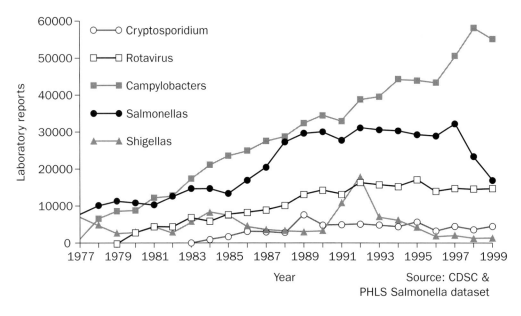

Figure 6.1 Laboratory reporting of selected enteric pathogens in England and Wales.

PATHOPHYSIOLOGY OF GASTROINTESTINAL INFECTION

Infections of the alimentary tract manifest as a variety of clinical syndromes. This provides a convenient way of classifying these diseases and also guides the clinician towards a working diagnosis that may assist in the development of empirical management strategies before microbiological assessment is complete (Table 6.1).

Infective oesophagitis and gastritis

Infective oesophagitis is predominantly a problem for the immunocomprised, the major opportunistic pathogens being *Candida albicans*, herpes simplex virus (HSV) and cytomegalovirus (CMV). These infections cause dysphagia and odynophagia as a result of intense inflammation and ulceration of the oesophageal mucosa. The most common cause of gastritis is now known to be infection with *Helicobacter pylori*. The pathophysiology and treatment of this infection is described in

Chapter 2. The parasite *Anisakis simplex*, which is transmitted by the ingestion of raw or inadequately cooked fish is particularly common in Japan, Holland and California. The symptoms of acute pain, nausea and vomiting are produced by inflammation of the gastric mucosa owing to direct invasion by the parasite.

Infectious diarrhoea

Infectious diarrhoea presents clinically as one of three major syndromes, namely:

1. Acute watery diarrhoea
2. Diarrhoea with blood (dysentery)
3. Persistent diarrhoea with or without evidence of intestinal malabsorption.

Acute infectious diarrhoea usually resolves within 5–10 days, while persistent diarrhoea is defined as diarrhoea that has continued for more than 14–21 days. In Table 6.2 are listed the common enteropathogens responsible for these clinical syndromes and an indication of where overlap can occur is given.

Table 6.1 Infections of the gastrointestinal tract: clinical syndromes.	
Clinical syndrome	**Infective agent**
Oesophagitis and gastritis	
Bacteria	*Candida albicans*
	Helicobacter pylori
Viruses	Herpes simplex virus
	Cytomegalovirus
Helminths	*Anisakis simplex*
Diarrhoea	
Acute watery	
Dysentery	See Table 6.2
Persistent	
Enteric fever	*Salmonella typhi*
	Salmonella paratyphi
Intestinal obstruction	
Bacteria	*Mycobacterium tuberculosis*
Helminths	*Schistosoma* spp.
Proctitis and perianal disease	
Bacteria	*Chlamydia trachomatis*
	Chlamydia trachomatis LGV
	Neisseria gonorrhoeae
	Treponema pallidum
	Mycobacterium tuberculosis
Viruses	Herpes simplex virus
	Cytomegalovirus
Helminths	*Schistosoma* spp.

LGV, lymphogranuloma venereum.

Diarrhoea occurs during intestinal infection as a result of two major disturbances of normal intestinal physiology, namely:

1. Increased intestinal secretion of fluid and electrolytes, predominantly in the small intestine; and
2. Decreased absorption of fluid, electrolytes and sometimes nutrients.

These disturbances can involve both the small intestine and the colon.

Increased intestinal secretion

Intestinal secretory processes in infective diarrhoea are generally activated by secretory enterotoxins. Cholera toxin (CT) is the prototype enterotoxin and its mechanism of action has been studied in great detail.[2,3] Until recently, the main focus of the action of cholera toxin has been on the enterocyte and the enzymic activity of the A_1 subunit of cholera toxin, which activates G_s—the catalytic unit of the enzyme adenylate cyclase. This results in an

Table 6.2 Enteropathogens responsible for infectious diarrhoea.

Enteropathogen	Acute watery diarrhoea	Dysentery	Persistent diarrhoea
Viruses			
Rotavirus	+	−	−
Enteric adenovirus (Types 40, 41)	+	−	−
Caliciviruses	+	−	−
Astrovirus	+	−	−
Cytomegalovirus	+	+	+
Bacteria			
Vibrio cholerae and other vibrios	+	−	−
ETEC	+	−	−
EPEC	+	−	+
EAggEC	+	−	+
EIEC	+	+	−
EHEC	+	+	−
Shigella spp.	+	+	+
Salmonella spp.	+	+	+
Campylobacter spp.	+	+	+
Yersinia enterocolitica	+	+	+
Clostridium difficile	+	+	+
Mycobacterium tuberculosis	−	+	+
Tropheryma whippelii	−	−	+
Protozoa			
Giardia intestinalis	+	−	+
Cryptosporidium parvum	+	−	+
Microsporidia	+	−	+
Isospora belli	+	−	+
Cyclospora cayetanensis	+	−	+
Entamoeba histolytica	+	+	+
Balantidium coli	+	+	+
Helminths			
Strongyloides stercoralis	−	−	+
Schistosoma spp.	−	+	+

ETEC, enterotoxigenic *Escherichia coli;* EPEC, enteropathogenic *Escherichia coli*; EAggEC, enteroaggregative *Escherichia coli;* EIEC, enteroinvasive *Escherichia coli;* EHEC, enterohaemorrhagic *Escherichia coli.*

increase in intracellular cyclic AMP, which, through a series of intermediate steps, results in phosphorylation of the transmembrane chloride channel protein, with opening of chloride channels in the apical membrane of the enterocyte.

There are other important bacterial enterotoxins, particularly those produced by *Escherichia coli*. *E. coli* heat-labile toxins (LT) are closely related structurally, functionally and immunologically to CT. Like CT, *E. coli* LT has A and B subunit structure and activates adenylate cyclase. Other bacterial enteropathogens produce LT-like toxins, including *Camplyobacter jejuni*, *Salmonella typhimurium*, *Salmonella enteritidis*, *Aeromonas* spp. and *Plesiomonas* spp. *E. coli* also produces a heat-stable toxin, which differs from LT and CT in that it activates guanylate cyclase. Heat-stable toxins (ST) are also produced by *Yersinia enterocolitica*, *Vibrio cholerae* non-O1 and enteroaggregative *E. coli*, which produces enteroaggregative *E. coli* heat-stable toxin 1 (EAST-1).[4] More recently, other enterotoxins have been characterized, including accessory cholera enterotoxin (ACE), which increases short-circuit current in Ussing chambers and causes fluid secretion,[5] and zonular occludens toxin (ZOT), which increases the permeability of the small intestinal mucosa by altering the structure of the intercellular tight junction (zonular occludens).[6]

It is now evident that secretory diarrhoea may be partly mediated by a variety of endogenous secretagogues, including prostaglandins, 5-hydroxytryptamine (5-HT) and substance P. Neuronal pathways have been shown to be involved in amplification of the effects of enterotoxins.[7] CT, for example, has been shown to release 5-HT from enterochromaffin cells,[8–10] which is thought to activate the afferent limb of a neuronal reflex by 5-HT_3 and possibly 5-HT_4 neuronal receptors. The effector limb of the neuronal reflux probably completes the neuronal pathway by releasing the neurotransmitter vasoactive intestinal polypeptide (VIP).[11] Interneurones appear to propagate the secretory effects of CT distally in the small intestine.

LT and ST also appear to activate neural secretory reflexes, although 5-HT is not involved in the secretory mechanism of either toxin.[12] Further work is required to delineate clearly the neural pathways involved in these reflexes and to identify the dominant neurotransmitters.

Decreased intestinal absorption

Impaired intestinal absorption is the other major mechanism by which enteropathogens cause diarrhoea; it is generally accompanied by macroscopic or microscopic injury to the intestine.[13,14] Diarrhoea resulting from impaired absorption can be related to:

- Impaired fluid, electrolyte and nutrient absorption in the small intestine
- Osmotic diarrhoea owing to the appearance of incompletely absorbed nutrients in the colon
- Impaired water and sodium retrieval by the colon owing to direct involvement of colonic absorptive processes

Intestinal injury can occur at many levels. It ranges from discrete damage to the microvillus membrane (such as occurs during the attachment process of enteropathogenic *E. coli* (EPEC) and *Cryptosporidium parvum*), to the mucosal inflammatory response to invasive pathogens (e.g. *Shigella* spp., *Salmonella* spp. and *Entamoeba histolytica*), usually involving the release of cytolethal cytotoxins, and which results in epithelial cell loss and ulceration. Rotavirus directly invades the epithelial cells in the mid and upper portion of the villus, with rapid epithelial cell death and acute villous atrophy.[15]

Invasive enteropathogens also produce an acute inflammatory response within the mucosa, with recruitment of pro-inflammatory mediators, such as prostaglandins and leukotrienes, which are secretagogues and will promote a pro-secretory state in the intestine.[13] Many invasive enteropathogens also promote the synthesis and release of chemokines, such as IL-8, by intestinal epithelial cells. IL-8 is a potent chemoattractant for polymorphonuclear leukocytes, which enhance the inflammatory cascade and produce further mucosal and epithelial damage by release of reactive oxygen species.

Although it is helpful to consider the patho-physiology of infectious diarrhoea under two broad headings, there are often situations in which these two pathophysiological disturbances co-exist.

Enteric fever

Enteric fever is primarily a systemic bacter-aemic infection with a gastrointestinal portal of entry and with important intestinal complications. Infection is classically with *Salmonella typhi* and *paratyphi* but enteric fever-like illnesses may also occur with other penetrating organisms such as *Campylobacter jejuni* and *Yersinia enterocolitica*. The systemic features of the illness result from the bacteraemia and systemic release of pro-inflammatory cytokines. Intestinal ulceration, particularly in the ileum may be complicated by bleeding or perforation.

Intestinal obstruction

Infections such as tuberculosis and schistosomiasis produce, in the small and large intestine, inflammatory lesions which frequently progress and heal with marked fibrosis.[16,17] This results in stricture formation, which can lead to subacute intestinal obstruction. The fibrotic consequences of these infections are also seen in other affected organs, such as the lungs, liver and renal tract. Obstruction may also occur in ascaris infection when worm burdens are heavy. The physical presence of a mass of worms, usually in the small intestine, can occlude the gut lumen and cause obstruction. Occasionally ascaris may also enter the bile duct and produce biliary obstruction with jaundice and cholangitis.

Proctitis and perianal disease

Several bacterial and virus infections can affect the rectum and perianal tissues (Table 6.3). The symptoms of infective proctitis are similar to those of non-specific inflammatory bowel disease (ulcerative colitis, Crohn's disease) and include the passage of blood and mucus, proctalgia, constipation and tenesmus. Some infections such as lymphogranuloma venereum and tuberculosis can produce Crohn's disease-like fistula formation and anorectal strictures.

TREATMENT RATIONALE

The primary aim of the management of gastrointestinal infections is to use appropriate supportive therapy while self-limiting infections resolve and, when necessary, to initiate diagnostic tests to enable a specific pathogen to be identified, thereby enabling the administration of an effective, safe antimicrobial chemotherapeutic agent. Many bacterial and viral infections cause relatively mild illnesses in immunocompetent individuals and will be cleared spontaneously without the use of antibiotics. In the immuno-compromised, however, this is often not the case, although the introduction of highly active anti-retroviral therapy (HAART) has confirmed that this intervention has had a major impact in controlling the natural history of intestinal infection in this setting.

Table 6.3	**Proctitis and perianal disease.**
Cause	**Organism responsible**
Bacteria	*Chlamydia trachomatis non-LGV*
	Chlamydia trachomatis LGV
	Neisseria gonorrhoeae
	Treponema pallidum
	Mycobacterium tuberculosis
Viruses	Herpes simplex virus
	Cytomegalovirus
Helminths	*Schistosoma mansoni*
	Schistosoma japonicum
	Schistosoma haematobium

LGV, lymphogranuloma venereum.

The diagnosis of intestinal infection relies heavily on faecal microscopy and culture, although mucosal biopsy is important for the diagnosis of CMV and serology for amoebiasis, schistosomiasis and strongyloidiasis. Faecal antigen ELISA testing is available for *Giardia intestinalis* and rotavirus; indeed, molecular biological approaches to diagnosis are gradually being introduced and have already proved to be of value in difficult infections such as tuberculosis and Whipple's disease.

TREATMENT REGIMENS

Infectious oesophagitis and gastritis

Oesophagitis
Candida oesophagitis occurs in immunocompromised patients, including those with HIV infection, diabetes mellitus, those receiving steroids or broad-spectrum antibiotics and anticancer chemotherapy. Candidiasis in immunocompetent individuals can be treated with nystatin suspension 1–3 million units orally four times daily or clotrimazole 10 mg orally five times daily; these regimens have similar efficacy. Systemic therapy is required for immunocompromised patients. The treatment of choice is oral fluconazole 100–200 mg daily, which will achieve endoscopic clearance in more than 90% of patients.[18] Fluconazole is clinically superior to ketoconazole and itraconazole in AIDS patients.[18,19] For fluconazole-resistant candida oesophagitis, combination therapy with itraconazole (100–200 mg daily) and flucytosine (100 mg/kg daily)[20] or intravenous amphotericin B 3–5 mg/kg daily, are equally effective options.[21]

In patients who are susceptible to recurrent candida oesophagitis, prophylaxis with either ketoconazole (200 mg daily) or fluconazole (50 mg daily) significantly reduces the risk of relapse and are well tolerated.[22]

Viral oesophagitis caused by HSV or CMV is found most commonly in individuals with HIV infection. These infections in the immunocompromised host require treatment with anti-viral agents. In severely symptomatic patients with HSV oesophagitis, aciclovir 5 mg/kg should be given intravenously every 8 hours for 7–10 days.[23] In these patients, oral maintenance therapy with 400 mg aciclovir orally twice daily should probably also be given. Milder infections may respond to oral aciclovir. When HSV is resistant to aciclovir an alternative therapy is foscarnet 40–60 mg/kg intravenously every 8 h for 2–3 weeks.[24]

CMV oesophagitis should be treated with ganciclovir 5 mg/kg intravenously twice daily for 3–6 weeks.[25] Maintenance therapy with oral ganciclovir 1000 mg orally three times daily may also be considered.[26] An alternative drug is foscarnet.[27]

Gastritis
Infection with *Anisakis simplex* cannot reliably be treated with anti-helminthic agents, although success has been reported with mebendazole. For severe infections, parasites may be removed physically from the gastric mucosa at endoscopy using grasping forceps. The treatment options for *H. pylori* are reviewed in Chapter 3.

Infectious diarrhoea

The treatment of infectious diarrhoea can be considered at three levels, namely:

1. General supportive therapy in the form of fluid and electrolyte replacement and then maintenance of hydration;
2. Symptomatic treatment to reduce bowel frequency and other symptoms such as abdominal pain; and
3. Specific therapeutic interventions in the form of antimicrobial chemotherapy, which might alter the natural history of the infection and thereby reduce the duration and severity of the illness.

Replacement of fluid and electrolyte losses
Whenever possible fluid and electrolyte losses should be replaced orally in the form of oral

rehydration therapy with a glucose-electrolyte oral rehydration solution (ORS).[28] The scientific rationale for oral rehydration therapy centres around the principle of active, carrier-mediated sodium-glucose co-transport. In this energy-dependent process, glucose and sodium are absorbed together by the same transporter, a process that then promotes the absorption of chloride ions and water. The co-transporter is active in all diarrhoeal states, irrespective of whether diarrhoea is enterotoxin-mediated or it occurs as a result of intestinal damage, such as in rotavirus infection.[29–32] ORS should be administered early during the course of acute diarrhoea, particularly in infants and young children, with the aim of preventing severe dehydration and acidosis (Table 6.4). In the developing world, the WHO-ORS (sodium concentration 90 mmol/l, osmolality 331 mOsm/kg) is still recommended, although there is increasing evidence that solutions with lower sodium concentrations (50–60 mmol/l) and lower osmolality (about 240 mOsm/kg) are equally effective as WHO-ORS in correcting dehydration and acidosis and have an added advantage in that they appear to be more effective in reducing faecal losses.[33–36]

Additional modifications that aim to improve efficacy have been made to the ORS. Replacing glucose with a glucose polymer such as rice starch has the dual advantage of produc-ing a low osmolality solution[37] while, at the same time, delivering increased amounts of substrate in the form of rice-starch polymer and also some protein, which will also drive active sodium absorption. Cereal-based ORS has been evaluated during randomized controlled trials in several acute diarrhoea settings but only appears to have a significant advantage over WHO-ORS in cholera.[38] More recently, resistant starch has been used as a substrate in ORS on the basis that it will be incompletely hydrolysed in the small intestine and with up to 30% enter-ing the colon; this will be subject to degradation by colonic bacteria, with the production of short-chain fatty acids, such as butyrate, which promote sodium and water absorption in the colon. A resistant starch-ORS has been subject to randomized controlled trial in cholera and shown to be significantly more effective in reducing faecal losses compared with WHO-ORS and a hypotonic glucose monomer ORS.[39] Oral rehydration solutions available in the UK are shown in Table 6.5.

Intravenous fluids may be required in infants and young children with more severe dehydra-tion (>5%) (Table 6.4). Although acidosis com-monly accompanies the more severe degrees of dehydration, administration of intravenous bicarbonate is usually not necessary since acid–base abnormalities are generally rectified by fluid replacement alone.

Table 6.4 Simplified guidelines for assessing the severity of dehydration.*	
% Dehydration	**Clinical signs**
2–3%	Thirst, mild oliguria
5%	Discernible alteration in skin tone, slightly sunken eyes, some loss of intraocular tension, thirst, oliguria. Sunken fontanelle in infants
7–8%	Very obvious loss of skin tone and tissue turgor, sunken eyes, loss of intraocular tension, marked thirst and oliguria. Often some restlessness or apathy
≥10%	All the foregoing, plus peripheral vasoconstriction, hypotension, cyanosis, and sometimes hyperpyrexia. Thirst may be lost at this stage

*Intravenous rehydration is recommended when % dehydration >5%.

Table 6.5 Composition (mmol/l) of oral rehydration solutions available in the UK in 2000.*

Oral rehydration solution	Na	K	Cl	HCO$_3$	Citrate	Glucose	Osmolality (calculated)
Powders							
WHO formulation	90	20	80	—	10	111	311
Diocalm Replenish	60	20	50	—	10	111	251
Dioralyte	60	25	45	—	20	90	240
Dioralyte Relief	60	20	50	—	10	—†	NS
Electrolade	50	20	40	30	—	111	251
Rehidrat	50	20	50	20	9	91‡	336
Effervescent tablets							
Dioralyte	60	25	45	—	20	90	240

*Data from British National Formulary, March 2000. NS, not stated.
†Contains cooked rice powder 6 g/sachet (30 g/l).
‡Also contains sucrose 94 mmol/l and fructose 1–2 mmol/l.

Food and oral fluids should be commenced as soon as the individual wishes to eat and drink. Breastfeeding should be continued throughout the illness in young infants. In adults, with acute diarrhoea, with the exception of cholera, formal ORT is often not required. It is usually sufficient to recommend an increase in oral fluids such as salty soups (for sodium), fruit juices (for potassium) and a source of carbohydrate (e.g. salty crackers, rice, bread, pasta, potatoes) to provide a glucose source for glucose-sodium co-transport.

Symptomatic anti-diarrhoeal therapy
Drugs such as loperamide and a diphenoxylate/atropine combination reduce bowel frequency and may have a modest effect on reducing faecal losses. These drugs act predominantly on intestinal motility by increasing transit time and thereby enhancing the potential for reabsorption of fluid and electrolytes. Although loperamide may have some antisecretory activity,[40] in clinical practice it seems likely that this is only a minor contributor to its clinical efficacy. Loperamide has been subjected to randomized control trials in comparison with placebo and other anti-diarrhoeal agents. In a recent randomized controlled trial (RCT), loperamide was superior to placebo in reducing stool frequency and duration of the illness.[41] However, several previous RCTs had failed to demonstrate benefit over placebo.[42–44] There is some evidence that combining loperamide with an antibiotic is advantageous,[45,46] although other studies have failed to confirm this apparent benefit.[47,48] These drugs continue to be the first-line treatment for self-therapy in travellers' diarrhoea but should not be given to infants and young children because of concerns about possible effects on the central nervous system such as respiratory depression.[49]

There is still controversy as to whether anti-diarrhoeal agents that act by reducing gut motility should be used in individuals with dysentery, although the clinical evidence on which these concerns are based is limited.[50] A more recent study suggests that loperamide is safe in bacillary dysentery,[46] although there have been concerns about colonic dilatation associated with infective colitis. Similarly, there have been concerns that anti-motility agents will increase faecal carriage of gut enteropathogens; again the evidence for this is poor.

Anti-secretory agents

For several decades, there has been a search for drugs that will directly inhibit secretory mechanisms in the intestine. Initially attention focused on intracellular signalling mechanisms, particularly those related to calcium and the calcium-binding protein, calmodulin. A calmodulin inhibitor, zalderide maleate has been developed and evaluated in phase III randomized controlled trials. However, its further development was discontinued because of the lack of additional benefit compared with standard anti-diarrhoeal agents.[51–53]

A promising new approach has been the development of an enkephalinase inhibitor, racecadotril, which has pro-absorptive activity through its ability to potentiate endogenous enkephalins in the intestine.[54,55] Randomized controlled trials in adults and children confirm that this is an effective agent for reducing stool weight and bowel frequency, without the unwanted effects of rebound constipation, which is commonly reported with anti-motility, anti-diarrhoeal agents.[56–58] Studies in children have shown that it is safe and superior in efficacy to loperamide.[58]

Anti-microbial chemotherapy

Intestinal infections can be considered in three categories depending on whether antimicrobial agents have been shown to be *definitely effective* in treating the infection, conditions in which these agents are *possibly effective* and finally, conditions in which antimicrobial agents are *probably not effective* (Table 6.6). Evidence that antibiotics can reduce the severity and duration of some intestinal infections, particularly those due to bacteria that produce acute watery diarrhoea, will be reviewed. Antibiotics are also effective when there is evidence of systemic involvement following infection with some invasive bacterial enteropathogens. Antibiotics are also effective in some causes of persistent diarrhoea, particularly those related to enteropathogenic protozoa.

In situations when there is doubt about the efficacy of antibiotics, this may not be simply the result of antibiotic failure but of problems with the design of the study; for example, antibiotics may be administered after a considerable delay, while the results of stool cultures were awaited. This means that the antibiotic is then commenced relatively late in the natural history of the illness, a time when natural resolution is occurring and thus, any benefit of early administration would be missed.

Acute watery diarrhoea

The viruses responsible for acute watery diarrhoea are managed in an exclusively supportive manner, there being no indication for the use of specific anti-viral agents.

Antibiotics are effective in the treatment of cholera, reducing both the severity and duration of diarrhoea (Table 6.6). Standard therapy is with tetracycline[59] for 3 days but equally effective alternatives include doxycycline, trimethoprim-sulphamethoxazole, norfloxacin and ciprofloxacin.[60–63] Single-dose ciprofloxacin has been shown to be equally effective as 3 days' treatment with doxycycline.[64,65]

Travellers' diarrhoea is a major cause of acute watery diarrhoea, about 80% of which is caused by bacterial enteropathogens.[66–68] The most frequently isolated organism is enterotoxigenic E. coli. Broad-spectrum antibiotics have been shown to be effective in treating this condition,[47,48] although the increasing resistance to trimethoprim-sulphamethoxazole and ampicillin make these agents less suitable for 'blind' self-therapy. The quinolone antibiotics are now the treatment of choice and, when used in standard doses for 3–5 days, will reduce the severity and duration of the illness by at least 50%.[69–71] Similar efficacy has also been demonstrated with single-dose regimens (Table 6.7).[72] The use of antibiotics for the treatment of travellers' diarrhoea, while being unequivocally effective, remains controversial. Many feel it is undesirable to use an antibiotic for what is generally a mild, non-fatal self-limiting illness

Table 6.6   Efficacy of antimicrobial chemotherapy in bacterial and protozoal diarrhoea.

Efficacy of antimicrobial	Bacteria*	Protozoa
Proven efficacy	*Vibrio cholerae*	*Giardia intestinalis*
	ETEC (travellers' diarrhoea)	*Encephalitozoon intestinalis*
	Shigella spp.	*Isospora belli*
	Salmonella spp. (dysentery, fever)	*Cyclospora cayetanensis*
	Clostridium difficile	*Entamoeba histolytica*
	Yersinia enterocolitica (septicaemia)	*Balantidium coli*
	Campylobacter jejuni (dysentery/sepsis)	
Possible efficacy	EPEC	*Cryptosporidium parvum*
	EIEH	*Enterocytozoon bieneusi*
	Campylobacter jejuni	
Doubtful efficacy	*Salmonella* spp. (enterocolitis)	
	EHEC	
	Yersinia enterocolitica (uncomplicated)	

*EPEC, enteropathogenic *E. coli*; EIEC, enteroinvasive *E. coli*; EHEC, enterohaemorrhagic *E. coli*.

Table 6.7   Antimicrobial chemotherapy for acute watery diarrhoea.

	Drug of choice	Alternative(s)
Viruses		
Rotavirus	Antiviral agents	
Enteric adenovirus	not indicated	
Calicivirus		
Astrovirus		
Bacteria		
Vibrio cholerae	Tetracycline 500 mg four times daily for 3 days[59]	TMP-SMX,† doxycycline, norfloxacin, ciprofloxacin, for 3 days[60–63] Ciprofloxacin 1000 mg, single dose[64,65]
ETEC* (travellers' diarrhoea)	Ciprofloxacin 500 mg,[69,70] twice daily for 3–5 days Norfloxacin 400 mg,[71] twice daily for 3–5 days	Ciprofloxacin 500 mg, single dose[72]

*ETEC, enterotoxigenic *E. coli*.
†TMP-SMX, trimethoprim-sulphamethoxazole.

since there are concerns about increasing antibiotic resistance and the fact that an individual could develop a life-threatening complication such as the Stevens-Johnson syndrome or pseudomembranous colitis. One would anticipate that these risks are diminished with single-dose regimens but risk analysis would need to be carried out in each individual case.

Bismuth sub-salicylate is also effective in the treatment of travellers' diarrhoea but it has a lower efficacy than antibiotic regimens.[73] Adverse effects are uncommon and bacterial resistance has not been reported.

Dysentery

Antibiotics are indicated for the treatment of dysenteric shigellosis,[74–79] *Clostridium difficile*-associated diarrhoea,[80–83] amoebiasis[84] and balantidiasis[85] (Table 6.8). Antibiotic therapy is also of value in *Yersinia* septicaemia and when there is associated bone and joint infections[86,87] but its value in milder forms of enteritis has not been established, again usually because the antibiotic has been administered late in the natural history of the infection.[88] Similarly, the role of antibiotic therapy in *Campylobacter* infection remains controversial[89,90] There is good evidence that antibiotics do not alter the natural history of the illness if treatment is begun more than 4 days after the onset of symptoms. One randomized controlled trial has shown that treatment with erythromycin early in the infection significantly reduces the duration of the illness in children,[91] although a second study failed to confirm these findings.[92]

A role for antibiotics in the treatment of enteroinvasive *E. coli* infection has not been established, although in severe cases with evidence of systemic involvement it would seem reasonable to treat along the same lines as those recommended for dysenteric shigellosis. There is a major controversy as to whether antibiotics should be used in EHEC infection, although the balance of evidence at present is that antibiotics, particularly when given after infection is well-established, do not significantly improve the outcome.[93] In addition, there is evidence that administration of antibiotics at this stage can promote the development of the haemolytic-uraemic syndrome[94,95] presumably because of lysis of organisms and release of Shiga-like toxins and endotoxin. Thus, current evidence suggests that antimicrobial chemotherapy should not be used in children with proven EHEC infection.

Anti-viral agents such as ganciclovir and foscarnet are effective in CMV colitis but prolonged courses may be required in the immunocompromised[96–98] (Table 6.9).

Persistent diarrhoea

Many of the organisms responsible for persistent diarrhoea are sensitive to antimicrobial chemotherapeutic agents and, for many, there is randomized controlled trial evidence that their use reduces the severity and duration of the illness (Table 6.9). *Cryptosporidium parvum* continues to be resistant to the majority of antimicrobial agents, although paromomycin has been shown to have some efficacy in an open study.[100] Recent evidence suggests that high-dose albendazole or the emerging agent, nitazoxanide, may also have a role in the treatment of *C. parvum* infection.[101] The microsporidia have variable sensitivity to antibiotics; albendazole is effective in treating *Encephalitozoon intestinalis* but not *Enterocytozoon bieneusi* infection,[102,103] although the latter may, in some cases, be suppressed by this agent. Other antibiotics that have been shown in small uncontrolled studies to suppress infection include atovaquone,[104] furazolidone,[105] furazolidone-albendazole combination[106] and thalidomide.[107] *Cyclospora cayetanensis* infection responds promptly and predictably to trimethoprim-sulphamethoxazole.[108]

Enteric fever

Although chloramphenicol, ampicillin and co-trimoxazole have been used for many years for the treatment of *Salmonella typhi* infection, the rapid worldwide spread of multi-drug-resistant strains of *Salmonella* means that antibiotic

Table 6.8 Antimicrobial chemotherapy for dysentery.

	Drug of choice	Alternative(s)
Bacteria		
Shigella spp.[g]	TMP-SMX 2 tablets twice daily for 5 days[74]	Short-term quinolone[75-79]
	[c]Ciprofloxacin 500 mg twice daily for 5 days[75]	[a]Cefixime 400 mg daily for 5–7 days
		Nalidixic acid 1 g four times daily for 5–7 days
Salmonella spp.[h]	[b,c]Ciprofloxacin 500 mg twice daily for 10–14 days	[f]TMP-SMX, ampicillin, amoxycillin
Campylobacter jejuni[i]	Erythromycin 250–500 mg four times daily for 7 days[89-92]	[c,d]Ciprofloxacin 500 mg twice daily for 5–7 days
		Azithromycin 500 mg daily for 3 days
Yersinia enterocolitica	[c]Ciprofloxacin 500 mg twice daily for 7–10 days[86,87]	Tetracycline 250 mg four times daily for 7–10 days[86,87]
Clostridium difficile	Metronidazole 400 mg three times daily[80] for 7–10 days	Vancomycin 125 mg four times daily for 7–10 days[80-82]
		Fusidic acid, teicoplanin[83]
[e]EIEC	? as *Shigella* spp.	
[e]EHEC	? see text	
Protozoa		
Entamoeba histolytica	Metronidazole 750 mg three times daily for 5 days[84]	Paromomycin 25–35 mg/kg three times daily for 7–10 days[84]
	Diloxanide furoate 500 mg three times daily for 10 days[84]	
Balantidium coli	Metronidazole 400 mg three times daily for 10 days[84,85]	Tetracycline 500 mg four times daily for 10 days[84,85]

[a]And other third-generation cephalosporins.
[b]Usually only for bacteraemia.
[c]And other fluoroquinolones such as ofloxacin, norfloxacin, fleroxacin and cinoxacin.
[d]Increasing resistance to quinolones being recognized.
[e]EIEC, enteroinvasive *E. coli*; EHEC, enterohaemorrhagic *E. coli*.
[f]TMP-SMX, Trimethoprim-sulphamethoxazole.
[g]Multiple resistance to tetracycline, TMP-SMX, ampicillin and chloramphenicol in South America, Greece, Spain and Thailand.
[h]Chronic carrier state, norfloxacin 400 mg twice daily for 28 days.
[i]May only shorten duration of illness when given early.

Table 6.9 Antimicrobial chemotherapy for persistent infectious diarrhoea.

Enteropathogen	Drug regimen	Alternative(s)
Virus		
Cytomegalovirus	Ganciclovir 5 mg/kg/12 hourly for 14–21 days[96,97]	Foscarnet 60 mg/kg/8-h (14–21 days)[93] Maintenance therapy may be required
Bacteria		
Tropheryma whippelii	[d]Benzylpenicillin 2.4 g daily i.v. plus streptomycin 15 mg/kg daily i.v. for 2 weeks Co-trimoxazole 960 mg twice daily for 1 year (See also Tables 6.2 and 6.7)	
Protozoa		
Giardia intestinalis	Metronidazole 400 mg three times daily for 7–10 days[84,99]	Tinidazole 2 g single dose[84,99]
Cryptosporidium parvum	? Paromomycin 500 mg four times daily[100]	Nitazoxanide[101]
Encephalitozoon intestinalis	Albendazole 400 mg twice Daily, 14–28 days[102,103]	
Enterocytozoon bieneusi	Atovaquone[104]	Furazolidone 100 mg four times daily for 20 days[105]
Isospora belli	[c]TMP-SMX 2 tablets four times daily for 10 days	
Cyclospora cayetanensis	[c]TMP-SMX 2 tablets twice daily for 7 days[108]	
Entamoeba histolytica	See Table 6.7	
Helminths		
Strongyloides stercoralis	Albendazole 400 mg daily for 3 days	Thiabendazole 25 mg/kg twice daily for 2–3 days Ivermectin 100–200 μg/kg once daily for 2 days
Schistosoma spp.	Praziquantel [a]40–[b]60 mg/kg/day in two to three doses on one day	
Capillaria philippinensis	Mebendazole 200 mg oral twice daily for 20 days	Albendazole 400 mg daily for 10 days
Trichinella spiralis	Mebendazole 200–400 mg three times daily for 3 days	± corticosteroids 400–500 mg three times daily for 10 days

[a]*Schistosoma mansoni* and *S. haematobium*.
[b]*Schistosoma japonicum*.
[c]TMP-SMX, trimethoprim-sulphamethoxazole.
[d]For penicillin allergy or CNS involvement, replace penicillin with ceftriaxone 2 g twice daily i.v.

therapy for enteric fever must be informed by sensitivity testing. Fluoroquinolones are now the treatment of choice and have been shown to be equally effective to parenteral therapy with a third-generation cephalosporin such as ceftriaxone.[109,110] Oral cefixime and cefuroxime have also been shown to be effective in patients with multi-drug-resistant infection.[111-113]

Intestinal obstruction

Abdominal tuberculosis has three major clinical presentations, namely:

1.   Gastrointestinal disease;
2.   Mesenteric lymphadenopathy; and
3.   Peritonitis.[16]

In the UK, ileocaecal disease accounts for 40–60% of patients with abdominal tuberculosis and commonly presents with stricture formation in the terminal ileum.[114] A mass may be palpable and there is often fever, diarrhoea and general malaise. Colonic and anorectal involvement is less common where ulceration and stricture formation also occurs. Anorectal disease may be accompanied by abscess and fistula formation.[115]

Oesophageal involvement may arise either from extrinsic compression from enlarged mediastinal lymph nodes or from a mass lesion within the oesophagus itself.[116] Discrete tuberculous ulcers may also be found in the oesophagus, and infection can be complicated by broncho-oesophageal fistula. Gastroduodenal involvement also occurs and is typically accompanied by gastric and duodenal ulceration resembling peptic disease.[117]

Mesenteric lymphadenopathy is most commonly found in the tropics and, initially, has an insidious onset with weight loss, intermittent low-grade fever and malaise. Abdominal swelling may be apparent later in the illness and a major complication is rupture of caseating lymph nodes into the abdominal cavity producing tuberculous peritonitis.

Peritoneal involvement accounts for 25–30% of abdominal tuberculosis in the tropics and may present either as progressive ascites or abdominal pain and subacute obstruction, as a result of tuberculous adhesions producing an adherent mass of small bowel and intestinal obstruction.[118]

The current recommendations of the British Thoracic Society for the treatment of extra pulmonary tuberculosis is that daily isoniazid (330 mg) and rifampicin (450–600 mg) should be given for 6 months, with pyrazinamide (20–30 mg/kg daily, maximum 3 g daily) included for the first 2 months.[119] A fourth drug, such as streptomycin or ethambutol, should be added initially if drug resistance is suspected, particularly in patients who may have imported the disease from a developing country. Major adverse reactions are uncommon, and liver biochemistry should be assessed before treatment starts.

The treatment of other causes of intestinal obstruction such as schistosomiasis and *Ascaris lumbricoidum* infection are described in Tables 6.9 and 6.10, respectively.

Proctitis and perianal disease

Infectious proctitis occurs as a result of a variety of bacterial, viral and helminth infections. Treatment of *Chlamydia trachomatis* infection is with doxycycline 100 mg twice daily for 1 week. Lymphogranuloma venereum also caused by one of three specific serovars of *Chlamydia trachomatis* is also treated with doxycycline but treatment should be continued for at least 3 weeks. Alternative regimens include erythromycin 500 mg four times daily or trimethoprim-sulphamethoxazole, two tablets twice daily.

Neisseria gonorrhoeae is also an important cause of bacterial proctitis, which is sexually transmitted. Gonorrhoea can be treated with a single intramusclar dose of ceftriaxone or a single oral dose of cefixime, ciprofloxacin or ofloxacin. A 1-week course of doxycyline is usually included with treatment for gonorrhoea because of concomitant infection with *C. trachomatis*.

Table 6.10 Anti-helminthic therapy for nematode and cestode infections that are often asymptomatic.

	Drug regimen	Alternative(s)
Nematodes		
Ascaris lumbricoides[a]	Albendazole 400 mg single dose Pyrantel pamoate 11 mg/kg single dose	Mebendazole 100 mg twice daily for 3 days
Ancylostoma duodenale[b]	Mebendazole 100 mg twice daily for 3 days	Pyrantel pamoate 11 mg/kg single dose
Necator americanus[b]	Mebendazole 100 mg twice daily for 3 days	Pyrantel pamoate 11 mg/kg daily for 3 days
Trichuris trichiura[c]	As for *Ascaris* and hookworm	
Enterobius vermicularis[d]	Mebendazole 100 mg single dose repeated in 2 weeks	Albendazole 400 mg single dose repeated in 2 weeks
Cestodes		
Taenia solium[e]	Praziquantel 25 mg/kg oral single dose	Albendazole 400 mg oral for 3 days
Taenia saginata	As for *T. solium*	As for *T. solium*
Diphyllobothrium latum	Praziquantel 25 mg/kg oral single dose	Niclosamide 2 g oral single dose

[a]May cause biliary or intestinal obstruction.
[b]Anaemia may be severe and symptomatic.
[c]May cause symptomatic 'colitis' and rectal prolapse in children.
[d]Pruritus ani.
[e]May be complicated by cysticercosis with systemic dissemination, including the CNS.

Infection with *Treponema pallidum* continues to be a common cause of anorectal ulceration. The chancre usually occurs within 21 days of infection and heals spontaneously within 3–6 weeks. As an early form of syphilis, this should be treated with benzathine penicillin G 2.4 million units orally as a single dose. Alternative regimens include aqueous procaine penicillin 600 000–900 000 units intramuscular daily for 10 days, tetracycline 500 mg four times daily orally for 15 days and doxycycline 100 mg twice daily orally for 15 days. The treatment for *Mycobacterium tuberculosis* (see p. 121), HSV and CMV (see p. 113) and schistosomal infections (Table 6.9) are described elsewhere in this chapter.

Carrier states and asymptomatic gastrointestinal infections

Prolonged carriage of an enteropathogen is well-recognized in bacterial, viral, protozoal and helminth intestinal infections. Asymptomatic carriage of *Salmonella* spp. is probably the most common example of carriage of a bacterial enteropathogen. In the majority of patients, stool cultures become negative within 12 weeks but, in some stool cultures, may remain positive for 6–12 months or longer. This human reservoir of infection is particularly important in food handlers, healthcare workers and workers in day-care centres. Eradication of

Salmonella spp. can be achieved in more than 80% of cases by administration of amoxycillin or a quinolone for 4–6 weeks at standard doses. Long-term asymptomatic carriage is also recognized to occur with many other bacterial enteropathogens including *Camplyobacter jejuni*, *Yersinia enterocolitica* and *Clostridium difficile*.

Long-term asymptomatic carriage is also recognized to occur with a variety of intestinal protozoal pathogens including *Giardia intestinalis*, *Cryptosporidium parvum* and *Entamoeba histolytica*. In highly endemic areas, attempts at eradication are usually not considered appropriate but in countries where these infections are uncommon—particularly the industrialized nations in the northern hemisphere, antimicrobial chemotherapy to clear the infection is usually given. Failure to clear these enteropathogens is common in the immunocompromised, particularly those with HIV infection. Symptomatic treatment may be the only option when antibiotic therapy fails.

DRUGS

Antifungal drugs

Nystatin
Mode of action
Nystatin preferentially binds to ergosterol, the major sterol of fungal cell membrane, altering membrane permeability and producing cytoplasmic disequilibrium.

Indications
Candidiasis; oral and mild oesophageal infection are indications for treatment.

Preparations/dose
Oral suspension 1000 U/l and tablets 500 000 U/tablet, 1–3 million U four times daily may be given.

Dynamics/kinetics
Nystatin is not absorbed from the gastrointestinal tract, thus it is for topical use only.

Adverse reactions
Nausea, vomiting and diarrhoea may occur at high doses. Oral irritation and sensitization, rash (including urticaria) and, rarely, Stevens-Johnson syndrome may occur.

Drug interactions
None are known.

Precautions and contraindications
For pregnancy and breastfeeding there is no information, although there is negligible absorption of nystatin from the gastrointestinal tract.

Fluconazole
Mode of action
Azoles block fungal ergosterol synthesis by preferentially inhibiting the cytochrome P_{450} system.

Indications
Severe oropharyngeal and oesophageal candidiasis are indications for treatment with fluconazole.

Preparations/dose
Capsules, oral suspension and intravenous infusion 100–200 mg daily may be taken orally for 7–30 days. For severe invasive infection and/or disseminated candidiasis, 400 mg initially and then 200–400 mg should be taken daily, orally or by intravenous infusion. For prophylaxis in immunocompromised patients, 50–400 mg daily should be taken but adjusted according to patient risk.

Dynamics/kinetics
Fluconazole is almost completely absorbed from the gastrointestinal tract. 90% excreted through kidneys with an elimination half-life of 25–30 h. This drug is widely distributed in tissues and body fluids including the cerebrospinal fluids.

Adverse reactions
Nausea, abdominal discomfort, diarrhoea and flatulence may occur; occasionally, abnormalities of liver enzymes. Headache, rash (rarely),

angio-oedema, anaphylaxis, bullous lesions, toxic epidermal necrolysis and Stevens-Johnson syndrome may also occur. Severe cutaneous reactions in AIDS patients have also been reported.

Drug interactions

Extensive interactions are generally related to multi-dose treatment. Imidazole anti-fungals interact with analgesics, antacids, quinidine, rifampicin, anticoagulants, the antidepressant reboxetine, sulphonylureas, phenytoin, antihistamines (terfenadine and mizolastine), the antipyschotic agents, sertindol and pimozide, antiviral agents, midazolam, calcium-channel blockers, digoxin, cyclosporin, cisapride, corticosteroids, vincristine, simvastatin and cerivastatin, sildenafil, tacrolimus, and theophylline.

Precautions and contraindications

Reduce the dose by 50% in mild–moderate renal failure, and avoid in pregnancy and during breastfeeding.

Ketoconazole

Mode of action

As for fluconazole.

Indications

As for fluconazole.

Preparations and dose

Tablets 200 mg should be taken once daily with food, usually for 14 days. A more prolonged course may be necessary in severe infections.

Dynamics/kinetics

There is variable oral absorption of ketoconazole. Its plasma half-life is 7–8 h.

Adverse reactions

As for fluconazole. Ketoconazole may also cause fatal liver damage, the risk of which is increased if the drug is used for longer than 14 days. Liver biochemistry should be monitored before and at 2–4-weekly intervals after starting treatment.

Drug interactions

As for fluconazole.

Precautions and contraindications

Ketoconazole contraindicated in hepatic impairment, and should be avoided in pregnancy and during breastfeeding.

Itraconazole

Mode of action

As for fluconazole.

Indications

As for fluconazole.

Preparations and dose

Capsules and liquid preparation are available, in 100–200 mg doses, which should be taken daily for 15 days.

Dynamics/kinetics

This drug has a variable oral absorption. 90% bound to plasma proteins with extensive tissue binding. Its plasma half-life is about 30 h.

Adverse reactions

As for fluconazole and ketoconazole. If peripheral neuropathy occurs, the drug must be discontinued. Prolonged use may produce hypokalaemia, oedema and hair loss.

Drug interactions

As for fluconazole and ketoconazole.

Precautions and contraindications

As for fluconazole and ketoconazole. Special caution should be taken in hepatic and renal impairment. Avoid in pregnancy and during breastfeeding.

Flucytosine

Mode of action

Flucytosine acts as an antimetabolite inhibiting DNA, RNA and protein synthesis.

Indications

Severe systemic candidiasis and other severe fungal infections are indications for treatment.

Preparations and dose
An intravenous infusion, of 100–200 mg/kg daily should be given in four divided doses, administered over 20–40 min.

Dynamics/kinetics
Flucytosine is well-absorbed with peak plasma levels at 1–2 h and a half-life of about 3–6 h. It is widely distributed in the body with low plasma protein binding.

Adverse reactions
These include nausea, vomiting, diarrhoea and rashes; less frequently, confusion, hallucinations, convulsions, headache, sedation and vertigo. Abnormalities of liver biochemistry indicating hepatitis and hepatic necrosis may occur, as may blood disorders including thrombocytopenia, leukopenia and aplastic anaemia.

Drug interactions
Other antifungal agent such as amphotericin can reduce renal excretion and increase cellular uptake. Cytotoxic drugs such as cytarabine may reduce plasma flucytosine concentrations.

Precautions and contraindications
Caution should be exercised in renal impairment, the elderly and those with blood disorders. Routine monitoring of liver, kidney and bone marrow function are required. Flucytosine is teratogenic in animals and thus should be avoided in pregnancy and breastfeeding.

Amphotericin
Mode of action
Amphotericin preferentially binds to ergosterol, the major sterol of fungal cell membrane, altering membrane permeability and producing cytoplasmic disequilibrium.

Indications
Severe candidiasis is an indication for its use.

Preparation and dose
Oral flucytosine should be given 100–200 mg four times daily or an intravenous infusion of 3–5 mg/kg daily for 7–14 days or longer as necessary.

Dynamics/kinetics
There is negligible absorption of this drug from the gastrointestinal tract. Extensive tissue binding after intravenous administration accounts for the terminal phase of the elimination half-life of 15 days.

Adverse reactions
Parenteral administration may produce anorexia, nausea, vomiting, diarrhoea and epigastric pain. Febrile reactions, headache, muscle and joint pain may also occur as may anaemia and disturbances of renal function. Cardiovascular toxicity including arrhythmias, blood disorders, neurological disorders including hearing loss, diplopia, convulsions and peripheral neuropathy and abnormal liver biochemistry may occur. Pain and thrombophlebitis may be experienced at the injection site. Anaphylaxis occurs rarely but a test dose is advisable before the first infusion.

Drug interactions
Close monitoring is required when given with nephrotoxic or cytotoxic drugs. There is increased risk of nephrotoxicity with aminoglycosides; other antifungal agents may antagonize the effect of amphotericin. There is increased toxicity of cardiac glycosides in the presence of hypokalaemia. The risk of nephrotoxicity is increased with cyclosporin and tacrolimus and there is increased risk of hypokalaemia with corticosteroids.

Precautions and contraindications
Caution should be exercised in renal and liver impairment with close monitoring of liver biochemistry, blood count and plasma electrolytes. Avoid this drug in pregnancy and during breastfeeding.

Antiviral drugs

Aciclovir
Mode of action
Aciclovir inhibits viral DNA polymerase and causes DNA-chain termination when incorporated into replicating DNA.

Indications

Herpes simplex virus (HSV) and varicella zoster infections are treated using aciclovir.

Preparation/dose

Oral tablets and intravenous infusions are available in severe HSV oesophagitis 5 mg/kg should be given intravenously every 8 h for 7–10 days. For milder infections 200–400 mg should be given 5 times daily for 5 days. Maintenance therapy should be given in immunocompromised patients at a dose of 400 mg twice daily.

Dynamics/kinetics

The oral bioavailability is 10–30%. Aciclovir has a rapid first-pass metabolism, with an elimination of half-life 1.5–6 h.

Adverse reactions

Skin rash, gastrointestinal disturbance and abnormalities of liver biochemistry, urea and creatinine may be seen. Haematological indices may be decreased. Other adverse reactions include headache, neurological reactions and fatigue; during intravenous infusion: confusion, hallucinations, agitation, tremors, somnolence, psychosis, convulsions and coma may occur. Co-administration with mycophenolate increases the plasma concentration of both drugs. Probenecid increases plasma concentration owing to reduced urinary clearance.

Precautions and contraindications

Maintain adequate hydration and reduce dose in renal impairment. Use in pregnancy only when its benefits outweigh potential harm. Significant amounts enter breast milk therefore avoid during breastfeeding.

Ganciclovir
Mode of action
As for aciclovir

Indication

This drug is used to treat life-threatening or sight-threatening CMV infections in immuno-compromised patients. Prevention of CMV disease in immunocompromised patients is another indication.

Preparations and dose

Intravenous infusion should be given 5 mg/kg every 12 h for 14–21 days, although longer treatment periods may be required. Maintenance treatment is 1 g three times daily with food or, in severe cases, intravenous infusion of 5 mg/kg daily.

Dynamics/kinetics

This drug has a poor oral bioavailability. Its elimination half-life is 2–4 h; 90% is eliminated unchanged in urine.

Adverse reactions

Bone marrow suppression, abnormal liver biochemistry, gastrointestinal symptoms (nausea, vomiting, mouth ulcers, dyspepsia, dysphagia, diarrhoea, anorexia and haemorrhage), neurological symptoms, cardiovascular disturbances (hypertension, hypotension, dyspnoea), renal impairment, decrease in blood glucose, and aspermatogenesis are all possible adverse reactions.

Drug interactions

There is an increased risk of myelosuppression with other myelosuppressive drugs. There are interactions with other antiviral agents, including didanosine and zidovudine. Probenecid reduces renal excretion.

Precautions and contraindications

Pregnancy and breastfeeding are contraindications. Barrier contraception is a precaution for men during and for 90 days after treatment. Low neutrophil or platelet counts are other contraindications.

Foscarnet
Mode of action
Foscarnet binds to pyrophosphate binding sites on viral DNA polymerases and reverse transcriptases.

Indication
It is indicated for treating CMV in AIDS

patients, and aciclovir resistant HSV infection.

Preparations and dose
An intravenous infusion of 40–60 mg/kg should be given every 8 h for 2–3 weeks; maintenance therapy of 60 mg/kg daily may be increased to 90–120 mg/kg daily if tolerated (usually only for CMV retinitis).

Dynamics/kinetics
Foscarnet has a poor oral bioavailability; 80% is excreted unchanged in urine.

Adverse reactions
Gastrointestinal, neurological and metabolic (impaired renal function, hypokalcaemia, abnormal liver biochemistry) adverse reactions may occur also myelosuppression.

Precautions and contraindications
Foscarnet should not be taken during pregnancy and breastfeeding.

Oral rehydration solutions (see Table 6.5)

Antidiarrhoeal drugs

Co-phenotrope
Co-phenotrope is a mixture of diphenoxylate hydrochloride and atropine sulphate.

Mode of action
Diphenoxylate hydrochloride is a synthetic opioid anti-motility drug that acts predominantly on opioid μ-receptors in gastrointestinal smooth muscle.

Indication
Co-phenotrope is used to treat acute diarrhoea in conjunction with rehydration therapy.

Preparation and dose
Tablets for diphenoxylate hydrochloride (2.5 mg), and atropine sulphate (25 μg) are available. Four tablets should be taken initially, followed by two tablets every 6 h until the diarrhoea is controlled.

Adverse reactions
Adverse reactions include nausea and vomiting, constipation and drowsiness. Large doses may produce respiratory depression and hypotension.

Drug interactions
Co-phenotrope enhances sedative and hypotensive effects of alcohol and other CNS depressants including antidepressants, antipsychotics, anxiolytics and hypnotics.

Precautions and contraindications
This drug is not recommended for use in children. Caution should be exercised in severe acute colitis whether due to infection or non-specific inflammatory bowel disease. Avoid in pregnancy and breastfeeding.

Loperamide hydrochloride
See Chapter 5.

Antibacterial drugs

Tetracyclines
Mode of action
Tetracyclines are bacteriostatic drugs that inhibit bacterial protein synthesis by interrupting ribosomal function (transfer RNA).

Indication
Cholera, yersiniosis, balantidiasis and travellers' diarrhoea are indications for treatment.

Preparation and dose
Tetracycline should be given 250–500 mg four times daily for 3–10 days (Tables 6.7 and 6.8).

Dynamics/kinetics
Tetracyclines are incompletely absorbed by the gastrointestinal tract. Peak plasma concentrations are reached at 2–4 h. Tetracyclines have plasma half-lives of 6–12 h; they are eliminated by the kidney and excreted in bile with the enterohepatic circulation.

Adverse reactions

Adverse reactions include:

- Nausea, vomiting, diarrhoea, oesophageal irritation
- Erythema and photosensitivity
- Headache and visual disturbances indicative of benign intracranial hypertension
- Hepatotoxicity, pancreatitis and antibiotic-associated colitis

Drug interactions

Tetracycline absorption is reduced by ACE inhibitors and angiotensin-II antagonists, antacids and absorbents, calcium salts and dairy products. Tetracyclines reduce the absorption of oral iron and plasma concentration of atovaquone.

Precautions and contraindications

Tetracyclines should be avoided in renal insufficiency; they may affect skeletal development in pregnancy and cause dental discoloration and should be avoided during breastfeeding.

Quinolones

Mode of action

Quinolones inhibit bacterial DNA synthesis by inhibiting DNA gyrase, the enzyme responsible for maintaining the superhelical twists in DNA.

Indications

These drugs are effective against a broad range of Gram-negative and some Gram-positive bacteria including *Shigella*, *Salmonella*, *Campylobacter*, *Yersinia* spp, enterovirulent *E. coli*, *Vibrio cholerae* and in travellers' diarrhoea.

Preparations

These include nalidixic acid, ciprofloxacin, norfloxacin, ofloxacin. See text (p. 116) and Tables 6.7 and 6.8 for dose regimens.

Dynamics/kinetics

Quinolones are well-absorbed with peak levels at 1–3 h. Their bioavailability is 50–95% and their plasma half-life is 3–5 h.

Adverse reactions

Quinolones may cause seizures in patients with or without a history of epilepsy. Use with caution in G_6PD deficiency. Quinolones may cause flatulence, dysphagia, tremor, altered prothrombin concentration, jaundice and hepatitis, renal failure, nephritis, vasculitis, erythema nodosum, petechiae, haemorrhagic bullae, tinnitus, tenosinovitis and tachycardia.

Drug interactions

Their absorption is reduced by antacids, adsorbants and calcium salts. There is an increased risk of convulsions with NSAIDS and theophylline. Ciprofloxacin possibly enhances activity of the antidiabetic glibenclamide and increases the plasma concentration of phenytoin. There is an increased risk of nephrotoxicity during cyclosporin therapy.

Precautions and contraindications

Caution should be exercised in children because of concerns about joints and the growth plate, although short-term use in children appears to be safe. Avoid exposure to excessive sunlight. Avoid in pregnancy.

Co-trimoxazole (sulpamethoxazole and trimethoprim)

Mode of action

Sulphonamides block thymidine and purine synthesis by inhibiting microbial folic acid synthesis. Trimethoprim prevents the reduction of dihydrofolate to tetrahydrofolate.

Indications

Although in the past co-trimoxazole has been recommended for a variety of intestinal infections including cholera, *Salmonella* and for the treatment and prevention of travellers' diarrhoea, current recommendations by the Committee on Safety of Medicines in the UK now indicate that its use should be limited because of adverse reactions (see text following). It is still appropriate to use the drug in infections caused by *Isospora belli*, *Cyclospora cayetanensis* and in Whipple's disease.

Preparation and dose
Two tablets (960 mg) should be given twice daily for 7–10 days (see Tables 6.8 and 6.9 and text, p. 116).

Dynamics/kinetics
Peak plasma concentrations occur at 2–4 h, with plasma half-lives of 11 h and 10 h for TMP and SMX, respectively.

Adverse reactions
These include:

- Nausea and vomiting
- Rash including Stevens-Johnson syndrome, toxic epidermal necrolysis and photosensitivity
- Blood disorders (including neutropenia, thrombocytopenia, rarely agranulocytosis and purpura)
- Rarely allergic reactions, diarrhoea, glossitis, stomatitis, anorexia, arthralgia and myalgia
- Liver damage, pancreatitis, antibiotic-associated colitis, eosinophilia, cough, pulmonary infiltrates, aseptic meningitis, headache, depression, convulsions, ataxia, tinnitus, megaloblastic anaemia (trimethoprim), electrolyte disturbances and renal disorders

Drug interactions
There is an enhanced effect of warfarin, sulphonylureas and intravenous anaesthetic agents (thiopental), also an increased risk of ventricular arrhythmias with amiodarone. Antifolate effects are enhanced when used with other antifolate drugs (e.g. phenytoin, pyrimethamine, methotrexate). There is an increased risk of nephrotoxity with cyclosporin.

Precautions and contraindications
Avoid in elderly patients. Discontinue immediately if blood disorders or rash develop. Avoid in pregnancy.

Erythromycin

Mode of action
Erythromycin inhibits protein synthesis by interrupting ribosomal function.

Indications
Erythromycin is used to treat *Campylobacter jejuni* infection (azithromycin, another macrolide antibiotic is also indicated, see Table 6.8).

Preparation and dose
Oral tablets in a dose of 250–500 mg should be taken every 6 h.

Dynamics/kinetics
The erythromycin base is incompletely absorbed from the gastrointestinal tract but esters are better absorbed. The peak plasma concentration occurs at 4 h. Clarithromycin and azithromycin are rapidly absorbed. Erythromycin is excreted in an active form in bile; its plasma half-life is 1.6 h.

Adverse reactions
Nausea, vomiting, abdominal discomfort, diarrhoea including antibiotic-associated colitis may occur with erythromycin. Allergic reactions including urticaria and rashes. Reversible hearing loss occurs after large doses. Cholestatic jaundice and cardiac effects are also reported.

Drug interactions
Erythromycin and other macrolides including clarithromycin have extensive interactions with analgesics, antiarrhythmics, anticoagulants, antidepressants, antiepileptics, antihistamines, antisycotics, antivirals, anxiolytics and hypnotics, calcium-channel blockers and cardiac glycosides. Interactions also occur with cyclosporin, corticosteroids, cytotoxics, dopaminergics, lipid-regulating drugs, tacrolimus and theophylline.

Precautions and contraindications
Avoid the use of erythromycin in hepatic and renal impairment. Caution should be exercised

in the presence of prolongation of Q–T interval and porphyria. Erythromycin is not known to be harmful in pregnancy and only small amounts appear in human milk. Erythromycin estolate is contraindicated in liver disease.

Metronidazole
Mode of action
After reduction of the nitro group to a nitroso-hydroxyl amino group by microbial enzymes, nitroimidazoles cause strand breaks in microbial DNA.

Indications
Metronidazole is used to treat anaerobic bacterial infections, particularly bacteroides. It is indicated for enteric protozoal infections (*Entamoeba histolytica*, *Balantidium coli* and *Giardia intestinalis*) and *Clostridium difficile* infection.

Preparation and dose
Oral tablets 400 mg should be taken three times daily for 5–10 days (Tables 6.8 and 6.9).

Dynamics/kinetics
Metronidazole is rapidly absorbed with peak plasma concentrations at 1 h. Its half-life in plasma is about 8 h.

There is good tissue penetration, and it is extensively metabolized in the liver.

Adverse reactions
These include:

- Nausea, vomiting and metallic taste
- Skin rash
- Rarely drowsiness, headache, dizziness, ataxia, erythema multiforme, pruritis, urticaria, angioedema and anaphylaxis
- Abnormal liver biochemistry, jaundice, thrombocytopenia, aplastic anaemia, myalgia and arthralgia
- Peripheral neuropathy, transient epileptiform seizures and leukopenia with prolonged or intensive therapy

Drug interactions
There is a disulfiram-like reaction with alcohol.

Anticoagulant effects are enhanced with concomitant use of metronidazole. Metronidazole inhibits metabolism of phenytoin and fluorouracil.

Precautions and contraindications
Avoid in pregnancy and breastfeeding.

Diloxanide furoate
Mode of action
This mode of action of this drug is unknown.

Indications
Diloxanide furoate is used to treat intraluminal amoebae.

Preparation and dose
Oral tablets 500 mg are taken three times daily for 10 days.

Dynamics/kinetics
Peak plasma concentrations occur at 1 h. Diloxanide furoate rapidly excreted in urine.

Adverse reactions
Vomiting, urticaria, pruritis are possible adverse reactions.

Drug interactions
No drug interactions have been reported

Precautions and contraindications
Avoid in pregnancy and breastfeeding.

Vancomycin
Mode of action
Vancomycin inhibits cell wall synthesis in sensitive bacteria by binding to the D-alanyl-D-alanine terminus of cell wall precursor units.

Indications
Used to treat *C. difficile* infection, Gram-positive cocci including multi-resistant staphylococci.

Preparations and dose
Capsules 125 mg may be taken every 6 h for 7–10 days. More prolonged courses may be required in recurrent and persistent infections.

Dynamics/kinetics
Vancomycin is poorly absorbed after oral administration.

Adverse reactions
No adverse reactions are seen when given orally.

Drug interactions
Vancomycin is antagonized by cholestyramine.

Precautions and contraindications
Oral administration usually does not result in significant systemic absorption.

Isoniazid
Mode of action
The mode of action of isoniazid is unknown but may relate to inhibitory effects on mycolic acid synthesis.

Indication
Isoniazid is used to treat tuberculosis.

Preparation and dose
Tablets or elixir 300 mg are given as a single daily dose.

Dynamics/kinetics
This drug is rapidly absorbed, with peak concentrations at 1–2 h.

It is mainly (75–95%) excreted in urine.

The rate of acetylation determines its half-life.

Adverse reactions
These include:

- Nausea, vomiting, peripheral neuritis with high doses (reduced by co-administration of pyridoxine 10 mg daily), optic neuritis, convulsions, psychotic episodes
- Hypersensitivity reactions including fever, erythema multiforme, purpura
- Agranulocytosis, hepatitis, SLE, pellagra, hyperglycaemia and gynaecomastia

Drug interactions
Hepatotoxicity is possibly potentiated by the anaesthetic isoflurane. There is reduced absorption with antacids. There may be enhanced effects of some antiepileptic agents, diazepam and theophylline.

Precautions and contraindications
Hepatic and renal impairment, increased risk of side effects in individuals with slow acetylator status. Caution should be exercised during pregnancy and breastfeeding.

Rifampicin
Mode of action
Rifampicin inhibits DNA-dependent RNA polymerase of mycobacteria and other microorganisms.

Indications
Used to treat tuberculosis, rifampicin is also useful in brucellosis, legionnaires disease and serious staphylococcal infections when combined with other drugs.

Preparations and dose
Capsules or syrup are available in a 600 mg single daily dose (a dose of 450 mg is available if body weight is below 55 kg).

Dynamics/kinetics
Peak plasma concentration is reached in 2–4 h. Rifampicin is eliminated in bile via the enterohepatic circulation. Its half-life varies from 1.5–5 h, but decreases as a result of induction of liver enzymes.

Adverse reactions
These include:

- Gastrointestinal symptoms, influenza-like symptoms, respiratory symptoms, collapse and shock, haemolytic anaemia, acute renal failure and thrombocytopenic purpura
- Abnormalities or liver biochemistry and jaundice
- Flushing, urticaria and rashes
- Oedema, muscular weakness, leukopenia, eosinophilia, menstrual disturbances
- Urine, saliva and other body secretions are coloured orange-red

Drug interactions

Many drug interactions involve a reduction in efficacy of other drugs given with rifampicin. There are interactions with ACE-inhibitors and angiotensin-II antagonists, antiarrhythmics, other antibacterial agents, anticoagulants, antidepressants, antidiabetic agents, antiepileptic agents, antifungal agents, antiviral agents, anxiolytics, beta-blockers, calcium-channel blockers, cardiac glycosides, cyclosporin, corticosteroids, cytotoxics, lipid-regulating drugs, estrogens and progestogens, tacrolimus and theophylline.

Precautions and contraindications

Reduce dose in liver impairment. Rifampicin may, however, be used during pregnancy and breastfeeding.

Pyrazinamide

Mode of action

Its mode of action is unknown.

Indications

Pyrazinamide is indicated in tuberculosis.

Preparation and dose

A dose of 2.5 g three times weekly is taken (for a body weight of less than 50 kg, 2 g is taken three times weekly).

Dynamics/kinetics

Pyrazinamide is well-absorbed, with peak plasma concentrations at 2 h. Excretion is via the kidney.

Adverse reactions

These include:

- Hepatotoxicity including fever, anorexia, hepatomegaly, jaundice, liver failure
- Nausea, vomiting, arthralgia, sideroblastic anaemia, urticaria

Drug interactions

Pyrazinamide antagonizes of the effect of probenecid.

Precautions and contraindications

Caution should be exercised in renal and hepatic impairment, diabetes and gout. Pyrazinamide may be used in pregnancy and during breastfeeding.

Antihelminthic drugs

Albendazole

Mode of action

Albendazole inhibits microtubule polymerization by binding to β-tubulin.

Indications

Strongyloidiasis, ascariasis, trichuriasis, threadworm and tapeworm infections, capillariasis, *Encephalitozoon intestinalis* infection and hydatid disease are indications for treatment.

Preparations and dose

A dose of 400 mg is taken twice daily for 3–28 days (see Tables 6.9 and 6.10 and text, p. 118).

Dynamics/kinetics

Albendazole has erratic absorption and low systemic bioavailability and has a plasma half-life of 8–9 h; 70% is bound to plasma proteins.

Drug interactions

No drug interactions are known.

Adverse reactions

These include:

- Gastrointestinal disturbances, headache, dizziness, abnormalities of liver biochemistry
- Reversible alopecia, rash, fever, blood disorders

Precautions and contraindications

Blood count and liver biochemistry should be monitored. It is contraindicated during pregnancy and breastfeeding.

Mebendazole

Mode of action
Its mode of action is as for thiabendazole.

Indications
Threadworm, roundworm, whipworm and hookworm infections are treated using mebendazole.

Preparation and dose
Oral tablets 100 mg are available as a single dose or 100–400 mg twice or three times daily for 3–20 days (Tables 6.9 and 6.10).

Dynamics/kinetics
Mebendazole has an erratic absorption and low systemic bioavailability; 95% is bound to plasma proteins and it is extensively metabolized.

Adverse reactions
Rarely abdominal pain and diarrhoea occur. Hypersensitivity reactions including rash, urticaria and angio-oedema may also be present.

Drug interactions
None are known.

Precautions and contraindications
Mebendazole is contraindicated in pregnancy. There is no information on safety in breastfeeding.

Thiabendazole

Mode of action
Its mode of action is as for thiabendazole.

Indications
Strongyloidiasis, cutaneous and visceral larva migrans, trichinosis, threadworm, hookworm, whipworm and roundworm infections are all indications for treatment.

Preparations and dose
Oral tablets are available 25 mg/kg to be taken twice daily for 2–3 days.

Dynamics/kinetics
Peak plasma concentration after 1 h.

Adverse reactions
These include:

- Anorexia, nausea, vomiting, dizziness, diarrhoea, headache, pruritis and drowsiness
- Hypersensitivity reactions including erythema multiforme and Stevens-Johnson syndrome
- Rarely tinnitus, collapse, visual disorders and liver damage

Drug interactions
Thiabendazole may increase plasma levels of theophylline.

Precautions and contraindications
Hepatic and renal impairment may occur in the elderly. Thiabendazole is contraindicated in pregnancy and breastfeeding.

Ivermectin

Mode of action
Ivermectin induces tonic paralysis of the parasite musculature through its effects on glutamate-gated chloride channels.

Indications
Strongyloidiasis, ascariasis, trichuriasis and enterobiasis are indications for treatment.

Preparation and dose
A dose of 100–200 μg/kg is taken once daily for 2 days.

Dynamics/kinetics
Peak plasma levels within 4 h. Long terminal half-life about 27 h. 93% bound to plasma proteins.

Adverse reactions
Rash and pruritis.

Drug interactions
None reported.

Precautions and contraindications

None reported.

Praziquantel

Mode of action

Praziquantel causes influx of calcium ions across the tegument of the adult worm, leading to tetanic contraction and vacuolization of the tegument that makes the parasite susceptible to immune destruction.

Indications

Schistosomiasis, tapeworm infections and liver flukes are indications for treatment.

Preparation and dose

Oral tablets 40–60 mg/kg in two or three divided doses are available on one day (see Tables 6.9 and 6.10).

Dynamics/kinetics

Maximal plasma levels are reached in 1–2 h. There is extensive first-pass metabolism resulting in a short plasma half-life of 0.8–2 h; this may be prolonged in severe liver disease.

Adverse reactions

No serious toxic effects have been reported.

Drug interactions

None have been reported.

Precautions and contraindications

None have been reported.

INFECTIONS OF THE LIVER AND BILIARY TRACT

The treatment of viral hepatitis is discussed in Chapter 11. There are a variety of other important infections of the liver including liver abscess, diffuse parenchymal infections, cholecystitis and cholangitis and schistosomiasis producing portal hypertension (Table 6.11).

TREATMENT RATIONALE

The primary aim of treatment for non-viral liver and biliary tract infections is eradication of the pathogen early in the course of the illness to

---

Table 6.11 Infections of the liver and biliary tract: clinical syndromes.

Clinical syndrome	Infective agent
Liver abscess	
Pyogenic	Polymicrobial
	Enterobacteriacae
	Enterococci
Amoebic	*Entamoeba histolytica*
Diffuse parenchymal infections	*Mycobacterium tuberculosis*
	Leptospira icterohaemorrhagiae
	Echinococcus granulosus
Cholangitis/cholecystitis	Bacterial infections
	Liver flukes
	Cryptosporidium parvum, *Microsporidium* spp.
Portal hypertension	*Schistosoma* spp.

avoid chronic complications. This is particularly important in schistosomiasis when long-standing infection often results in irreversible liver fibrosis, portal hypertension and its complications particularly variceal bleeding. Similarly, eradication of liver flukes early in the course of the illness is important to avoid irreversible biliary tract fibrosis with its septic complications, and possibly secondary biliary cirrhosis. Liver abscesses usually present with a typical clinical syndrome and thus chronic complications are usually avoided. However, drainage procedures may be required in addition to antimicrobial chemotherapy when there is associated biliary obstruction or with large and multi-locular liver abscesses. Similarly, the cystic disease associated with echinococcus infection almost always requires a combination of antimicrobial agents and drainage; the precise method remains controversial but may be surgical or percutaneous.

TREATMENT REGIMENS

Liver abscess

Pyogenic abscess
Bacteria can reach the liver via the portal vein, systemic circulation, biliary tree or directly following trauma. A mixed population of bacteria is often involved including enterobacteriacae, entrococci and anaerobic bacteria.[120] *Streptococcus milleri* is commonly isolated from pyogenic abscesses. Pyogenic abscesses may require drainage either by needle aspiration or percutaneous catheter drainage. Owing to the polymicrobial nature of these abscesses, broad-spectrum antimicrobial agents are required usually initially given intravenously. Standard regimens include combinations of gentamicin and amoxycillin-clavulanic acid or ticarcillin-clavulanic acid combined with metronidazole.

Amoebic abscess
Although it is possible to manage many amoebic liver abscesses using drug therapy alone, large abscesses should be aspirated,[121] particularly those in the left lobe beneath the diaphragm because of the danger of rupture into the thorax or pericardium.[122,123] Treatment is with metronidazole 800 mg three times daily for 10 days or tinidazole 2 g daily for 5 days. The nitroimidazole derivative should be followed by diloxanide furoate 500 mg three times daily for 10 days to clear luminal amoebic cysts.[122]

Diffuse parenchymal infections

The liver is often involved in miliary tuberculosis and, when severe, can cause liver failure. Standard antimycobacterial therapy should be given.[124] Leptospirosis caused by *Leptospira icterohaemorrhagiae* is a multi-system disease often with liver involvement presenting with jaundice and hepatomegaly. The majority of infections are mild but when there is extensive multi-organ disease, the treatment of choice is high-dose intravenous penicillin.

Hydatid infection with the *Echinococcus* tapeworm continues to be an important infection in sheep-farming areas of the world including Europe, parts of the Mediterranean, Asia and South America. Although the management of hepatic hydatid disease remains controversial, it is generally accepted that antihelminthic therapy with albendazole, mebendazole or praziquantel is insufficient alone and should usually be combined with a drainage procedure. Typical drug regimens include albendazole 10–15 mg/kg/day for 6–8 weeks or mebendazole 100 mg/kg/day for 6–12 months. Cysts may disappear in up to 30% of patients and in another 30–50% of cysts will degenerate or show significant size reduction. Cysts remain morphologically unchanged in 20–40% of patients.

Cholangitis and cholecystitis

Gallbladder and bile duct infections are most commonly associated with impaired biliary drainage, usually as a result of gallstones or obstructing parasites such as liver flukes. Benign and malignant bile duct strictures also impair biliary drainage and predispose to infection.[125,126]

Bacterial infections in the biliary tract generally involve Gram-negative bacilli, enterococci and anaerobes. Cephalosporins and quinolones alone are inadequate to cover enterococci and should be combined with amoxycillin, piperacillin or ticarcillin. Alternative regimens include ticarcillin or piperacillin in combination with an aminoglycoside (such as gentamicin) and metronidazole. When there is associated obstruction of the biliary tract, an appropriate drainage procedure should accompany antimicrobial chemotherapy.

The liver flukes, *Clonorchis sinensis* and *Fasciola hepatica* reside within the biliary tract and produce inflammatory and fibrotic reactions, leading to biliary obstruction, often complicated by bacterial cholangitis.[127] The treatment of choice for both flukes is praziquantel given as three oral doses of 25 mg/kg during one day. The benzimidazole drugs, mebendazole and albendazole also have activity against these liver flukes, although more prolonged courses of treatment are required. Endoscopic or surgical intervention is often required to provide biliary drainage.

Cryptosporidiosis and microsporidiosis have been implicated as a cause of the sclerosing cholangitis-like syndrome, which occurs in individuals with HIV infection. Treatment of these infections is described on p. 118.

Portal hypertension

Fibrotic liver disease is a classic feature of infection with *Schistosoma mansoni* and *Schistosoma japonicum* and can also occur with *Schistosoma haematobium*. The granulomatous inflammatory reaction within the liver progresses over many years to produce portal fibrosis and portal hypertension.[128]

The treatment of choice is praziquantel given orally as a single 40 mg/kg dose.[128] Improved cure rates for all forms of schistosomiasis have been obtained by giving praziquantel 60 mg/kg as three divided doses over an 8-h period. This is, however, a more difficult regimen to administer in the field. An alternative regimen is oxamniquine given as a single dose of 15 mg/kg up to a total 60 mg/kg over 2–3 days. Metriphonate is only effective against *S. haematobium*.

REFERENCES

1. Wheeler JG, Sethi D, Cowden JM, *et al.* Study of infectious intestinal disease in England: rates in the community, presenting to general practice, and reported to national surveillance. *Brit Med J* 1999; **318**: 1046–1050.
2. Rao MC. Molecular mechanisms of bacterial toxins. In: *Enteric Infection.* MJG Farthing, GT Keusch (Eds), Chapman & Hall, London, 1989, 87–104.
3. Field M, Fao M, Chang EB. Intestinal electrolyte transport and diarrheal disease. *N Engl J Med* 1989; **321**: 879–883.
4. Savarino SJ, Fasano A, Watson J, *et al.* Enteroaggregative *Escherichia coli* heat-stable enterotoxin 1 represents another subfamily of *E. coli* heat-stable toxin. *Proc Natl Acad Sci USA* 1993; **90**: 3093–3097.
5. Trucksis M, Galen JE, Michalski J, Fasano A, Kaper JB. Accessory cholera enterotoxin (ACE), the third toxin of a *Vibrio cholerae* virulence cassette. *Proc Natl Acad Sci USA* 1993; **90**: 5267–5271.
6. Fasano A, Baudry B, Pumplin DW, *et al. Vibrio cholerae* produces a second enterotoxin, which affects intestinal tight junctions. *Proc Natl Acad Sci USA* 1991; **88**: 5242–5246.
7. Jodal M. Neuronal influence on intestinal transport. *J Intern Med* 1990; **228**: 125–132.
8. Munck LK, Mertz-Nielson A, Westh H, Bukhave K, Beubler E, Rask-Madsen J. Prostaglandin E_2 is a mediator of 5-hydroxtryptamine induced water and electrolyte secretion in the human jejunum. *Gut* 1988; **29**: 1337–1341.
9. Beubler E, Kollar G, Saria A, Bukhave K, Rask-Madsen J. Involvement of 5-hydroxytryptamine, prostaglandin E_2 and cyclic adenosine monophosphate in cholera toxin-induced fluid secretion in the small intestine of the rat *in vivo*. *Gastroenterology* 1989; **96**: 368–376.

10. Bearcroft CP, Perrett D, Farthing MJG. 5-hydroxytryptamine release into human jejunum by cholera toxin. *Gut* 1996; **39:** 528–531.

11. Cassuto J, Fahrenkrug J, Jodal M, Tuttle R, Lundgren O. Release of vasoactive intestinal polypeptide from the cat small intestine exposed to cholera toxin. *Gut* 1981; **22:** 958–963.

12. Turvill JL, Mourad FH, Farthing MJG. Crucial role for 5-HT in cholera toxin but not *Escherichia coli* heat-labile enterotoxin-intestinal secretion in rats. *Gastroenterology* 1998; **115:** 883–890.

13. Farthing MJG. Pathophysiology of infective diarrhoea. *Eur J Gastroenterol Hepatol* 1993; **5:** 796–807.

14. Farthing MJG. Acute diarrhea: Pathophysiology. In: *Diarrhoeal Disease.* M Gracey, JA Walker-Smith (Eds), Lippincott-Raven Publishers, Vevey, 1997, 55–71.

15. Salim AFM, Phillips AD, Walker-Smith JA, Farthing MJG. Sequential changes in small intestinal structure and function during rotavirus infection in neonatal rats. *Gut* 1995; **36:** 231–238.

16. Farthing MJG. Mycobacterial disease of the gut. In: *Modern Coloproctology.* RKS Phillips, JMA Northover (Eds), Edward Arnold, London, 1992, 174–189.

17. Farthing MJG. Tropical coloproctology. In: *Surgery of the Anus, Rectum and Colon.* MRB Keighley, NS Williams (Eds), WB Saunders, London, 1993, 2223–2261.

18. Laine L, Dretler RH, Conteas CN, *et al.* Fluconazole compared with ketoconazole for the treatment of *Candida* esophagitis in AIDS. A randomized trial. *Ann Intern Med* 1992; **117:** 655–660.

19. Barbaro G, Barbarini G, Calderon W, Grisorio B, Alcini P, Di Lorenzo G. Fluconazole versus itraconazole for *Candida* esophagitis in acquired immunodeficiency syndrome. *Gastroenterology* 1996; **111:** 1169–1177.

20. Barbaro G, Barbarini G, Di Lorenzo G. Fluconazole vs itraconazole-flucytosine association in the treatment of esophageal candidiasis in AIDS patients. A double-blind, multicenter placebo-controlled study. *Chest* 1996; **110:** 1507–1514.

21. Brockmeyer NH, Hantschke D, Olbricht T, Hengge UA, Goos M. Comparative study of the therapy of *Candida* esophagitis in HIV$_1$ infected patients with fluconazole or amphotericin B and flucytosine. *Mycoses* 1991; **34:** 83–86.

22. Parente F, Ardizzone S, Cernuschi M, *et al.* Prevention of symptomatic recurrences of esophageal candidiasis in AIDS patients after the first episode: a prospective open study. *Am J Gastroenterol* 1994; **89:** 416–420.

23. Genereau T, Lortholary O, Bouchaud O, *et al.* Herpes simplex eosophagitis in patients with AIDS: report of 34 cases. *Clin Infect Dis* 1996; **22:** 926–931.

24. Safrin S, Crumpacker C, Chatis P, *et al.* A controlled trial comparing foscarnet with vidarabine for acyclovir-resistant mucocutaneous herpes simplex in the acquired immunodeficiency syndrome. *N Engl J Med* 1991; **325:** 551–555.

25. Wilcom CM, Straub RF, Schwartz DA, Cytomegalovirus esophagitis in AIDS: a prospective evaluation of clinical response to ganciclovir therapy, relapse rate, and long-term outcome. *Am J Med* 1995; **98:** 169–176.

26. Whitley RJ, Jacobson MA, Friedberg DN, *et al.* Guidelines for the treatment of cytomegalovirus disease in patients with AIDS in the era of potent anti-retroviral therapy: recommendations of an international panel. *Arch Intern Med* 1998; **158:** 957–969.

27. Parente F, Bianchi Porro G. Treatment of cytomegalovirus esophagitis in patients with acquired immune deficiency syndrome: a randomized controlled study of foscarnet versus ganciclovir. *Am J Gastroenterol* 1998; **93:** 317–322.

28. Farthing MJG. History and rationale of oral rehydration and recent developments in formulating an optimal solution. In: Advances in Oral Rehydration Seminar in Print. *Drugs* 1988; **36 (Suppl. 4):** 89–90.

29. Mahalanabis D, Choudhuri AB, Bagchi NG, *et al.* Oral fluid therapy of cholera among Bangladesh refugees. *Johns Hopkins Med J* 1973; **132:** 197–205.

30. Pizarro D, Posada G, Mata L. Treatment of 242 neonates with dehydrating diarrhoea with an oral glucose-electrolyte solution. *J Pediatr* 1983; **102:** 153–156.

31. Pizarro D, Posada G, Levine MM. Hypernatremic diarrheal dehydration treated with 'slow' (12-hour) oral rehydration therapy: a preliminary report. *J Pediatr* 1984; **104:** 316–319.

32. Finberg L. The role of oral electrolyte-glucose solutions in hydration for children: international and domestic aspects. *J Pediatr* 1980; **96:** 51–54.

33. Rautanen T, El-Radhi S, Vesikari T. Clinical experience with a hypotonic oral rehydration solution in acute diarrhoea. *Acta Paediatr* 1993; **92**: 52–54.

34. International Study Group on Reduced-Osmolality ORS solutions. Multicentre evaluation of reduced-osmolality oral rehydration salts salutation. *Lancet* 1995; **346**: 282–285.

35. Santosham M, Fayad I, Abu Zikri M, *et al.* A double-blind clinical trial comparing World Health Organization oral rehydration solution with a reduced osmolality solution containing equal amounts of sodium and glucose. *J Pediatr* 1996; **128**: 45–51.

36. Rautanen T, Kurki S, Vesikari T. Randomised double-blind study of hypotonic oral rehydration solution in diarrhoea. *Arch Dis Child* 1997; **76**: 272–274.

37. Thillainayagam AV, Hunt JB, Farthing MJG. Enhancing clinical efficacy of oral rehydration therapy: is low osmolality the key? *Gastroenterology* 1998; **114**: 197–210.

38. Gore SM, Fontaine O, Pierce NF. Impact of rice-based oral rehydration solution on stool output and duration of diarrhoea: meta-analysis of 13 clinical trials. *Br Med J* 1992; **304**: 287–291.

39. Ramakrishna BS, Venkataraman S, Srinivasan P, Dash P, Young GP, Binder HJ. Amylase-resistant starch plus oral rehydration solution for cholera. *N Engl J Med* 2000; **342**: 308–313.

40. Beubler E, Badhri P, Schirgi-Degen A. Antisecretory activities of orally administered loperamide and loperamide oxide on intestinal secretion in rats. *Lancet* 1994; **344**: 1520–1521.

41. Kaplan MA, Prior MJ, McKonly KI, DuPont HL, Temple AR, Nelson EB. A multicentre randomized controlled trial of a liquid loperamide product versus placebo in the treatment of acute diarrhea in children. *Clin Pediatr* 1999; **38**: 579–591.

42. Owens JR, Broadhead R, Hendrickse RG, Jaswal OP, Gangal RN. Loperamide in the treatment of acute gastroenteritis in early childhood. Report of a two centre, double-blind, controlled clinical trial. *Ann Trop Paediatr* 1981; **1**: 135–141.

43. Bergstrom T, Alestig K, Thoren K, Trollfors B. Symptomatic treatment of acute infectious diarrhoea: loperamide versus placebo in a double-blind trial. *J Infect* 1986; **12**: 35–38.

44. Bowie MD, Hill ID, Mann MD. Loperamide for treatment of acute diarrhoea in infants and young children. A double-blind placebo-controlled trial. *S Afr Med J* 1995; **85**: 885–887.

45. Ericsson CD, Nicholls-Vasquez I, DuPont HL, Mathewson JJ. Optimal dosing of trimethoprim-sulfamethoxazole when used with loperamide to treat traveller's diarrhea. Antimicrob Agents Chemother 1992; **36**: 2821–2824.

46. Murphy GS, Bodhidatta L, Echeverria P, *et al.* Ciprofloxacin and loperamide in the treatment of bacillary dysentery. *Ann Intern Med* 1993; **118**: 582–586.

47. Taylor DN, Sanchez JL, Candler W, Thornton S, McQueen C, Echeverria P. Treatment of traveler's diarrhoea: ciprofloxacin plus loperamide compared with ciprofloxacin alone. A placebo-controlled, randomized trial. *Ann Intern Med* 1991; **114**: 731–739.

48. Petruccelli BP, Murphy GS, Sanchez JL, *et al.* Treatment of traveler's diarrhea with ciprofloxacin and loperamide. *J Infect Dis* 1992; **165**: 557–560.

49. Motala C, Hill ID, Mann MD, Bowie MD. Effect of loperamide on stool output and duration of acute infectious diarrhea in infants. *J Pediatr* 1990; **117**: 467–471.

50. DuPont HL, Hornick RB. Adverse effects of lomotil therapy with shigellosis. *J Am Med Assoc* 1973; **226**: 1525–1528.

51. DuPont HL, Ericsson CD, Mathewson JJ, Marani S, Knellwolf-Cousin A-L, Martinez-Sandoval FG. Zaldaride maleate, an intestinal calmodulin inhibitor, in the therapy of traveler's diarrhea. *Gastroenterology* 1993; **104**: 709–715.

52. Silberschmidt G, Schick MT, Steffen R, *et al.* Treatment of travellers' diarrhoea: zaldaride compared with loperamide and placebo. *Eur J Gastro Hepatol* 1995; **7**: 871–875.

53. Okhuysen PC, DuPont HL, Ericsson CD, *et al.* Zaldaride maleate (a new calmodulin antagonist) versus loperamide in the treatment of traveler's diarrhea: randomized, placebo-controlled trial. *Clin Infect Dis* 1995; **21**: 341–344.

54. Turvill JL, Farthing MJG. Enkephalins and enkephalinase inhibitors in intestinal fluid and electrolyte transport. *Eur J Gastro Hepatol* 1997; **9**: 877–880.

55. Farthing MJG. Enkephalinase inhibition: a rationale approach to anti-secretory therapy for acute diarrhoea. *Aliment Pharmacol Ther* 1999; **13 (Suppl. 6)**: 1–2.

56. Roge J, Baumer P, Berard H, Schwartz JC, Lecomte JM. The enkephalinase inhibitor, acetorphan, in acute diarrhoea. A double-blind,

controlled clinical trial versus loperamide. *Scand J Gastroenterol* 1993; **28:** 352–354.

57. Hamza H, Khalifa HB, Baumer P, Berard H, Lecomte JM. Racecadotril versus placebo in the treatment of acute diarrhoea in adults. *Aliment Pharmacol Ther* 1999; **13 (Suppl. 6):** 15–19.

58. Turck D, Berard H, Fretault N, Lecomte JM. Comparison of racecadotril and loperamide in children with acute diarrhoea. *Aliment Pharmacol Ther* 1999; **13 (Suppl. 6):** 27–32.

59. Greenough W, Rosenberg I, Gordon RS, Davies BI, Benenson AS. Tetracycline in the treatment of cholera. *Lancet* 1964; **1:** 355.

60. Alam AN, Alam NH, Ahmed T, Sack DA. Randomised double blind trial of single dose doxycycline for treating cholera in adults. *Brit Med J* 1990; **300:** 1619–1621.

61. Grados P, Bravo N, Battilana C. Comparative effectiveness of co-trimoxazole and tetracycline in the treatment of cholera. *Bull Pan Am Health Organ* 1996; **30:** 36–42.

62. Dutta D, Bhattacharya SK, Bhattacharya MK, *et al*. Efficacy of norfloxacin and doxycycline for treatment of *Vibrio cholerae* O139 infection. *J Antimicrob Chemother* 1996; **37:** 575–581.

63. Khan WA, Begum M, Salam MA, Bardhan PK, Islam MR, Mahalanabis D. Comparative trial of five antimicrobial compounds in the treatment of cholera in adults. *Trans Roy Soc Trop Med Hyg* 1995; **89:** 103–106.

64. Khan WA, Bennish ML, Seas C, *et al*. Randomised controlled comparison of single-dose ciprofloxacin and doxycycline for cholera caused by *Vibrio cholerae* 01 or 0139. *Lancet* 1996; **348:** 296–300.

65. Usubutun S, Agalar C, Diri C, Turkyilmaz R. Single-dose ciprofloxacin in cholera. *Eur J Emerg Med* 1997; **4:** 145–149.

66. Farthing MJG. Prevention and treatment of travellers' diarrhoea. *Aliment Pharmacol Ther* 1991; **5:** 15–30.

67. Farthing MJG, DuPont HL, Guandalini S, *et al*. Treatment and prevention of travellers' diarrhoea. *Gastroenterol Internat* 1992; **5:** 162–175.

68. DuPont HL, Ericsson CD. Prevention and treatment of traveler's diarrhea. *N Engl J Med* 1993; **328:** 1821–1827.

69. Pichler HE, Diridl G, Stickler K, Wolf D. Clinical efficacy of ciprofloxacin compared with placebo in bacterial diarrhoea. *Am J Med* 1987; **82:** 329–332.

70. Ericsson CD, Johnson PC, DuPont HL, Morgan DR, Bitsura JA, de a Cabada FJ. Ciprofloxacin or trimethoprim-sulfamethoxazole as initial therapy for traveler's diarrhea. A placebo-controlled, randomized trial. *Ann Intern Med* 1987; **106:** 216–220.

71. Mattila L, Peltola H, Siitonen A, Kyronseppa H, Simula I, Kataja M. Short-term treatment of traveler's diarrhea with norfloxacin: a double-blind, placebo-controlled study during two sessions. *Clin Infect Dis* 1993; **17:** 779–782.

72. Salam I, Katelaris P, Leigh-Smith S, *et al*. A randomised placebo-controlled trial of single dose ciprofloxacin in treatment of travellers' diarrhoea. *Lancet* 1994; **344:** 1537–1539.

73. Steffen R. Worldwide efficacy of bismuth subsalicylate in the treatment of traveler's diarrhea. *Rev Infect Dis* 1990; **12 (Suppl. 1):** 80–86.

74. Tauxe RV, Puhr ND, Wells JG, Hargrett-Bean N, Blake PA. Antimicrobial resistance of *Shigella* isolates in the USA: the importance of international travelers. *J Infect Dis* 1990; **162:** 1107–1111.

75. Bennish ML, Salam MA, Haider R, Barza M. Therapy for shigellosis. II. Randomized, double-blind comparison of ciprofloxacin and ampicillin. *J Infect Dis* 1990; **162:** 711–716.

76. Khan WA, Seas C, Dhar U, Salam MA, Bennish ML. Treatment of shigellosis: V. comparison of azithromycin and ciprofloxacin. A double-blind, randomized, controlled trial. *Ann Intern Med* 1997; **126:** 697–703.

77. Bassily S, Hyams KG, el-Masry NA, *et al*. Short-course norfloxacin and trimethoprim-sulfamethoxazole treatment of shigellosis and salmonellosis in Egypt. *Am J Trop Med Hyg* 1994; **51:** 219–223.

78. Gotuzzo E, Oberhelman RA, Maguina C, *et al*. Comparison of single-dose treatment with norfloxacin and standard 5-day treatment with trimethoprim-sulfamethoxazole for acute shigellosis in adults. *Antimicrob Agents Chemother* 1989; **33:** 1101–1104.

79. Bennish ML, Salam MA, Khan WA, Khan AM. Treatment of shigellosis III. Comparison of one or two-dose ciprofloxacin with standard 5-day therapy. A randomized, blinded trial. *Ann Intern Med* 1992; **117:** 727–734.

80. Teasley DG, Gerding DN, Olson MM, *et al*. Prospective randomised trial of metronidazole versus vancomycin for *Clostridium difficile*-associated diarrhoea and colitis. *Lancet* 1983; **2:** 1043–1046.

81. Wilcox MH, Howe R. Diarrhoea caused by *Clostridium difficile*: response time for treatment with metronidazole and vancomycin. *J Antimicrob Chemother* 1995; **35**: 673–679.

82. Young GP, Ward PB, Bayley N, *et al*. Antibiotic-associated colitis due to *Clostridium difficile*: double-blind comparison of vancomycin with bacitracin. *Gastroenterology* 1985; **89**: 1038–1045.

83. Wenisch C, Parschalk B, Hasenhundl M, Hirschl AM, Graninger W. Comparison of vancomycin, teicoplanin, metronidazole and fusidic acid for the treatment of *Clostridium difficile*-associated diarrhea. *Clin Infect Dis* 1996; **22**: 813–818.

84. Kelly MP, Farthing MJG. Infections of the gastrointestinal tract. In: *Antibiotic and Chemotherapy, 7th Edn*. F O'Grady, HP Lambert, RG Finch, D Greenwood (Eds). Churchill Livingstone, London, 1997, 708–720.

85. Garcia-Laverde A, de Bonilla L. Clinical trials with metronidazole in human balantidiasis. *Am J Trop Med Hyg* 1975; **24**: 781–783.

86. Gayraud M, Scavizzi MR, Mollaret HJH, Guillevin L, Hornstein MJ. Antibiotic treatment of *Yersinia enterocolitica* septicemia: a retrospective review of 43 cases. *Clin Infect Dis* 1993; **17**: 405–410.

87. Crowe M, Ashford K, Ispahani P. Clinical features and antibiotic treatment of septic arthritis and osteomyelitis due to *Yersinia enterocolitica*. *J Med Microbiol* 1996; **45**: 302–309.

88. Pai CH, Gillis F, Tuomanen E, Marks MI. Placebo-controlled double-blind evaluation of trimethoprim-sulfamethoxazole treatment for *Yersinia enterocolitica* gastroenteritis. *J Pediatr* 1984; **104**: 308–311.

89. Anders BJ, Lauer BA, Paisley JW, Reller LB. Double-blind placebo controlled trial of erythromycin for treatment of *Campylobacter* enteritis. *Lancet* 1982; **1**: 131–132.

90. Mandal BK, Ellis ME, Dunbar EM, Whale K. Double-blind placebo-controlled trial of erythromycin in the treatment of clinical *Campylobacter* infection. *J Antimicrob Chemother* 1984; **13**: 619–623.

91. Salazar-Lindo E, Sack RB, Chea-Woo E, *et al*. Early treatment with erythromycin of *Campylobacter jejuni*-associated dysentery in children. *J Pediatr* 1986; **109**: 355–360.

92. Williams MD, Schorling JB, Barrett LJ, *et al*. Early treatment of *Campylobacter jejuni* enteritis. *Antimicrob Agents Chemother* 1989; **33**: 248–250.

93. Prouix F, Turgeon JPJ, Delage G, Lafleur L, Chicoine L. Randomized, controlled trial of antibiotic therapy for *Escherichia coli* O157:H7 enteritis. *J Pediatr* 1992; **121**: 299–303.

94. Carter AO, Borczyk AA, Carlson JA, *et al*. A severe outbreak of *Escherichia coli* O157-H7-associated hemorrhagic colitis in a nursing home. *N Engl J Med* 1987; **317**: 1496–1500.

95. Wong CS, Jelacic S, Habeeb RL, Watkins SL, Tarr PI. The risk of the hemolytic-uremic syndrome after antibiotic treatment of *Escherichia coli* O157:H7 infections. *N Eng J Med* 2000; **342**: 1930–1936.

96. Dieterich DT, Kotler DP, Busch DF, *et al*. Ganciclovir treatment of cytomegalovirus colitis in AIDS: a randomized, double-blind, placebo-controlled multicenter study. *J Infect Dis* 1993; **167**: 278–282.

97. Nelson MR, Connolly GM, Hawkins DA, Gazzard BG. Foscarnet in the treatment of cytomegalovirus infection of the esophagus and colon in patients with the acquired immune deficiency syndrome. *Am J Gastroenterol* 1991; **86**: 876–881.

98. Salzberger B, Stoehr A, Jablonowski H, *et al*. Foscarnet 5 versus 7 days a week treatment for severe gastrointestinal CMV disease in HIV-infected patients. *Infection* 1996; **24**: 121–124.

99. Vesy CJ, Peterson WL. Review article: the management of giardiasis. *Aliment Pharmacol Ther* 1999; **13**: 843–850.

100. Bissuel F, Cotte L, Rabodonirina M, Rougier P, Piens MA, Trepo C. Paromomycin: an effective treatment for cryptosporidial diarrhea in patients with AIDS. *Clin Infect Dis* 1994; **18**: 447–449.

101. Farthing MJG. Clinical aspects of human cryptosporidiosis. *Contrib Microbiol* 2000; **6**: 50–74.

102. Molina JM, Castang C, Goguel J, *et al*. Albendazole for treatment and prophylaxis of microsporidiosis due to *Encephalitozoon intestinalis* in patients with AIDS: a randomized double-blind controlled trial. *J Infect Dis* 1998; **177**: 1373–1377.

103. Leder K, Ryan N, Spelman D, Crowe SM. Microsporidial disease in HIV-infected patients: a report of 42 patients and review of the literature. *Scand J Infect Dis* 1998; **30**: 331–338.

104. Anwar-Bruni DM, Hogan SE, Schwartz DA, Wilcox CM, Bryan RT, Lennox JL. Atovaquone is effective treatment for the symptoms of gas-

trointestinal microsporidiosis in HIV-1 infected patients. *AIDS* 1996; **10**: 619–623.

105. Dionisio D, Sterrantino G, Meli M, Trotta M, Mil D, Leoncini F. Use of furazolidone for the treatment of microsporidiosis due to *Enterocytozoon bieneusi* in patients with AIDS. *Recent Prog Med* 1995; **86**: 394–397.

106. Dionisio D, Manneschi LI, Di Lollo S, *et al.* Persistent damage to *Enterocytozoon bieneusi* with persistent symptomatic relief after combined furazolidone and albendazole in AIDS patients. *J Clin Pathol* 1998; **51**: 731–736.

107. Sharpstone D, Rowbottom A, Francis N, *et al.* Thalidomide: a novel therapy for microsporidiosis. *Gastroenterology* 1997; **112**: 1823–1829.

108. Hoge CW, Shlim DR, Ghimire M, *et al.* Placebo-controlled trial of co-trimoxazole for *Cyclospora* infections among travellers and foreign residents in Nepal. *Lancet* 1995; **345**: 691–693.

109. Lasserre R, Sangaalang RP, Santiago. Three-day treatment of typhoid fever with two different doses of ceftriaxone, compared to 14-day therapy with chloramphenicol. *J Antimicrob Chemother* 1991; **28**: 765–772.

110. Smith MD, Duong NM, Hoa NT, *et al.* Comparison of ofloxacin and ceftriaxone for short-course treatment of enteric fever. *Antimicrob Agents Chemother* 1994; **38**: 1716–1720.

111. Memon IA, Billoo AG, Memon HI. Cefixime: an oral option for the treatment of multidrug-resistant enteric fever in children. *South Med J* 1997; **90**: 1204–1207.

112. Deshpande AK, Joshi SR, Lal HM, Cooverji ND, Ajay S. Cefuroxime axetil in the treatment of *Salmonella typhi* infection (enteric fever) in adults. *J Assoc Physicians India* 1996; **44**: 786–789.

113. Girgis NI, Butler T, Frenck RW, *et al.* Azithromycin versus ciprofloxacin for treatment of uncomplicated typhoid fever in a randomized trial in Egypt that included patients with multidrug resistance. *Antimicrob Agents Chemother* 1999; **43**: 1441–1444.

114. Wells AD, Northover JMA, Howard ER. Abdominal tuberculosis: still a problem today? *J Roy Soc Med* 1986; **79**: 149–153.

115. Balikian JP, Uthman SM, Kabakian HA. Tuberculous colitis. *Am J Proctol* 1977; **28**: 75–79.

116. McNamara M, Williams CE, Brown TS, Gopichandra TD. Tuberculosis affecting the oesophagus. *Clin Radiol* 1987; **38**: 419–422.

117. Mandal BK, Schofield PF. Abdominal tuberculosis in Britain. *Practitioner* 1976; **216**: 686–689.

118. Bastani B, Shariatzdesh MR, Dehdasti F. Tuberculous peritonitis—report of 30 cases and review of the literature. *Quart J Med* 1985; **56**: 549–57.

119. Joint Tuberculosis Committee of the British Thoracic Society. Chemotherapy and management of tuberculosis in the United Kingdom: recommendations 1998. *Thorax* 1998; **54**: 536–548.

120. Huang CJ, Pitt HA, Lipsett PA, *et al.* Pyogenic hepatic abscess. Changing trends over 42 years. *Ann Surg* 1996; **223**: 600–607.

121. Tandon A, Jain AK, Dixit VK, Agarwal AK, Gupta JP. Needle aspiration in large amoebic liver abscess. *Trop Gastroenterol* 1997; **18**: 19–21.

122. Thompson JE, Forlenza S, Verma R. Amoebic liver abscess: therapeutic approach. *Rev Infect Dis* 1985; **7**: 171–179.

123. Van Sonnenberg E, Mueller PR, Schiffman HR, *et al.* Intrahepatic amoebic abscesses: indications for and results of percutaneous catheter drainage. *Radiology* 1985; **156**: 631–635.

124. Essop AR, Posen JA, Hodkinson J, Segal I. Tuberculous hepatitis: a clinical review of 96 cases. *Quart J Med* 1984; **53**: 465–477.

125. Strasberg SM. Cholelithiasis and acute cholecystitis. *Baillières Clin Gastroenterol* 1997; **11**: 643–661.

126. Leese T, Neoptolemos JP, Baker AR, Carr-Locke DL. Management of acute cholangitis and the impact of endoscopic sphincterotomy. *Br J Surg* 1986; **73**: 988–992.

127. Chan CW, Lam SK. Diseases caused by liver flukes and cholangiocarcinoma. *Baillière's Clin Gastroenterol* 1987; **1(2)**: 297–318.

128. Degrémont A. Parasitic diseases of the liver. *Baillière's Clin Gastroenterol* 1987; **1(2)**: 251–272.

7

Motility disorders

Ralph RSH Greaves

INTRODUCTION

The motility disorders of the gut represent a heterogeneous group of conditions associated with different parts of the gastrointestinal tract. Although investigative techniques are becoming more sophisticated, the exact relationship between gut dysmotility and gut symptoms is far from clear. In addition, there is a marked overlap, not only between apparently discrete motility conditions but also between these conditions and the normal population. This chapter discusses the separate motility disorders, adopting an anatomical, aboral route.

ACHALASIA

Introduction

Achalasia is a primary motor disorder of the oesophagus, characterized by a failure of relaxation at the lower oesophageal sphincter (LOS), and aperistalsis of the oesophageal body.[1] This leads to the cardinal symptoms of dysphagia, regurgitation and chest pain.

Pathophysiology

The exact pathogenesis of achalasia is still poorly understood. The primary pathophysiological lesion is at the LOS, where there is a failure of relaxation. This is mediated by an imbalance between loss of inhibitory nitrergic[2] and vasoactive intestinal peptide (VIP)ergic neurones[3] with maintenance of cholinergic constrictor tone.[4] The reason for this selective neuropathy is unclear; it neither appears to be familial nor genetic.[5] Neurotropic viral damage to the oesophageal myenteric plexus has been suggested as having a pathogenic role in achalasia, and patients with achalasia have higher antibody titres to measles[6] and herpes varicella zoster virus;[7] however, polymerase chain reaction techniques have provided conflicting evidence for virus involvement in this condition.[7,8]

Therapeutic approaches—rationale

Until its exact pathogenesis is fully understood, the ideal treatment is likely to remain elusive. Present first-line treatment modalities include surgical cardiomyotomy or endoscopic pneumatic dilatation of the LOS (Fig. 7.1), both of which aim to forcibly disrupt LOS function.[9,10]

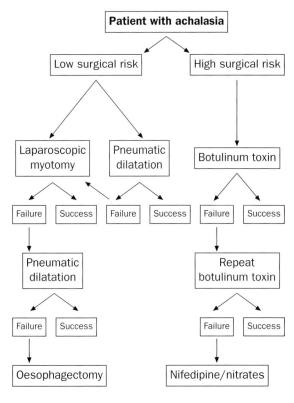

Figure 7.1 Suggested algorithm for the treatment of achalasia. Redrawn from Vaezi MF and Richter JE 1998.[31]

Effective pharmacological therapies that have been used to reduce the LOS pressure include calcium-channel blockers and nitrates. Although anticholinergic agents, β-adrenergic agonists and theophylline has been shown to reduce LOS pressure, this has not translated into clinical efficacy.[11–14] Nifedipine, the most widely-studied calcium-channel blocker in achalasia, is efficacious in the treatment of mild achalasia,[15–17] where its efficacy is equivalent to pneumatic dilatation (Table 7.1).[18] Although isosorbide dinitrate is effective in achalasia, with a response rate of 76%, its efficacy is limited by the 30% incidence of headaches.[19] In the only published comparative study between these drugs, isosorbide dinitrate was slightly more effective than nifedipine.[20] At present, calcium-channel blockers and nitrates should be used in patients in whom endoscopic dilatation or myotomy might be hazardous, or in patients awaiting definitive treatment.

Recently, direct injection of botulinum neurotoxin into the LOS has been introduced as a useful treatment for achalasia (Table 7.1). The toxin of *Clostridium botulinum* acts by irreversibly binding to presynaptic cholinergic neurones and preventing the release of acetylcholine into the synaptic cleft.[21–24] This potency has led to its use in conditions of skeletal muscle overactivity, such as hemifacial spasm and blepharospasm.[25] The use of botulinum toxin has been extended to conditions of gastrointestinal smooth muscle overactivity, as is seen at the LOS in achalasia. Several groups have now demonstrated the efficacy and safety of intrasphincteric botulinum toxin (Botox®, Allergan, USA) in achalasia.[26–29] Intrasphincteric botulinum toxin is reported as having an efficacy of approximately 65% lasting between 6 months and 1 year,[27–30] and presents a safe and repeatable technique. Recent work using Dysport® (Speywood Pharmaceuticals, UK) has been less encouraging, although this might

Table 7.1 Drug regimens for the treatment of achalasia.

Drug	Regimen
Nifedipine	10–30 mg sublingually 30–45 min before meals
Isosorbide dinitrate	5 mg sublingually 5–10 min before meals
Intrasphincteric botulinum toxin	Botox® 20–25 units/Dysport® 80–160 units into each quadrant of the LOS

represent a dosage problem.[32] Older patients and those with vigorous achalasia are likely to have a more sustained response.[26] In comparative trials, Annese and colleagues described equivalent results in a randomized trial of intrasphincteric botulinum toxin and pneumatic dilatation in patients with achalasia with a 6-month follow-up;[28] Vaezi and colleagues demonstrated more recently a distinct superiority of pneumatic dilatation over Botox® (Allergan Inc. USA) at 12 months.[30]

Pharmacology of major drugs

Nifedipine
Mode of action
Nifedipine is a calcium-channel blocker.

Adverse reactions
Headaches, flushing, tachycardia, oedema may occur.

Drug interactions
With concomitant use with beta-blockers, hypotension may occur; with theophylline there is an enhanced effect.

Contraindications
Advanced aortic stenosis and unstable angina are contraindications for its use.

Isosorbide dinitrate
Mode of action
Isosorbide dinitrate acts by nitric oxide donation, relaxation of vascular and non-vascular smooth muscle.

Adverse reactions
Headache, flushing and tachycardia may occur.

Drug interactions
With sildenafil the hypotensive effect is significantly enhanced, so concomitant use should be avoided.

Contraindications
Hypotension, hypertrophic obstructive cardiomyopathy, aortic stenosis are all contraindications for its use.

Botulinum toxin
Mode of action
Botulinum toxin inhibits cholinergic neurotransmission at the LOS.

Dynamics/kinetics
Its effect lasts up to 3 months.

Adverse reactions
Paralysis of distant muscles and antibody formation may occur.

Drug interactions
Its effects are enhanced by aminoglycosides.

Contraindications
Myasthenia gravis, pregnancy and breastfeeding are all contraindications.

CHAGAS' DISEASE

Introduction

Chagas' disease (American trypanosomiasis) is a zoonosis caused by the protozoon *Trypanosoma cruzi*. It is widespread in North and South America, where approximately 20 million people are infected. The subsequent inflammatory response affects the heart and the gut, predominantly causing a cardiomyopathy and a gut myopathy, respectively.

Pathophysiology

The infective metacyclic trypanosomes are introduced through the skin when the insect vector (Reduiviid) feeds on a human. The non-proliferative forms invade muscle and nerve cells of the heart and gastrointestinal tract. The parasites differentiate to trypomastigotes that destroy the host cell and enter the bloodstream. Tissue damage results from both the direct parasitic action and the ensuing inflammatory response. The consequences in the gastrointestinal tract are dilatation of the oesophagus and colon.

Therapeutic approaches—rationale

There have been significant advances in the control of vectorial and transfusional transmission of this parasitosis but direct chemotherapy remains unsatisfactory. Benznidazole have been used in acute cases but its use in chronic cases is unproven. The symptomatic treatment of Chagasic megaoesophagus follows a similar approach to the treatment of achalasia (see previous text), and the treatment of Chagasic megacolon is similar to that of idiopathic megacolon (see later text).

DIFFUSE OESOPHAGEAL SPASM

Introduction

Diffuse oesophageal spasm (DOS) is a rare syndrome characterized by intermittent symptoms of retrosternal pain and dysphagia. In the past, diagnosis was made on a typical clinical picture with associated radiographic changes on barium swallow examination.[33] With the advent of oesophageal manometry, the diagnosis now includes 'two or more simultaneous contractions interspersed with normal peristalsis in a series of 10 wet swallows'.[34] This section describes the pathophysiology and drug therapies for this challenging condition.

Pathophysiology

The pathophysiology of DOS is obscure. There is no consistent evidence of a neuropathic defect.[35,36] The oesophagus, however, appears to be particularly sensitive to a variety of stimuli including cholinergic drugs,[37,38] α-adrenergic agents,[39,40] distension,[41] acid instillation.[42] Furthermore, anxiety and affective disorders are more prevalent in patients with DOS compared with a control population.[43]

Therapeutic approaches—rationale

A summary of treatment regimens is given in Table 7.2.

The aim of treatment is to reduce the symptoms of pain and dysphagia. Several agents have been studied, with variable effect.

Both short- and long-acting nitrates reduce symptoms and improve manometric findings.[44–48]

The calcium-channel blockers have a more variable effect in the treatment of DOS. Uncontrolled studies demonstrate the efficacy of nifedipine in the treatment of DOS.[49,50]

Antidepressants may alter visceral pain sensation. Trazodone, a tricyclic-related antidepressant, has been shown, in low doses, to

---

Table 7.2 Treatment regimens for diffuse oesophageal spasm.

Drug	Regimen
Isosorbide dinitrate	5 mg sublingually 5–10 min before meals
Nifedipine	10–30 mg sublingually 30–45 min before meals
Diltiazem	60 mg orally four times daily
Trazodone	100–150 mg orally each day
Intrasphincteric botulinum toxin	Botox® 20–25 units/Dysport® 80–160 units into each quadrant of the LOS

relieve the chest pain of DOS,[51] although the manometric effects were inconsistent.

Intrasphincteric botulinum toxin, as used in achalasia, has also been demonstrated in uncontrolled trials to relieve the symptoms of DOS.[52]

Pharmacology of major drugs

Nifedipine
See previous text (p. 145).

Diltiazem
Mode of action
Diltiazem is a calcium-channel blocker.

Adverse reactions
Headaches, flushing, bradycardia and oedema may occur.

Drug interactions
As for nifedipine.

Contraindications
Bradycardia and heart failure and contraindications.

Trazodone
Mode of action
Trazodone reduces visceral sensitivity.

Adverse reactions
Dry mouth, constipation and arrhythmias may occur with its use.

Drug interactions
Alcohol: enhances sedative effect; amiodarone: increases risk of ventricular arrhythmias; anxiolytics and hypnotics: enhances sedative effect; antiepileptics: antagonism.

Contraindications
Recent myocardial infarction and arrhythmias are contraindications to treatment.

Intrasphincteric botulinum toxin
See previous text (p. 145).

GASTROPARESIS

Introduction

Gastroparesis is defined as delayed gastric emptying resulting from abnormal gastric motility in the absence of mechanical gastric outflow obstruction. Gastroparesis is a common cause of morbidity. Although approximately one-third of cases are caused by diabetes, several other conditions are associated with this condition. Patients typically present with nausea, vomiting, heartburn, early satiety or postprandial discomfort. This section reviews the pathophysiology, therapeutic approaches, treatment regimens and pharmacology of the major drug groups in relation to this challenging condition.

Pathophysiology

One of the major functions of the stomach is the production of chyme from ingested foodstuffs, and the subsequent delivery of the chyme to the duodenum. This requires co-ordination of motility in the antrum and fundus. Gastric motility is divided into two patterns, the fasting state and the postprandial state. In the fasting state, periods of quiescence (Phase I) are punctuated by periods of activity. A burst of irregular activity (Phase II) is soon followed by a co-ordinated tonic contraction (Phase III). Phase III contractions in the stomach, have a frequency of three times/min. Phase III corresponds to the migrating motor complex (MMC). The MMC carries a propulsive wave from the proximal stomach to the ileum, and lasts approximately 100 min. In the postprandial stomach, the fundus of the stomach firstly undergoes receptive relaxation to accommodate the foodstuffs. Subsequently, a gradual increase in fundal tone forces foodstuffs into the body and antrum. Particles less than 1 mm pass through the pyloric sphincter. Larger particles are propelled backwards by antral contraction—known as retropulsion.[53] A series of irregular high-amplitude contractions gradually break down these particles. Chyme enters the duodenum at a rate of 2–3 ml per peristaltic contraction. The stomach has extensive extrinsic and intrinsic innervation for neural control of gastric emptying. The autonomic nervous system provides extrinsic regulation via the vagus nerve and the splanchnic plexus. The vagus nerve supplies the stomach with parasympathetic fibres for excitatory stimulation, while the splanchnic plexus furnishes the sympathetic innervation for inhibitory regulation.

Many disorders are known to cause gastroparesis. Diabetes mellitus is the most common cause of gastroparesis, accounting for up to one-third of cases of delayed gastric emptying. It occurs more frequently in insulin-dependent diabetics and is associated with the presence of autonomic neuropathy, retinopathy and renal disease.[54] Up to one-half of all diabetic patients show scintigraphic or ultrasonographic evidence of delayed gastric emptying. Multiple mechanisms have been postulated to explain diabetic gastroparesis, including hyperglycaemia,[55] vagal neuropathy[56] and abnormal neuroendocrine profiles.[54,57] Further causes of gastroparesis are as follows:

- Metabolic and endocrine
  —Diabetes mellitus
  —Thyroid disorders
  —Renal failure
- Iatrogenic
  —Postsurgical
  —Drugs
  —Postirradiation
- Neurological disorders
  —Cerebral tumours
  —Stroke
  —Multiple sclerosis
- Psychogenic
  —Anorexia nervosa/bulimia
- Inflammatory
  —Viral gastritis
  —Atrophic gastritis
  —Pernicious anaemia
- Rheumatological
  —Scleroderma
  —Systemic lupus erythematosus
  —Amyloidosis

- Paraneoplastic syndrome
- Idiopathic causes

Therapeutic approaches—rationale

The first line of therapy in patients with gastroparesis is dietary modification and treatment of any underlying condition. Patients should be instructed to eat frequent, small meals throughout the day. Meals should be low in fat and fibre since both these components will delay gastric emptying. Since liquids exit the stomach quicker than solids, liquid or puréed foods are recommended. Several agents are available that enhance gastric emptying; however, comparative studies between these treatments are rare. In practical terms, these agents should be tried for 1 month to assess efficacy and acceptability. Ideally, formal documentation of emptying with scintigraphy should be tried, although the correlation between symptoms and documented gastroparesis is poor.[58]

Metoclopramide has been demonstrated to improve gastric emptying in patients with gastroparesis;[59,60] however, results have been inconsistent.[61]

Cisapride has been demonstrated in a variety of studies to improve objective measurements of gastric emptying and symptoms in patients with gastroparesis.[61–63] In other studies, the effects on symptoms has been less impressive.[64,65]

Erythromycin has been shown to improve gastric emptying in patients with diabetic gastroparesis.[66] Its effect on idiopathic gastroparesis has not been described.

Pharmacology of major drugs

The treatment regimens for gastroparesis are listed in Table 7.3.

Metoclopramide
Mode of action
Metoclopramide is a dopamine receptor antagonist, serotonin receptor antagonist, and it sensitizes muscarinic receptors.

Table 7.3 Treatment regimens for gastroparesis.	
Drug	**Regimen**
Metoclopramide	5–20 mg orally before meals and at night
Domperidone	10–30 mg orally four times daily
Cisapride	5–20 mg orally before meals
Bethanecol	25 mg orally four times daily
Erythromycin	1–2 mg/kg orally four times daily

Dynamics/kinetics
It acts both peripherally and centrally.

Adverse reactions
Dystonic reactions (especially in young females), drowsiness, hallucinations, hyperprolactinaemia may occur.

Drug interactions
With concomitant use with antipsychotics there is an increased risk of extrapyramidal reactions.

Domperidone
Mode of action
Domperidone is a peripheral dopamine receptor antagonist.

Dynamics/kinetics
Domperidone acts at peripheral sites in the oesophagus and stomach. It does not cross the blood–brain barrier.

Adverse reactions
Dystonia (rarely) and hyperprolactinaemia may occur.

Drug interactions
These are as for metoclopramide.

Cisapride*
The product licence for this drug has been withdrawn in the UK and USA.

Mode of action
Cisapride is a $5HT_4$ agonist, and a $5HT_3$ antagonist, it increases acetylcholine release throughout gastrointestinal tract.

Dynamics/kinetics
Its effects last after drug withdrawal.

Adverse reactions
Abdominal cramps, diarrhoea, prolongation of the Q–T interval and arrhythmias may occur.

Drug interactions
Concomitant administration of the following drugs may lead to elevated blood cisapride levels and is contraindicated:

- Antibiotics: erythromycin, clarithromycin
- Antifungals: fluconazole, itraconazole, miconazole, ketoconazole
- Protease inhibitors, e.g. indinavir.

Contraindications
Cisapride is also contraindicated with drugs that are known to increase the QT interval on the ECG such as terfenadine, some anti-arrhythmic drugs, halofantrine, amitriptyline, thioridazine, chlorpromazine, haloperisol and lithium.

Bethanecol
Mode of action
Bethanecol is a muscarinic agonist.

Adverse reactions
Abdominal cramps, flushing, sweating, lacrimation, salivation and bronchoconstriction.

Drug interactions

Bethanecol antagonizes the effects of antimuscarinic agents and with concomitant use of β-blockers, the risk of arrhythmias is increased.

Erythromycin

Mode of action

Erythromycin stimulates motilin receptors in the stomach, small bowel and large bowel.

Adverse reactions

It may cause abdominal cramps, diarrhoea, cholestatic jaundice, prolongation of the Q–T interval and arrhythmias.

Drug interactions

Erythromycin interacts with amiodarone, warfarin, carbamazepine, digoxin, cisapride and theophylline.
*Product licence withdrawn in USA and UK

CHRONIC IDIOPATHIC INTESTINAL PSEUDO-OBSTRUCTION

Introduction

Chronic idiopathic intestinal pseudo-obstruction (CIIP) is a disorder of gastrointestinal motility that is characterized by the failure of the intestine to propel its contents through an unobstructed lumen. The first description of this condition was in a series of patients with clinical signs of intestinal obstruction, where laparotomy was normal.[67] More recently, a consensus group has defined CIIP as 'a rare, severe, disabling disorder characterized by repetitive episodes or continuous symptoms and signs of bowel obstruction, including radiographic documentation of dilated bowel with air-fluid levels, in the absence of a fixed, lumen-occluding lesion.[68]

Pathophysiology

As in the stomach (see earlier text, pp. 147–148), motility in the small bowel is divided into two phases:

1. The fasting state
2. The post-prandial state.

In the fasting state, periods of quiescence (Phase I) are punctuated by periods of irregular activity (Phase II). Soon after, co-ordinated contraction occurs (Phase III). Phase III constitutes the migrating motor complex. Phase III waves have a frequency of approximately 12/min in the duodenum, decreasing to 7/min in the ileum.

In adults, pseudo-obstruction is often secondary to a systemic disease. As with gastroparesis, diabetes and systemic sclerosis are the most common predisposing disorders in clinical practice. Other associated conditions include the visceral myopathies, hypothyroidism, amyloidosis, herpes virus infections and the paraneoplastic syndromes.

CIIP is a heterogeneous group of conditions with several causes. A point mutation of mitochondrial DNA has been described in a child with pseudo-obstruction.[69] Furthermore, a T-cell mediated inflammatory response against enteric neurones, leading to aganglionosis and pseudo-obstruction has also been described.[70]

Patients with CIIP can present at any age with abdominal pain, distension and radiographic evidence of an obstructed gut. Patients with small bowel involvement may develop bacterial overgrowth, leading to diarrhoea and steatorrhea. Patients with colonic involvement tend to present with constipation. Manometric studies of the small bowel demonstrate a reduced or absent migrating motor complex (MMC).

Therapeutic approaches—rationale

CIIP remains challenging to treat. The goal of treatment is to restore normal intestinal propulsion; however, most treatment is supportive—chiefly to improve hydration and nutrition. If bacterial overgrowth is diagnosed or suspected, antibiotics such as tetracycline, amoxycillin or metronidazole should be administered. Unfortunately prokinetic drugs are rarely effective. In patients with an irreversibly dilated bowel, no drug can restore normal motility.

Metoclopramide and domperidone appear ineffective in the treatment of CIIP.[71,72] In contrast, cisapride has been shown to be partially effective in the management of CIIP.[64,73,74]

Treatment regimens

Based on present evidence, only cisapride has been demonstrated to have a therapeutic effect on patients with CIIP (see p. 149 for regimen and pharmacology).

SYSTEMIC SCLEROSIS

Introduction

Systemic sclerosis (SS) is a multisystem disorder that affects the skin, the gastrointestinal tract, the lung, the heart and the kidney. It can be divided into a diffuse or limited cutaneous form, according to clinical and biochemical parameters. SS can affect all parts of the gastrointestinal tract, although the oesophagus is most often affected, in up to 80% of cases.[75] The pathogenesis of SS is incompletely understood, therefore therapeutic efforts are limited to treatment of complications.

Pathophysiology

The primary feature of SS is likely to be an early neuropathic event, followed by smooth muscle atrophy.[76] The close relationship between Raynaud's phenomenon and oesophageal dysmotility suggests a disorder of autonomic nervous function,[77] and this has been supported by manometric investigations.[78] Histological examination of the gastrointestinal tract reveals marked fibrosis in the submucosa.

The oesophagus is the most frequently involved gastrointestinal organ, with up to 80% of patients showing involvement. SS of the oesophagus produces reduced peristaltic stripping waves and a hypotensive LOS. These combine to produce gastro-oesophageal reflux, occasionally progressing to stricturing.

Stomach and small intestine involvement is seen in approximately one-half of patients with SS. Clinically, this presents with gastroparesis and intestinal pseudo-obstruction.

Involvement of the colon is seen in approximately 50% of patients with SS.[79] Muscle fibrosis and atrophy leads to diverticula formation and an atonic colon.[80] Colonic transit is delayed, with ensuing constipation.[81]

Therapeutic approaches—rationale

Oesophagus
Treatment regimens for SS-associated reflux are as for severe GORD (see Chapter 1), although patients with SS are likely to require higher maintenance doses of a PPI than expected.[82]

The evaluation of prokinetic drugs such as metoclopramide,[83] cisapride[84–86] and erythromycin[87] in patients with SS of the oesophagus been generally disappointing. These drugs may have an effect on the early stages of the disorder but are likely to be unhelpful when muscle atrophy and fibrosis predominate.

Stomach and small intestine
An uncontrolled study demonstrated dramatic effects of octreotide, a somatostatin analogue, in patients with SS, intestinal pseudo-obstruction and bacterial overgrowth.[88] Here, administration of octreotide 50 μg/day for 3 weeks normalized the migrating motor complex, reduced bacterial overgrowth and improved symptoms in this group of patients. Long-term, controlled trials are awaited (see Chapter 13, p. 303 for pharmacology).

Colon
Treatment of SS-associated constipation is similar to that of functional constipation (see later text, pp. 152–154).

FUNCTIONAL CONSTIPATION

Introduction

Constipation is a common complaint that physicians encounter. It affects up to 20% of the population at any one time.[89] A satisfactory definition remains a challenge. Health care professionals typically define constipation in terms of a reduction in bowel frequency, whereas patients consider constipation to be the passage of hard stools or associated straining.[90] Epidemiological studies show that 90% of the population have a bowel movement between three times a day, to three times a week.[91] Therefore health care professionals often define constipation as less than three bowel movements a week. The recent Rome II consensus group on functional gastrointestinal disorders defined functional constipation as two or more of the following factors for at least 12 weeks:

- Straining in more than one out of four defaecations
- Lumpy or hard stools in more than one out of four defaecations
- Sensation of incomplete evacuation in more than one out of four defaecations
- Sensation of anorectal obstruction/blockade in more than one out of four defaecations
- Manual manoeuvres to facilitate in more than one out of four defaecations
- Less than three defaecations/week

The term 'functional' indicates that no secondary cause for the symptoms can be identified.[92]

Secondary causes for constipation include medication-induced causes, irritable bowel syndrome, systemic causes (e.g. endocrine, neurological) or structural causes (e.g. benign and malignant stricturing). This section discusses the role of colonic motility and its relationship to functional constipation.

Pathogenesis

Colonic motility is complex, since it serves three roles:

1. Aboral propulsion of stool
2. Adequate mixing of luminal contents
3. Storage and defaecation at socially acceptable times.

Manometric studies over 24 h demonstrate that colonic motility in the basal state comprises segmental contractions, with waves of 2–20 mmHg. These serve to slow colonic transit, thus enhancing mucosal absorption, and improve oral and aboral mixing of luminal contents. Colonic propagated events are divided into low-amplitude propagated contractions (LAPCs) and high-amplitude propagated contractions (HAPCs).[93] The role of LAPCs is imperfectly understood. HAPCs, previously known as migrating movements, produce an aboral shift of considerable amounts of colonic content and the creation of a pressure gradient able to initiate defaecatory mechanisms. HAPCs occur approximately six times per day. The basic mechanisms regulating LAPCs and HAPCs are poorly understood. Patients with constipation will usually demonstrate a decrease in the number of HAPCs.[93]

Colonic transit is now easily studied by the ingestion of radio-opaque markers[94] or scintigraphy.[95] Normal colonic transit ranges from 18–72 h (mean 35 h). Patients with slow transit constipation (STC) have transit times higher than 72 h. There is increasing evidence for an underlying neuromuscular disorder.[96]

Normal defaecation requires co-ordinated relaxation of the internal and external anal sphincters, with straightening of the anorectal angle secondary to relaxation of the puborectalis. Accurate diagnosis requires anorectal manometry, occasionally with defaecating proctography. Anorectal manometric studies measure rectal and anal sphincter pressures, and also the anorectal reflex. Anismus is the association of a high resting pressure in the anal canal with failure of relaxation during defaecation. The puborectalis syndrome describes the inability of the puborectalis sling to relax appropriately. There is considerable overlap between these features; they are now best described together as 'functional outflow obstruction'.

Therapeutic approaches—rationale

General measures
The first intervention in the management of

functional constipation is to increase the intake of dietary fibre. The majority of patients will respond to this simple measure. A gradual increase to 25–30 g per day is suggested. Some patients will experience bloating, but this can be minimized by a gradual increase in fibre intake of 5 g per day each week.

Second-line therapy would involve the addition of an osmotic laxative such as lactulose or magnesium salts (Table 7.4). Further therapy would include bowel stimulants such as bisacodyl, senna or sodium picosulphate. Stool softeners such as docusate sodium are unpredictable in their effects. In severe cases, rectal enemata such as sodium phosphate or sodium citrate may be beneficial. A recent meta-analysis of differing pharmacological therapies in constipation found a paucity of well-conducted randomized controlled trials. It concluded, however, that both fibre and laxatives increase bowel frequency. Fibre improved the associated symptoms of pain, whereas cisapride and lactulose improved stool consistency. There was no convincing evidence of the superiority of fibre over laxatives, or whether one class of laxatives was superior to another.[97]

Slow-transit constipation

Prokinetic drugs have some benefit in the treatment of slow transit constipation (STC). Cisaparide has been demonstrated in a variety of studies to improve colonic transit and

Table 7.4   Treatment regimens for functional constipation.

Treatment	Regimen
Fibre	
Ispaghula	3.5 g orally up to two times daily
Methylcellulose	1–3 g orally twice daily
Sterculia	5–10 ml orally twice daily
Bran	1–3 tablespoons orally up to three times daily
Osmotic laxatives	
Lactulose	5–60 ml orally up to two times daily
Lactitol	10–20 g orally once daily
Polyethylene glycol	2–3 sachets orally once daily
Magnesium hydroxide	25–50 ml orally twice daily
Magnesium sulphate	5–10 g orally up to twice daily
Sodium phosphate	20–45 ml orally not more than once a week
Sodium phosphate suppositories	1–2 rectally each day
Sodium phosphate enema	1–2 rectally each day
Sodium citrate enema	1–2 rectally each day
Stool softeners	
Docusate sodium	100–200 mg orally up to twice daily
Liquid paraffin	10–30 ml orally at night
Arachis oil enema	130 mg rectally at night

improve symptoms in patients with constipation.[98–100]

Functional outflow obstruction

The most effective treatment of paradoxical spasm of the puborectalis and anismus is retraining of the pelvic floor muscles with biofeedback.[101] However, much of the reported experience is from short-term studies, and the long-term follow-up is unclear.

Botulinum toxin injection into the puborectalis muscle has been attempted in patients with paradoxical contraction of the puborectalis.[102] Short-term results were encouraging but the work has not been replicated. Here, it has a similar effect to the intrasphincteric injection of botulinum toxin into the LOS of patients with achalasia (see previous text, pp. 144–145).

Pharmacology of major drugs

Lactulose/lactitol

Mode of action

Lactulose or lactitol are non-absorbable, semi-synthetic disaccharides producing an osmotic diarrhoea.

Adverse reactions

Abdominal cramps may occur.

Magnesium hydroxide/sulphate

Mode of action

These agents are osmotic laxatives.

Adverse reactions

Abdominal cramps may occur.

Contraindications

Renal impairment and hepatic impairment are contraindications for use.

Sodium salts

Mode of action

These are stimulant and osmotic laxatives.

Adverse reactions

Abdominal cramps and sodium and water retention may occur.

MEGACOLON/MEGARECTUM

Introduction

Patients with severe constipation can be divided into those who have a normal diameter colon and rectum, and those who have gut dilatation. The latter include Hirschprung's disease, chronic idiopathic intestinal pseudo-obstruction and idiopathic megacolon or megarectum. Idiopathic megacolon and megarectum are uncommon and poorly understood. This section describes the pathophysiology of these conditions and gives a guide to treatment.

Pathophysiology

Patients with idiopathic megacolon typically present in adulthood, and rarely develop faecal impaction. In contrast, patients with idiopathic megarectum have a dilated rectum but the colon is of normal calibre. Patients typically present in childhood and faecal impaction is common. The pathophysiology is imperfectly understood. The enteric innervation is generally intact,[103] although some studies have demonstrated neuronal loss.[104] The majority of studies on smooth muscle abnormalities in these conditions demonstrate muscle hypertrophy.[103,105] Patients with idiopathic megarectum demonstrate a maximum anal resting pressure below normal, implying sphincter damage.[103] Both groups of patients show an altered rectal sensitivity to distension, implying impaired sensory function.[103]

Therapeutic approaches—rationale

The aim of treatment in these patients is to restore bowel frequency and reduce episodes of faecal impaction. Although the majority of patients are controlled with laxatives, some will require surgical intervention.

Treatment regimens

Randomized controlled trials of these rare disorders are lacking. For management, see sections on chronic idiopathic pseudo-obstruction (p. 150) and slow-transit constipation (pp. 153–154).

POSTOPERATIVE ILEUS

Introduction

The motility of the gastrointestinal tract is temporarily impaired after surgery. The effect that an abdominal operation has on gastrointestinal motility is referred to as 'postoperative ileus', denoting disruption of the normal co-ordinated movement of the gut, and failure of propulsion of intestinal contents. Postoperative ileus involves delay in gastric, small intestinal and large intestinal motility. The cause is multifactorial, and treatments remain far from ideal.

Pathophysiology

Several factors contribute to the aetiology of postoperative ileus. Early studies supported the hypothesis that postoperative ileus is a result of stress-induced sympathetic hyperactivity.[106] Later work demonstrated that manipulation of the intestine increases noradenaline release from noradrenergic nerve terminals in the gut wall.[107] In addition, other inhibitory neuroendocrine agents such as substance P[108] and motilin[109] have also been implicated in the pathogenesis of postoperative ileus.

Intraoperative handling of the stomach and intestines also results in a reduction in gastrointestinal motility postoperatively,[106] possibly as a result of alterations to the gastric pacemaker. More recent work, however, suggests that prolonged exposure and handling of abdominal contents is not so important a factor as previously thought.[110,111]

The advent of laparoscopic surgical techniques has changed several perceptions of surgical recovery. Proponents of laparoscopic surgery claim that less intraoperative handling of bowel contents might hasten the return of normal gastrointestinal motility.[112] Although an early trial demonstrated an earlier return of gastrointestinal function after laparoscopy compared with laparotomy, the study was biased towards the laparoscopic group with earlier feeding and less opiate analgesia.[113] Whether laparoscopic surgery *per se* reduces postoperative ileus compared with laparotomy is not yet proven.

Electrolyte imbalances have long been associated with postoperative ileus. Hypokalaemia, hypochlorhydria, hypomagnesemia and hyponatraemia have been demonstrated to delay the return of normal postoperative gastric motility.

Several anaesthetic and analgesic agents used in surgery will adversely affect gastrointestinal motility. Most volatile agents inhibit gastrointestinal motility but the effects are best characterized with nitrous oxide, which appears to delay the recovery of normal postoperative gastrointestinal motility.[114] Opiates inhibit gastrointestinal motility. Typically fentanyl has the most prolonged effect, followed by morphine, with alfentanyl having the shortest effect.

Therapeutic approaches—rationale

Prevention of postoperative ileus requires precise anaesthetic and surgical techniques, including the minimum of gut handling. Swifter control of peritonitis has led to a reduction in the number of patients developing severe postoperative ileus. Increasing preoperative dietary fibre in patients undergoing elective abdominal surgery has significantly reduced the time to resolution of postoperative ileus compared with placebo.[115]

The mainstay of treatment of established postoperative ileus is supportive. Intravenous hydration and correction of any metabolic abnormalities are vital. Nasogastric intubation remains the only effective therapy.[116] No specific drug therapy has been shown to be effective in double-blind trials.

Given the role of sympathetic hyperactivity in postoperative ileus, both parasympathomimetic and adrenergic receptor-blocking agents have been used in the treatment of post-operative ileus. Bethanecol, a muscarinic agonist, has improved postoperative ileus but its use is limited by its effects on the heart.[117] Propranolol—a non-selective β-blocker—has also demonstrated a reduction on postoperative ileus after colonic surgery.[118]

The role of metoclopramide in postoperative ileus is controversial. A randomized double-blind study of metoclopramide in patients undergoing laparotomy demonstrated no difference in postoperative ileus; however, metoclopramide reduced symptoms of nausea, and hastened the introduction of a solid diet.[119] In a further trial, metoclopramide was unexpectedly shown to increase the duration of postoperative ileus.[120] In this situation, metoclopramide may be more effective given intravenously rather than orally.[121]

The efficacy of cisapride in postoperative ileus is variable. Intravenous cisapride has a beneficial effect on postoperative ileus,[122] whereas the rectal route showed no improvement compared with placebo.[123]

Erythromycin has been demonstrated to have no significant effect on postoperative ileus compared with placebo.[124]

Treatment regimens

In patients with acute colonic pseudoobstruction from a variety of causes, neostigmine is efficacious. Neostigmine, a reversible acetyl-cholinesterase inhibitor, will produce rapid colonic decompression at a dose of 2 mg intravenously over 3–5 minutes. Contraindications include mechanical intestinal obstruction, bradycardia and extreme caution in asthmatics and patients with a history of ischaemic heart disease.

SPHINCTER OF ODDI DYSFUNCTION

Introduction

The sphincter of Oddi is a complex muscular structure surrounding the distal common bile duct, pancreatic duct and ampulla of Vater. Its major role is to regulate the delivery of bile and pancreatic juice into the duodenum. It also serves to prevent the reflux of duodenal contents into the pancreatobiliary tree. Sphincter of Oddi dysfunction is a controversial topic. Although an increasing amount is known about the physiology and pathophysiology of this structure, understanding is far from complete.

The basal pressure of the sphincter of Oddi is 15–30 mmHg, using manometric techniques. Phasic contractions of amplitude 50–150 mmHg are superimposed over this, at a frequency of approximately 5/min. In the fasting state, the human gallbladder rhythmically contracts and relaxes, emptying up to 20% of its contents via the sphincter of Oddi into the duodenum every hour. This occurs in close association with the migrating motor complex.[125] After food, sphincter of Oddi motility increases, allowing delivery of bile in to the duodenum in a co-ordinated fashion.[125]

Pathophysiology

The clinical picture of sphincter of Oddi dysfunction is incompletely understood, and limited by imprecise definition. Sphincter of Oddi dysfunction should be suspected in patients with biliary or pancreatic pain, with no demonstrable cause after conventional investigation. Hogan and Geenen have proposed a widely-accepted classification of sphincter of Oddi dysfunction, using clinical, biochemical and radiological criteria, known as the Milwaukee Biliary Group Classification[126] (Table 7.5). A similar classification has been proposed for pancreatic pain.[127]

The true prevalence of sphincter of Oddi dysfunction in the general population is unknown. In an uncontrolled group of patients with a clinical suspicion of sphincter of Oddi dysfunction, manometric confirmation was documented in 29% of patients.[128]

Biliary manometry has improved understanding of sphincter of Oddi dysfunction. It is,

Table 7.5   Milwaukee Biliary Group classification of sphincter of Oddi dysfunction.

	Biliary type pain	Abnormal liver biochemistry[a]	Dilated common bile duct[b]	Delayed drainage[c]
Type I	+	+	+	+
Type II	+	One or two of above		
Type III	+	None of above		

[a]Aspartate transaminase and alkaline phosphatase levels more than two times normal on at least two occasions.
[b]More than 12 mm on ultrasonography or 10 mM on ERCP.
[c]More than 45 min on ERCP.

however, invasive, and carries an appreciable risk of pancreatitis. In addition, the patient needs to be sedated, and the influence of sedation on the sphincter of Oddi is incompletely understood. Raised basal pressure of the sphincter (more than 40 mmHg) is the most reliable guide to diagnosing sphincter of Oddi dysfunction.[129]

Therapeutic Approaches—rationale

The objective of treatment of sphincter of Oddi dysfunction is to improve biliary and pancreatic drainage into the duodenum. Treatment can be pharmacological, endoscopic or surgical.

Nifedipine, a calcium-channel blocker, has been demonstrated to reduce sphincter of Oddi pressure and improve symptoms in patients with sphincter of Oddi dysfunction in controlled trials.[130,131] It is reasonable to give patients with sphincter of Oddi dysfunction a trial of nifedipine before embarking on more invasive treatments.

Definitive treatment of patients with Type I and Type II sphincter of Oddi dysfunction is endoscopic sphincterotomy.[132,133] Little benefit is seen in patients with Type III dysfunction.[133]

Treatment regimens

Nifedipine is used to treat sphincter of Oddi dysfunction. See Table 7.1.

Pharmacology of major drugs

The pharmacology of nifedipine is outlined on p. 145.

REFERENCES

1. Katz PO. Achalasia. In: *Esophageal Motility Testing.* DO Castell, J Richter, C Dalton (Eds), Elsevier, New York, 1987: 107–117.
2. Mearin F, Mourelle M, Guarner F, *et al.* Patients with achalasia lack nitric oxide synthase in the gastro-oesophageal junction. *Eur J Clin Invest* 1993; **23**: 724–728.
3. Aggestrup S, Uddman R, Sundler F, *et al.* Lack of vasoactive intestinal peptide nerves in achalasia. *Gastroenterology* 1983; **84**: 924–927.
4. Holloway RH, Dodds WJ, Helm JF, Hogan WJ, Dent J, Arndorfer RC. Integrity of cholinergic innervation to the lower esophageal sphincter in achalasia. *Gastroenterology* 1986; **90**: 924–929.
5. Mayberry JF, Atkinson M. A study of swallowing difficulties in first-degree relatives of patients with achalasia. *Thorax* 1985; **40**: 391–393.

6. Jones DB, Mayberry JF, Rhodes J, Munro J. Preliminary report of an association between measles virus and achalasia. *J Clin Pathol* 1983; **36:** 655–657.

7. Robertson CS, Martin BAB, Atkinson MA. Varicella-zoster virus DNA in the oesophageal myenteric plexus in achalasia. *Gut* 1993; **34:** 299–302.

8. Nimawoto H, Okamoto E, Fujimoto J, Takeuchi M, Furuyama J-I, Yamamoto Y. Are human herpes viruses or measles virus associated with esophageal achalasia? *Dig Dis Sci* 1995; **40:** 859–864.

9. Csendes A, Braghetto I, Henriquez A, Cortes C. Late results of a prospective randomised study comparing forceful dilatation and oesophago-myotomy in patients with achalasia. *Gut* 1989; **30:** 299–304.

10. Eckhardt VF, Aignherr C, Bernhard G. Predictors of outcome in patients with achalasia treated by pneumatic dilatation. *Gastroenterology* 1992; **103:** 1732–1738.

11. Wong RK, Maydonovitch CL, Garcia JE, Johnson LF, Catell DO. The effect of terbutaline sulphate, nitroglycerin and aminophylline on lower oesophageal sphincter pressure and radionuclide esophageal emptying in patients with achalasia. *J Clin Gastroenterol* 1987; **9:** 386–389.

12. DiMarino AJ, Cohen S. Effect of an oral beta$_2$ adrenergic agonist on lower esophageal sphincter pressure in normal subjects and in patients with achalasia. *Dig Dis Sci* 1982; **27:** 1063–1066.

13. Marzio L, Grossi L, DeLaurentis MF, Cennamo L, Lapenna D, Cuccurollo F. Effect of cimetropium bromide on esophageal motility and transit in patients affected by primary achalasia. *Dig Dis Sci* 1994; **39:** 1389–1394.

14. Penagini R, Bartesaghi B, Negri G, Bianchi P. Effect of loperamide on lower esophageal sphincter pressure in idiopathic achalasia. *Scand J Gastroenterol* 1994; **29:** 1057–1060.

15. Traube M, Dubovik S, Lamge RC, McCallum RW. The role of nifedipine therapy in achalasia: results of a randomized, double-blind, placebo-controlled study. *Am J Gastroenterol* 1989; **84:** 1259–1262.

16. Bortolotti M, Labo G. Clinical and manometric effects of nifedipine in patients with esophageal achalasia. *Gastroenterology* 1981; **80:** 39–44.

17. Triadafilopoulos G, Aaronson M, Sackel S, Bukaroff R. Medical treatment of esophageal achalasia. A double-blind crossover study with oral nifedipine, verapamil and placebo. *Dig Dis Sci* 1991; **84:** 1259–1264.

18. Cocchia G, Bortolotti M, Michetti P, Dodero M. Prospective clinical and manometric study comparing pneumatic dilatation and sublingual nifedipine in the treatment of oesophageal achalasia. *Gut* 1991; **32:** 604–606.

19. Gelfond M, Rozen P, Keren S, Gilat T. Effect of nitrates on LOS pressure in achalasia: a potential therapeutic aid. *Gut* 1981; **22:** 312–318.

20. Gelfond M, Rozen P, Gilat T. Isosorbide dinitrate and nifedipine treatment of achalasia: a clinical, manometric and radionuclide evaluation. *Gastroenterology* 1982; **83:** 963–969.

21. Simpson LL. The origin, structure and pharmacological activity of botulinum toxin. *Pharmacol Rev* 1981; **33:** 155–188.

22. DasGupta BR. The structure of botulinum neurotoxin. In: *Botulinum Neurotoxin and Tetanus Toxin*. LL Simpson (Ed.), Academic Press, San Diego, 1989: 53–66.

23. Melling J, Hambleton P, Shone CC. *Clostridium botulinum* toxins: nature and preparation for clinical use. *Eye* 1988; **2:** 16–23.

24. Simpson LL. Peripheral actions of the botulinum toxins. In *Botulinum Neurotoxin and Tetanus Toxin*. LL Simpson (Ed.), Academic Press, San Diego, 1989: 153–178.

25. Jankovics J, Brin MF. Therapeutic uses of botulinum toxin. *N Engl J Med* 1991; **324:** 1186–1194.

26. Pasricha PJ, Rai R, Ravich WJ, Hendrix TR, Kalloo AN. Botulinum toxin for achalasia: long-term outcome and predictors of response. *Gastroenterology* 1996; **110:** 1410–1415.

27. Pasricha PJ, Ravich WJ, Hendrix TR, Sostre S, Jones B, Kalloo AN. Intrasphincteric botulinum toxin for the treatment of achalasia. *N Engl J Med* 1995; **322:** 774–778.

28. Annese V, Basciani M, Perri F, *et al.* Controlled trial of botulinum toxin injection versus placebo and pneumatic dilatation in achalasia. *Gastroenterology* 1996; **111:** 1418–1424.

29. Cuilliere C, Ducrotte P, Zerbib F, *et al.* Achalasia: outcome of patients treated with intrasphincteric injection of botulinum toxin. *Gut* 1997; **41:** 87–92.

30. Vaezi MF, Richter JE, Wilcox CM, *et al.* Botulinum toxin versus pneumatic dilatation in the treatment of achalasia: a randomised trial. *Gut* 1999; **44:** 231–239.

31. Vaezi MF, Richter JE. Current therapies for achalasia. *J Clin Gastroenterol* 1998; **27**: 21–35.

32. Greaves RRSH, Mulcahy HE, Patchett SE, *et al.* Early experience with intrasphincteric botulinum toxin in the treatment of achalasia. *Aliment Pharmacol Ther* 1999; **13**: 1221–1225.

33. Schmidt HW. Diffuse spasm of the lower half of the esophagus. *Am J Dig Dis* 1939; **6**: 693.

34. Castell DO, Richter JE, Dalton CB (Eds). *Esophageal Motility Testing.* Elsevier, New York, 1987.

35. Friesen DL, Henderson RD, Hanna W. Ultrastructure of the esophageal muscle in achalasia and diffuse esophageal spasm. *Am J Clin Pathol* 1983; **79**: 319–324.

36. Gillies M, Nicks R, Skyring A. Clinical, manometric and pathological studies in diffuse esophageal spasm. *Br Med J* 1967; **2**: 527–530.

37. Mellow M. Symptomatic diffuse esophageal spasm. Manometric follow-up and response to cholinergic stimulation and cholinesterase inhibition. *Gastroenterology* 1977; **73**: 237–241.

38. Norstrant TT, Sams J, Huber T. Bethanecol increases the diagnostic yield in patients with esophageal chest pain. *Gastroenterology* 1986; **91**: 1141–1145.

39. London RL, Ouyang A, Snape WJ, Goldberg S, Hirschfield JW, Cohen S. Provocation of esophageal pain by ergonovine or edrophonium. *Gastroenterology* 1981; **81**: 10–14.

40. Koch KL, Curry RC, Feldman RL, Pepine CJ, Long A, Mathias JR. Ergonovine-induced esophageal spasm in patients with chest pain resembling angina pectoris. *Dig Dis Sci* 1982; **27**: 1073–1076.

41. Richter JE, Barish CF, Castell DO. Abnormal sensory perception in patients with esophageal chest pain. *Gastroenterology* 1986; **91**: 845–850.

42. Richter JE, Johns DN, Wu WC, Castell DO. Are esophageal motility abnormalities produced during the intra-esophageal acid perfusion test. *J Am Med Assoc* 1985; **253**: 1914–1919.

43. Clouse RE, Eckert TC. Gastrointestinal symptoms of patients with esophageal contraction abnormalities. *Dig Dis Sci* 1986; **31**: 236–239.

44. Orlando RC, Bozymski EM. Clinical and manometric effects of nitroglycerin in diffuse esophageal spasm. *N Engl J Med* 1973; **289**: 23–25.

45. Swamy N. Esophageal spasm: clinical and manometric response to nitroglycerine and long acting nitrates. *Gastroenterology* 1977; **72**: 23–25.

46. Parker WA, McKinnon GL. Nitrites in the treatment of diffuse esophageal spasm. *Drug Intell Clin Pharm* 1981; **15**: 806–809.

47. Mellow MH. Effect of isosorbide and hydralazine in painful primary esophageal motility disorders. *Gastroenterology* 1982; **83**: 364–367.

48. Konturek JW, Gillesen A, Domschke W. Diffuse esophageal spasm: a malfunction that involves nitric oxide? *Scand J Gastroenterol* 1995; **30**: 1041–1045.

49. Nasrallah SM, Tommaso CL, Singleton RT, Backhaus EA. Primary esophageal motor disorders: clinical response to nifedipine. *South Med J* 1985; **78**: 312–314.

50. Cargill G, Theodore C, Paolaggi JA. Nifedipine for relief of esophageal chest pain? *N Eng J Med* 1982; **307**: 187–190.

51. Clouse RE, Lustman PJ, Eckert TC, Ferney DM, Griffith LS. Low-dose trazodone for symptomatic patients with esophageal contraction abnormalities; a double-blind, placebo-controlled trial. *Gastroenterology* 1987; **92**: 1027–1031.

52. Miller LS, Parkman HP, Schiano TD, Cassidy MJ, Ter RB, Dabezies MA, *et al.* Treatment of symptomatic nonachalasia esophageal motor disorders with botulinum toxin injection at the lower esophageal sphincter. *Dig Dis Sci* 1996; **41**: 2025–2031.

53. Webb WW, Fogel RP. Gastroparesis: current management. *Compr Ther* 1995; **21**: 741–745.

54. Nillson PH. Diabetic gastroparesis: a review. *J Diabetes Complications* 1996; **10**: 113–122.

55. Fraser RJ, Horowitz M, Maddox AF. Hyperglycaemia slows gastric emptying in type I (insulin-dependent) diabetes mellitus. *Diabetologia* 1990; **33**: 675–680.

56. Campbell JW, Heading RC, Tothill P. Gastric emptying in diabetic autonomic neuropathy. *Gut* 1977; **18**: 462–467.

57. Horowitz M, Fraser RLJ. Gastroparesis: diagnosis and management. *Scand J Gastroenterol* 1995; **30 (Suppl.):** 7–16.

58. Enck P, Frieling T. Pathophysiology of diabetic gastroparesis. *Diabetes* 1997; **49 (Suppl.):** S77–S80.

59. Fink SM, Lange RC, McCallum RW. Effect of metoclopramide on normal and delayed gastric emptying in gastroesophageal reflux patients. *Dig Dis Sci* 1983; **28**: 1057–1061.

60. Mimami H, McCallum RW. The physiology and pathophysiology of gastric emptying in humans. *Gastroenterology* 1984; **86**: 1592–1610.

61. McHugh S, Lico S, Dimant NE. Cisapride *vs.* metoclopramide; an acute study in diabetic gastroparesis. *Dig Dis Sci* 1992; **37:** 997–1001.

62. McCallum RW. Cisapride: a new class of prokinetic agent. *Am J Gastroenterol* 1991; **86:** 135–149.

63. DePonti F, Malegelada J. Functional gut disorders: from motility to sensitivity disorders. *Pharmacol Ther* 1998; **80:** 49–88.

64. Camilleri M, Malegelada JR, Abell TL, Brown ML, Hench V, Zinsmeister AR. Effect of six weeks of treatment with cisapride in gastroparesis and intestinal pseudo-obstruction. *Gastroenterology* 1989; **96:** 704–712.

65. Richards RD, Valenzuela GA, Davenport KG, Fisher KL, McCallum RW. Objective and subjective results of a randomised, double-blind, placebo-controlled trial using cisapride to treat gastoparesis. *Dig Dis Sci* 1993; **38:** 811–816.

66. Janssens J, Peeters TL, VanTrappen G, *et al.* Improvement of gastric emptying in diabetic gastroparesis by erythromycin. *N Engl J Med* 1990; **322:** 1028–1031.

67. Dudley HF, Sinclair ISR, McLaren IF, McNair TJ, Newsam JE. Intestinal pseudo-obstruction. *J R Coll Surg Edinb* 1958; **3:** 206–217.

68. Rudolph CD, Hyman PE, Altshuler SM, *et al.* Diagnosis and treatment of chronic intestinal pseudo-obstruction in children. *J Pediatr Gastroenterol Nutr* 1997; **24:** 102–112.

69. Verma A, Piccoli DA, Bonilla E, Berry GT, DiMauro S, Moraes CT. A novel mitochondrial G8313A mutation associated with initial gastrointestinal symptoms and progressive encephaloneuropathy. *Pediatr Res* 1997; **42:** 448–454.

70. Smith VW, Gregson N, Foggensteiner L, Neale G, Milla PJ. Acquired intestinal aganglionosis and circulating antibodies without neoplasia or other neural involvement. *Gastroenterology* 1997; **112:** 1366–1371.

71. Lipton A, Knauer C. Pseudo-obstruction of the bowel: therapeutic trial of metoclopramide. *Am J Dig Dis* 1977; **22:** 263–267.

72. Turgeon D. Domperidone in chronic intestinal pseudo-obstruction. *Gastroenterology* 1990; **99:** 1194.

73. Cohen N, Booth I, Parshar K, Corkery J. Successful management of idiopathic intestinal pseudo-obstruction with cisapride. *J Pediatr Surg* 1988; **23:** 229–234.

74. Reyntjens A, Verlinden M, Schuermans V. Cisapride in the treatment of chronic intestinal pseudo-obstruction. *Gastroenterology* 1990; **28 (Suppl. 1):** 79.

75. Poirier TJ, Rankin GB. Gastrointestinal manifestations of progressive systemic scleroderma based on a review of 364 cases. *Am J Gastroenterol* 1972; **58:** 30–44.

76. Treacy WL, Baggenstoss AH, Slocumb CH. Scleroderma of the esophagus. A correlation of histological and physiological findings. *An Intern Med* 1963; **59:** 351–356.

77. Belch JJF, Land D, Park RHR. Decreased esophageal blood flow in patients with Raynaud's phenomenon. *Br J Rheumatol* 1988; **27:** 426–430.

78. Greydanus MP, Camilleri M. Abnormal postcibal antral and small bowel motility due to neuropathy or myopathy in systemic sclerosis. *Gastroenterology* 1989; **96:** 110–115.

79. Cohen S, Laufer I, Snape WJ. The gastrointestinal manifestations of scleroderma. *Gastroenterology* 1980; **79:** 155–166.

80. Basilico G, Barbera R, Vanoli M. Anorectal dysfunction and delayed colonic transit in patients with progressive systemic sclerosis. *Dig Dis Sci* 1993; **38:** 1525–1529.

81. Whitehead WE, Taitelbaum G, Wigley FM. Rectosigmoid motility and myoelectric activity in progressive systemic sclerosis. *Gastroenterology* 1989; **96:** 428–432.

82. Hendel L, Hage E, Hendel J. Omeprazole in the treatment of severe gastroesophageal reflux disease in patients with systemic sclerosis. *Aliment Pharmacol Ther* 1992; **6:** 565–577.

83. Johnson DA, Drane WE, Curran J. Metoclopramide response in patients with progressive systemic sclerosis. *Arch Intern Med* 1987; **147:** 1597–1601.

84. Kahan A, Chaussade S, Gaudric M. The effect of cisapride on gastro-oesophageal dysfunction in systemic sclerosis. *Br J Clin Pharmacol* 1991; **31:** 683–687.

85. Limburg AJ, Smit AJ, Kleibeuker JH. Effects of cisapride on the esophageal motor function of patients with progressive systemic sclerosis or mixed connective tissue disease. *Digestion* 1993; **49:** 156–160.

86. Horowitz M, Maddern GJ, Maddox A. Effects of cisapride on gastric and esophageal emptying in progressive systemic sclerosis. *Gastroenterology* 1987; **93:** 311–315.

87. Fiorrucci S, Distrutti E, Bassotti G. Effect of erythromycin administration on upper gastroin-

testinal motility in scleroderma patients. *Scand J Gastroenterol* 1994; **29:** 807–813.

88. Soudah HC, Hasler WL, Owyang C. Effect of octreotide on intestinal motility and bacterial overgrowth in scleroderma. *N Eng J Med* 1991; **325:** 1461–1467.

89. Talley NJ, Weaver AL, Zinsmeister AR, Melton LJ III. Functional constipation and outflow delay: a population-based study. *Gastroenterology* 1993; **105:** 781–790.

90. Johanson JF, Sonnenberg A, Koch TR. Clinical epidemiology of chronic constipation. *J Clin Gastroenterol* 1989; **11:** 525–536.

91. Drossman DA, Sandler RS, McKee DC, Lovitz AJ. Bowel patterns among subjects not seeking health care. Use of a questionnaire to identify a population with bowel dysfunction. *Gastroenterology* 1982; **83:** 529–534.

92. Rome II: a multinational consensus document on functional gastrointestinal disorders. *Gut* 1999; **45 (Suppl. 2):** II43–II47.

93. Bassotti G, Iantorno G, Fiorella S, Bustos-Fernandez L, Bilder C. Colonic motility in man: features in normal subjects and in patients with chronic idiopathic constipation. *Am J Gastroenterol* 1999; **94:** 1760–1767.

94. Metcalf A, Phillips S, Zinsmeister A. Simplified assessment of segmental colonic transit. *Gastroenterology* 1987; **92:** 40–47.

95. Kamm MA, Lennard-Jones, Thompson DG. Dynamic scanning defines colonic defect in severe idiopathic constipation. *Gut* 1988; **29:** 1085–1092.

96. Schouten WR, Ten Kate FJW, De Graaf EJR. Visceral neuropathy in slow transit constipation. *Dis Colon Rectum* 1993; **36:** 1112–1117.

97. Tramonte SM, Brand M, Mulrow C, Amato MG, O'Keefe ME, Ramirez G. The treatment of chronic constipation in adults. *J Gen Intern Med* 1997; **12:** 15–24.

98. Muller-Lissner SA. Treatment of chronic constipation with cisapride and placebo. *Gut* 1987; **28:** 1033–1038.

99. Verheyen K, Vervaeke M, Demyttenaere P, Van Mierlo J. Double-blind comparison of two cisapride dosage regimens with placebo in the treatment of functional constipation. *Curr Ther Res* 1987; **41:** 978–985.

100. Muller-Lissner SA. Cisapride in chronic idiopathic constipation: can the colon be re-educated? Bavarian Constipation study. *Eur J Gastroenterol Hepatol* 1995; **4:** 69–73.

101. Enck P. Biofeedback training in disordered defaecation: a critical review. *Dig Dis Sci* 1993; **38:** 1953–1960.

102. Hallan RI, Williams NS, Melling J. Treatment of anismus in intractable constipation with botulinum A toxin. *Lancet* 1988; **ii:** 714–717.

103. Gattuso JM, Kamm MA, Talbot IC. Pathology of idiopathic megarectum and megacolon. *Gut* 1997; **41:** 252–257.

104. Barnes PRH, Lennard-Jones JE, Hawley PR, Todd IP. Hirschprung's disease and idiopathic megacolon in adults and adolescents. *Gut* 1986; **27:** 534–541.

105. Stabile G, Kamm MA, Hawley PR, Lennard-Jones JE. Colectomy for idiopathic megarectum and megacolon. *Gut* 1991; **32:** 1538–1540.

106. Cannon WB, Murphy FT. Physiological observations on experimentally produced ileus. *J Am Med Assoc* 1907; **49:** 840–843.

107. Dubois A, Kopin IJ, Pettigrew KD. Chemical and histochemical studies of postoperative sympathetic activity in the digestive tract of rats. *Gastroenterology* 1974; **66:** 403–407.

108. Holzer P, Lippe IT. Inhibition of gastrointestinal transit due to surgical trauma or peritoneal irritation is reduced in capsaicin-treated rats. *Gastroenterology* 1986; **91:** 360–363.

109. Rennie JA, Christofides ND, Mitchenere P. Neural and humoral factors in postoperative ileus. *Br J Surg* 1980; **67:** 694–698.

110. Wilson JP. Postoperative motility of the large intestine in man. *Gut* 1975; **16:** 689–692.

111. Graber JN, Schulte WJ, Condon RE. Relationship of duration of postoperative ileus to extent and site of operative dissection. *Surgery* 1982; **92:** 87–92.

112. Phillips EH, Franklin M, Carroll BJ. Laparoscopic colectomy. *Ann Surg* 1992; **216:** 703–707.

113. Senagore AJ, Luchtefeld MA, Mackeigan JM. Open colectomy versus laparoscopic colectomy: are there differences? *Am Surg* 1993; **59:** 549–554.

114. Scheinin B, Lindgren L, Scheinin TM. Peroperative nitrous oxide delays function after colonic surgery. *Eur J Anaesthesiol* 1990; **64:** 154–158.

115. Sculati O, Gaimpiccoli G, Gozzi B. Bran diet for an earlier resolution of postoperative ileus. *J Int Med Res* 1982; **10:** 194–197.

116. Livingston EH, Passaro EP. Postoperative ileus. *Dig Dis Sci* 1990; **35:** 121–132.

117. Furness JB, Costa M. Adynamic ileus, its patho-genesis and treatment. *Med Biol* 1974; **52:** 82–89.

118. Hallerback B, Carlsen E, Carlsson K. Beta-adrenoceptor blockade in the management of postoperative adynamic ileus. *Scand J Gastoenterol* 1987; **22:** 149–155.

119. Davidson ED, Hersh T, Brinner RA. The effects of metoclopramide on postoperative ileus: a randomised double-blind study. *Ann Surg* 1979; **190:** 27–30.

120. Jepsen S, Klaerke A, Nielsen PH. Negative effect of metoclopramide in postoperative ady-namic ileus: a prospective, randomised, double-blind study. *Br J Surg* 1986; **73:** 290–291.

121. McNeill MJ, Ho ET, Kenney GN. Effect of IV metoclopramide on gastric emptying after opioid premedication. *Br J Anaesth* 1990; **64:** 450–452.

122. Boghaert A, Haesaert B, Mourisse P. Placebo-controlled trial of cisapride in postoperative ileus. *Acta Anaesthesiol Belg* 1987; **38:** 195–199.

123. Benson ML, Roberts JP, Wingate DL. Small bowel motility following major intra-abdominal surgery: the effect of opiates and rectal cis-apride. *Gastroenterology* 1994; **106:** 924–936.

124. Bonacici M, Quiasson S, Reynolds M. Effect of intravenous erythromycin on postoperative ileus. *Am J Gastroenterol* 1993; **88:** 208–211.

125. Coelho JC, Wiederkehr JC. Motility of Oddi's sphincter: recent developments and clinical applications. *Am J Surg* 1996; **172:** 48–51.

126. Hogan WJ, Geenen JE. Biliary dyskinesia. *Endoscopy* 1988; **20 (Suppl. 1):** 1125–1129.

127. Sherman S, Troiano FP, Hawes RH, O'Connor KW, Lehman GA. Frequency of abnormal sphincter of Oddi manometry compared with the clinical suspicion of Oddi dysfunction. *Am J Gastroenterol* 1991; **86:** 586–590.

128. Meshinkapour H, Mollot M. Bile duct dyskine-sia and unexplained abdominal pain: a clinical and manometric study. *Gastroenterology* 1987; **92:** 1533A.

129. Gilbert DA, DiMarino AJ, Jensen DM, Katon R, Kimmey MB, Laine LA. Status evaluation: sphincter of Oddi manometry. *Gastrointest Endosc* 1992; **38:** 757–759.

130. Guelrud M, Mendoza S, Rossiter G, Ramirez L, Barkin J. Effect of nifedipine on sphincter of Oddi motor activity: studies in healthy volun-teers and patients with biliary dyskinesia. *Gastroenterology* 1988; **95:** 1050–1055.

131. Khuroo MS, Zargar SA, Tattoo GN. Efficacy of nifedipine therapy in patients with sphincter of Oddi dysfunction: a prospective, double-blind, randomised, placebo-controlled, cross-over trial. *Br J Clin Pharmacol* 192; **33:** 477–485.

132. Tzovaras G, Rowlands BJ. Diagnosis and treat-ment of sphincter of Oddi dysfunction. *Br J Surg* 1998; **85:** 588–595.

133. Wehrmann T, Wiemer K, Lebcke B, Caspary WF, Jung M. Do patients with sphincter of Oddi dysfunction benefit from endoscopic sphinc-terotomy? A 5-year prospective trial. *Eur J Gastroenterol Hepatol* 1996; **8:** 251–256.

8

Functional abdominal disorders

Bernard Coulie, Michael Camilleri

*Physicians of the outmost fame were called at
    once,
and when they came they answered,
as they took their fees,
"There is no cure for this disease"*

Hillaire Belloc

INTRODUCTION

There is still no category of gastrointestinal disease that fosters a greater sense of frustration in physicians and patients than functional gastrointestinal disorders. This frustration reflects the paucity of effective medications, and is only tempered for the physician by the knowledge the diagnosis is most often correct and patients do not develop significant complications or die from these disorders. Regrettably, the patients experience impaired quality of life, and utilize health care resources extensively as they seek better 'solutions' (including unnecessary repeated investigations or even surgery). From a societal standpoint, there is also a significant economic burden estimated for 1998 at $41 billion for the eight most industrialized countries (namely Australia, Sweden, USA, Canada, Germany, France, Japan and UK); two-thirds of this burden reflects absenteeism from work and the indirect costs.

During recent years, a greater understanding of the pathophysiology of these disorders and a surge of interest in this challenge among pharmacologists, basic scientists, and clinical investigators have led to novel insights and promising therapies.

This chapter will review the evidence to support current therapies in non-ulcer dyspepsia and irritable bowel syndrome (IBS), and will introduce the reader to the novel therapeutic approaches that are on the threshold to clinical application. Prokinetic and antisecretory agents are currently the mainstays of the initial treatment of non-ulcer dyspepsia. Eradication of *Helicobacter pylori* in non-ulcer dyspepsia remains controversial, although recent evidence shows lack of benefit; the recent trials therefore contradict recommendations of the American Gastroenterological Association. Based on new insights into the origin of symptoms in non-ulcer dyspepsia, novel therapeutic agents are being explored intensively for correction of underlying pathophysiology and relief of dyspepsia symptoms.

In the treatment of IBS, therapeutic choices are based on the predominant symptoms: fiber for constipation; loperamide for diarrhea; smooth muscle relaxants for pain; psychotropic agents for depression, diarrhea and pain; and psychological treatments.

NON-ULCER DYSPEPSIA

Pathophysiology

Non-ulcer dyspepsia is a symptom complex characterized by postprandial upper abdominal discomfort or pain, early satiety, nausea, vomiting, abdominal distension, bloating, and anorexia in the absence of organic disease.[1] It is characterized by chronic or recurrent symptoms of the upper gut, with no identifiable organic or systemic disease.[1] Non-ulcer dyspepsia is one of the most common clinical problems encountered by gastroenterologists.

Currently, six major factors are considered etiologically important in the pathogenesis of non-ulcer dyspepsia:

1. Abnormal gastric emptying (possibly associated with vagal efferent dysfunction and abnormal intestinal reflexes);
2. Impaired fundus relaxation in response to a meal;
3. Increased gastric sensitivity (possibly associated with psychosocial or mechanosensory factors or both);
4. *Helicobacter pylori* infection;
5. Abnormal acid clearance and increased acid sensitivity of the duodenum; and
6. Psychosocial factors.

These mechanisms are discussed briefly in the text following.

Gastric motor abnormalities
Motor functions studied in patients with non-ulcer dyspepsia include interdigestive motor complexes,[2] gastric emptying, small bowel transit,[3,4] gastric receptive relaxation,[5–7] and gastric antral motility and myoelectric signals.[8] Antral hypomotility or impaired gastric emptying of solids has been observed in 30–50% of patients with non-ulcer dyspepsia, studied in clinics or tertiary referral centers worldwide.[3,4,9–14] In a recent meta-analysis of the role of impaired gastric emptying in non-ulcer dyspepsia, nearly 40% of patients had delayed gastric emptying of solids, and gastric emptying was 1.5 times slower in dyspeptic patients than in healthy controls.[15] Two recent studies also suggested that intragastric distribution of a solid meal is abnormal.[16,17] Although impaired motor function is not ubiquitous in patients with non-ulcer dyspepsia, current evidence strongly supports the view that motor function is impaired in some patients. A strong argument in favor of impaired motor function as an important factor in non-ulcer dyspepsia is the fact that treatment designed to correct the impaired motor function diminishes symptoms.[10,11,18]

Few studies have addressed the underlying mechanism for the impaired motor function. A reduced pancreatic polypeptide response to sham feeding in seven out of nine patients suggests the presence of efferent vagal dysfunction in patients with abnormal upper gut transit, and in those with normal transit but increased visceral perception.[3] These data were confirmed by Holtman *et al.*[19] However, a recent study in 17 patients with non-ulcer dyspepsia showed that vagal dysfunction was a rare finding.[6]

Thus, the hypothesis suggesting a role for motor abnormalities in non-ulcer dyspepsia is well-founded but the abnormalities are not universal. Further studies are needed to understand the mechanisms completely and to relate them to other pathophysiologic malfunctions in dyspepsia, such as sensory dysfunctions.

Gastric accommodation and compliance in non-ulcer dyspepsia
Several studies indicate that non-ulcer dyspepsia patients have reduced postcibal gastric accommodation compared with controls.[5,6] Among 40 consecutive non-ulcer dyspeptic patients who underwent measurement of gastric accommodation, early satiety and weight loss were significantly more frequent in patients with impaired compared with those with normal accommodation.[5] Since fasting gastric compliance is normal, these data suggest heightened gastric sensitivity with modulation of hypothalamic or other satiety centers.

Indirect evidence for impaired fundus response to a meal includes accelerated proximal gastric emptying of a liquid meal in non-ulcer dyspepsia patients.[20] Troncon and associates also showed intragastric maldistribution of the meal in patients with dyspepsia.[17] This maldistribution may result from either decreased proximal accommodation or increased distal accommodation of the meal.[17]

Data on the fasting gastric compliance as measured by the gastric barostat show that there are no differences in compliance in patients with non-ulcer dyspepsia in comparison with healthy control subjects.[6,21,22]

Altered gastric sensation

Patients with functional dyspepsia are hypersensitive to isobaric and isovolumetric balloon distention of the proximal stomach relative to controls, that is, the thresholds for first perception and discomfort are lower in dyspeptic patients.[22,23] Hypersensitivity to gastric distention is a feature of functional but not of organic dyspepsia.[24] It is unclear whether gastric sensory thresholds are correlated with current or recent symptom severity or whether hypersensitivity is associated with specific symptoms in functional dyspepsia patients. A preliminary study reported that almost one-half of the functional dyspepsia patients have hypersensitivity to gastric distention, and that postprandial pain is significantly more prevalent in these patients.[25] However, one can question the relevance of fasting perception thresholds as a biological marker for functional dyspepsia, which is, by definition, a symptom complex that occurs in the postprandial period. Patients who report pain during fasting gastric distensions are potentially more prone to report postprandial pain; increased sensation during the postprandial period may, especially with pressure-induced stimuli, be a better marker for functional dyspepsia.[6,26]

These visceral abnormalities do not extend to the somatic sensory system, since somatic sensitivity is normal in patients with non-ulcer dyspepsia.[19,21,27] The interactions between impaired accommodation and visceral hypersensitivity and dyspepsia symptoms remain unclear. Thus, the contribution of compliance and tone to mechanosensory function must be considered when evaluating visceral sensory perception.

Pharmacological data obtained in healthy subjects suggest that gastric tone determines almost one-half of the variance in the perception of intragastric distention.[28] Similar studies are clearly needed in patients with non-ulcer dyspepsia to ascertain the contribution of local motor responses and sensory mechanisms in the increased sensitivity of the stomach.

Non-ulcer dyspepsia and H. pylori: evidence from therapeutic trials

The association of *H. pylori* infection and gastritis, and peptic ulcer are well-established.[29] Although approximately 30% of patients with non-ulcer dyspepsia also have *H. pylori* infection,[30,31] it remains controversial whether *H. pylori* infection or gastritis is associated with non-ulcer dyspepsia or with delayed gastric emptying.[32–34]

Therapeutic trials assessing the efficacy of eradication of *H. pylori* in the treatment of non-ulcer dyspepsia reported divergent results, which may be partly explained by the lack of uniformity of patient characteristics.[32] Three recent, well-designed clinical trials assessing the effect of eradication of *H. pylori* on symptoms in patients with non-ulcer dyspepsia showed conflicting results.[35–37] Talley *et al.* and Blum *et al.* did not find any benefit of eradication *H. pylori* in patients with non-ulcer dyspepsia.[35,36] Conversely, McColl and colleagues documented a small symptomatic benefit in non-ulcer dyspepsia from eradication.[37]

Acid clearance and increased duodenal sensitivity to acid

The role of gastric acid secretion in non-ulcer dyspepsia is unproven on the basis of formal measurements of basal and peak acid output.[38,39] On meta-analysis, the best evidence for a role of acid is provided by the 20% mean therapeutic advantage of H_2 receptor blockers in comparison with placebo in controlling symptoms associated with non-ulcer dyspepsia.[40,41] A recent report provides a potential rationale for the use of antacids as a first empiric therapeutic strategy in non-ulcer dyspepsia patients.[42] Samsom *et al.*[42] demonstrated that clearance of exogenous acid from the duodenal bulb in dyspeptic patients is decreased. This is accompanied by a decrease in duodenal motor activity. Moreover, the duodenal bulb in these patients is hypersensitive to acid infusion, which causes nausea. In clinical practice, acid suppression is probably most effective in relieving the reflux component that frequently overlaps with the dyspeptic symptoms, that may not be easily differentiated by the patient.

Psychosocial factors

There is no unique personality profile identifiable in patients with non-ulcer dyspepsia, but such patients have more anxiety, neuroticism, and depression than healthy subjects.[43] Factors such as advanced age, male gender, unmarried status, and social incongruity are associated with greater frequency and severity of symptoms but not with health-care seeking behavior.[43] It appears that there is a higher prevalence of non-ulcer dyspepsia in men and a higher prevalence of lower gut functional disorders (irritable bowel syndrome) in women; the reason for this gender-difference is unclear. More fundamental studies are needed and the influence of heartburn on the estimated prevalence of dyspepsia in men needs to be evaluated because of the potential overlap.

The presence of non-ulcer dyspepsia is linked with increased need for absenteeism from work; a mean 2.6-fold increase compared with that for a control population.[44] Symptoms or complaints leading to absenteeism are often related to musculoskeletal rather than to abdominal symptoms.[44] This and other observations suggest that psychologic processes play a substantial role in non-ulcer dyspepsia.[45] Haug and associates[46] documented increased association of non-ulcer dyspepsia with psychologic features, such as anxiety, general psychopathology, lower general level of functioning, and multisystem complaints, in comparison with healthy control subjects and patients with duodenal ulcer.

Psychosensory arousal and autonomic stimuli can alter visceral perception of distention and tone within the gastrointestinal tract.[47,48]

Although only demonstrated in the colon of healthy volunteers, it is plausible that psychosensory arousal also influences the sensitivity of the stomach and that psychosocial factors affect motor and sensory functions of the stomach in patients with non-ulcer dyspepsia. Bennett and colleagues[49] showed that prolonged gastric emptying in 28 patients with non-ulcer dyspepsia was associated with attempts to resist, control, suppress, and hold in anger; efforts to adopt a 'fighting' spirit while dealing with chronic stressors; and with manifest unhappiness. Carefully controlled studies are needed to assess the role of behavioral approaches such as psychotherapy, stress management, and hypnosis or low doses of antidepressants in the treatment of non-ulcer dyspepsia; such strategies have been successfully applied to irritable bowel syndrome.[50]

Several questions related to the pathogenesis of non-ulcer dyspepsia remain unanswered. While a considerable portion of patients with non-ulcer dyspepsia have unequivocal evidence of impaired gastric emptying, it does not always seem to be the cause of their symptoms. Decreased perception thresholds to an unphysiological distension with a balloon have been observed in non-ulcer dyspepsia during fasting, and postprandially. Abnormal postcibal gastric accommodation may account for symptoms in dyspepsia. Improved pharmacological approaches are needed to modulate sensation by altering gastric tone or afferent function at one or more levels of the pathway, from the mechanoreceptors in the wall to the dorsal horn neurons or supraspinal centers. These concepts are being studied intensively in small numbers of patients, but larger clinical trials are required. Two large trials have shown that *H. pylori* eradication is generally ineffective in non-ulcer dyspepsia and the role of psychopharmacology needs to be clarified.

Therapeutic approaches—rationale

Despite the abundance of data on the treatment of non-ulcer dyspepsia, one definite treatment approach remains to be established. Treatment approaches that have been tested extensively include antisecretory agents, prokinetic agents, and *H. pylori* eradication. These therapies have been reviewed in an excellent meta-analysis,[51] and the American Gastroenterological Association (AGA) medical position statement on dyspepsia will be discussed briefly.[52]

Antisecretory agents
In general, antisecretory agents provide little benefit in the treatment of non-ulcer dyspepsia. Symptom improvement has been reported to vary between 35% and 80% of patients receiving acid-suppressing agents, compared with 30–60% improvement with placebo.[51,53] Omeprazole provides symptom improvement in up to 40% of patients versus 25% in the placebo-treated group.[54] Since acid output in non-ulcer dyspepsia is not significantly different from that of controls, symptom improvement may reflect either the overlap of heartburn, which responds to antisecretory agents, or relief of abnormal duodenal acid clearance in a subgroup of non-ulcer dyspepsia patients.[42]

Prokinetic agents
A majority of clinical trials has shown a benefit of prokinetic agents (e.g. metoclopramide, cisapride, and domperidone) over placebo in the treatment of non-ulcer dyspepsia.[51,53] A multicenter study in Switzerland showed that prokinetic agents are more effective than acid-suppressing agents.[55] However, the margin of benefit over placebo is relatively small, and prokinetics are probably reserved for patients with delayed gastric emptying.[56,57] The availability of valid, non-invasive approaches to measure gastric emptying in referral centers has led many to restrict relatively expensive prokinetics to those patients with documented gastric emptying delay. With the recent introduction of the ^{13}C-octanoic acid and Spirulina breath tests to measure gastric emptying of solids, it will be possible to measure gastric emptying with the same accuracy as the scintigraphic gastric emptying test, but

in the setting of a primary care physician's practice.[58,59]

Eradication of H. pylori
Well-designed clinical trials determining the effect of eradication of *H. pylori* on symptoms in patients with non-ulcer dyspepsia showed conflicting results. Talley *et al.* and Blum *et al.* were unable to show any benefit of eradicating *H. pylori* in patients with non-ulcer dyspepsia.[35,36] Conversely, McColl and colleagues documented a small symptomatic benefit in non-ulcer dyspepsia from eradication.[37] Differences may reflect lack of uniformity of patients in these studies.

Recent recommendations in a position paper commissioned by the AGA suggest that, in new patients who are younger than 45 years and without any alarm symptoms, a validated non-invasive *H. pylori* test (e.g. serology or urea breath test) should be performed, and when *H. pylori* infection is documented, an empiric trial for *H. pylori* eradication should be initiated (Fig. 8.1).[52] If symptoms fail to respond, or the patient is older than 45 years or presents with alarm symptoms, patients should be referred for early upper endoscopy. Two observations question these recommendations:

1. The lack of efficacy of *H. pylori* eradication in non-ulcer dyspepsia;
2. The availability of small-diameter endoscopes to facilitate transnasal, unsedated endoscopy at markedly reduced cost and inconvenience to the patient.

The latter approach also provides one of the most effective strategies to patient management . . . reassurance!

Psychotropic agents
The benefit of selected psychotropic agents such as tricyclics, selective serotonin reuptake inhibitors (SSRIs), and anxiolytic agents has been substantiated in different functional disease states, including irritable bowel syndrome and fibromyalgia.[60] However, there are no data available from controlled studies of these agents in the treatment of non-ulcer dyspepsia.

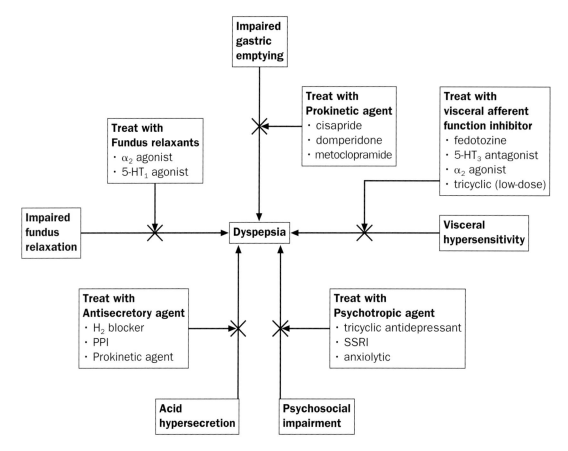

Figure 8.1 Therapy algorithm for patients presenting with dyspepsia based on new insights into the pathophysiology of non-ulcer dyspepsia.

Gorelich *et al.* showed that amitryptiline did not alter gastric compliance or sensory thresholds;[61] a very small study by Mertz *et al.* showed that the benefit of this medication was not related to any gastric effects but more likely to improve sleep habits while on therapy![62] Further studies are needed to address the potential benefit of such an approach in non-ulcer dyspepsia.

New treatment options
Visceral hypersensitivity and impaired fundus relaxation are currently receiving much attention as potential targets for new drug development in non-ulcer dyspepsia. Agents that are inhibitors of visceral afferent function such as low-dose tricyclic antidepressants, kappa-

opioid agonists (e.g. fedotozine), 5-HT$_3$ antagonists (e.g. ondansetron, alosetron), somatostatin analogues (e.g. octreotide), and alpha$_2$ adrenergic agonists (e.g. clonidine) may have therapeutic potential in the treatment of non-ulcer dyspepsia.[53,63] Fedotozine has been investigated in clinical trials and showed some benefit in the treatment of dyspepsia.[64] For alosetron, which appears effective for treatment of diarrhea-predominant irritable bowel syndrome, there are no clinical or experimental data in non-ulcer dyspepsia. Alosetron does not alter gastric compliance or gastric sensation in response to distension in healthy subjects.[65]

Several lines of evidence confirm the role of reduced postprandial gastric accommodation in non-ulcer dyspepsia patients.[5,6] Fundus-relaxing drugs were proposed as potentially beneficial in non-ulcer dyspepsia.[5,6,66] It has been shown that 5-HT$_{1A}$ agonists relax the fundus pre- and postprandially, thereby ameliorating sensation scores during gastric distension in both healthy subjects and non-ulcer dyspepsia patients.[6,66] A small double-blind, placebo-controlled clinical trial of the 5-HT$_{1A}$ agonist buspirone on symptoms in patients with non-ulcer dyspepsia, revealed a significant symptomatic benefit compared with placebo.[67] Larger clinical trials with drugs belonging to these classes of molecules are needed.

In addition to its fundus-relaxing properties, the alpha$_2$ adrenergic agonist clonidine reduces experimental pain from gastric distension without altering gastric emptying (in contrast to 5-HT$_{1A}$ agonists).[63] This combination of effects may well constitute the pharmacological profile of the 'ideal' dyspepsia drug but proper trials in dyspepsia are still to be performed.

Treatment regimens

A treatment algorithm for patients presenting with dyspepsia is provided in Fig. 8.1.

Pharmacology of major drugs

Pharmacology of the major drugs used in the empiric treatment of non-ulcer dyspepsia is described in the respective chapters pertaining to the use of these drugs. Cisapride, domperidone and metoclopramide in Chapter 7— *Motility disorders*, drug regimens for *H. pylori* eradication in Chapter 2—Peptic ulcer disease, and antisecretory agents in Chapter 1—Gastro-oesophageal reflux disease, and Chapter 4—Gastrointestinal bleeding.

IRRITABLE BOWEL SYNDROME

Pathophysiology

Irritable bowel syndrome (IBS) is defined as 'a functional bowel disorder in which abdominal pain is associated with defecation or a change in bowel habit, with features of disordered defecation and distention'. The consensus definition and criteria for IBS have been formalized in the 'Rome criteria', which are based on Manning's criteria.[68]

1. Pain relieved by defecation
2. More frequent stools at the onset to pain
3. Looser stools at the onset of pain
4. Visible abdominal distention
5. Passage of mucus
6. Sensation of incomplete evacuation.

Manning's criteria have diagnostic value in the many patients with suspected IBS, particularly female patients;[69] whereas, the Rome criteria have been widely used in clinical research.[70] Validation of these criteria has, however, been hampered by the lack of any biological marker for IBS. The Rome criteria have come to be accepted as the 'state-of-the-art' criteria for research studies; they have recently been refined and simplified for IBS to focus on the essential elements of abdominal pain and alteration of bowel habits.[71]

Unfortunately, the Rome and Manning criteria still appear to disregard features of IBS that are recognized in clinical practice,[72] such as:

1. Urgency and abdominal pain or diarrhea in the postprandial period; thus, a subgroup of patients displays a prominent 'gastro-colonic' response to feeding. This can be assessed by specific questions and has clear physiological correlates (postprandial high-amplitude propagated contractions) that can be shown objectively using colonic manometry.
2. Functional, painless diarrhea, which may be associated with postprandial urgency and borborygmi, with a sense of incomplete rectal evaluation. Owing to the absence of

abdominal pain, these patients would not be included in IBS on the basis of the Rome criteria, contrary to conventional clinical practice.

Symptoms in IBS have a physiological basis but there is no single physiological mechanism responsible for symptoms of IBS. Proposed pathophysiological mechanisms (and there is interaction between mechanisms) for IBS are summarized as follows:

- Abnormal motility
- Abnormal visceral perception
- Psychologic distress
- Luminal factors irritating small bowel or colon
    - Lactose, other sugars
    - Bile acids, short-chain fatty acids
    - Food allergens
- Post-infectious neuromodulation

Some dysfunction may predominate, but it is conceivable that more than one operates in any individual.[73] IBS is thus considered to be a biopsychosocial disorder in which both altered motility or sensation in the small bowel or colon are modulated by input from the central nervous system.[72,73] A prior infectious gastroenteritis may be a precipitating factor in about one-quarter of patients.[74] Persistence of symptoms in these patients is at least partly related to psychological factors. It is hoped that identification and better understanding of the mechanisms of IBS will lead to the development of more effective therapeutic strategies.

Abnormal motor function in IBS patients
Based on data obtained from a multitude of studies, which addressed the role of abnormal gastrointestinal motor patterns and functions in IBS patients, the following intestinal and colonic motor alterations may operate in IBS:[72,73]

- Psychologic and physical stress increase colonic contractions.[75–77]
- Patients with a clinically-prominent gastrocolonic reflex display increased postprandial distal colonic contractions.[78]
- Abnormal motor patterns in the small

bowel have been implicated in the generation of symptoms in IBS. Clustered contractions in the upper small intestine and ileal propagated giant contractions were observed during episodes of abdominal colic.[79,80]
- Symptom subgroups of IBS based on bowel habit alterations, are reflected by motor abnormalities. The number of fast colonic and propagated contractions is increased with diarrhea[81,82] and decreased in constipation-predominant IBS;[83] patients with IBS and diarrhea have accelerated whole-gut,[84] and specifically ascending and transverse colon, transit, which is positively correlated with stool weight.[85] Patients with idiopathic constipation, normal colonic diameter and normal anorectal and pelvic floor function have overall delays in colonic transit.[86]

Among constipation-predominant IBS patients with excessive straining or sense of incomplete evacuation, it is essential to exclude a rectal evacuation disorder (e.g. anismus, pelvic floor dyssynergia) for which re-training rather that pharmacotherapy is the treatment of choice.

Enhanced visceral perception
Abnormal visceral perception (or visceral hyperalgesia) has been demonstrated in patients with IBS by rectosigmoid, ileal and anorectal balloon distention.[87–89] Diarrhea-predominant IBS patients exhibit lower thresholds for sensation of gas, stool, discomfort and urgency when elicited by progressive rectal balloon distention, this is also accompanied by the development of excessive reflex contractile activity in the rectum. Patients with constipation-predominant IBS develop discomfort at greater distention volumes than healthy controls.[89,90] These observations indicate that excessive sensation and motor responsiveness are closely related. Similar to non-ulcer dyspepsia, IBS patients have normal or even increased thresholds for somatic pain stimuli, suggesting that hyperalgesia in these patients is confined to the abdominal viscera.[91]

It has been hypothesized that altered peripheral functioning of visceral afferents (e.g. recruitment of silent nociceptors, increased excitability of dorsal horn neurons) and/or the central processing of afferent information are important in the altered somatovisceral sensation and motor dysfunction in patients with functional bowel disease.[92] Vagal nerve dysfunction and abnormal sympathetic adrenergic function have been demonstrated in subgroups of patients with constipation- and diarrhea-predominant IBS, respectively.[93]

The development of current and new treatment approaches for IBS is based on the increased understanding of the mediators involved in these sensory pathways and what causes visceral afferent dysfunction. Novel drugs are aimed at suppressing excessive visceral perception or the reflex motor responses that may not require conscious perception of gut sensation.

Psychosocial factors

Stress and emotions affect gastrointestinal function and cause symptoms to a greater degree in IBS patients compared with healthy controls. Psychologic symptoms such as somatization, anxiety, hostility, phobia and paranoia are more common in patients with IBS.[73,94] At the time of presentation, almost one-half of the IBS patients demonstrate one or more of these symptoms. Since psychosocial symptoms modulate the experience of somatic symptoms, they contribute to the greater illness behavior, doctor consultations and reduced coping capability, that are common among IBS patients.[95] The role of physical and sexual abuse in the development of the psychosocial factors that are manifested by patients with functional gastrointestinal disease is controversial. If identified, abuse requires specific and expert care.[96]

Patients who frequently seek medical care have a higher frequency of psychological disturbances, regardless of the underlying medical condition. Life-event stressors and hypochondriasis are important determinants of the patients with postinfectious diarrhea who develop the full picture of IBS at 3 months.[74]

Luminal irritants, infection, inflammation

Rather than being etiologic factors in IBS, luminal factors appear to aggravate IBS symptomatology.[97] They include dietary components (e.g. malabsorbed sugars such as lactose and fructose)[98–102] and possibly endogenous chemicals involved in the digestive process such as short-chain fatty acids.[103,104] However, the prevalence of sugar malabsorption among patients with IBS does not differ from the prevalence in healthy controls.[105] Experimental data suggest that food allergens may also be important in IBS.[106] One clinical trial showed that 40% of patients with IBS persistently improved with dietary exclusions.[107] The role of dietary exclusion and bacterial fermentation in the colon in IBS is still controversial.

Ileal malabsorption of bile acids may induce choleric enteropathy with diarrhea; bile acid malabsorption may account for few patients with unexplained 'functional diarrhea' attributed to IBS.[108,109] Short- or median-chain fatty acids, which might reach the right colon in patients with borderline absorptive capacity or rapid transit in the small bowel, induce rapidly propagated, high-pressure waves in the right colon. These waves propel colonic content extremely effectively and may result in pain or diarrhea.[103,104]

There is epidemiological evidence that infectious diarrhea sometimes precedes the onset of IBS symptoms.[74,110] In some series, up to one-quarter of patients with chronic IBS symptoms report such a history.[74] It is not clear whether persistent symptoms reflect a physiological response to a previous infectious episode, even in the absence of demonstrable inflammation of the gut. Some have hypothesized that microscopic inflammatory changes such as infiltration of the enteric nervous system contribute to the development of IBS. Gwee et al.[74] have shown that about one-quarter of patients with infectious diarrhea IBS continue to experience symptoms after 3 months. Nevertheless, it appears that the 'mind' plays a greater role than 'matter' since life-event stress and hypochondriasis are predictive factors in the persistence of IBS; in contrast, physiological parameters such as whole-gut transit time and sensory thresholds are not different in patients with or without IBS symptoms at 3 months after the episode of 'infectious' diarrhea.[74] A confounding factor with interpretation of the predominant effect of psychological factors is the well-known presentation of the psychological disorder at the time of health-care seeking in IBS. Regrettably, the antecedent psychological profile is not available in these patients, and hence it cannot be concluded definitively that psychological trait determines postinfectious IBS.

Therapeutic approaches

Data of single trials and meta-analyses of pharmacotherapies for IBS have been evaluated in several excellent reviews.[73,111,112] We will focus on a more clinical and practical appraisal of effectiveness and present an empirical therapeutic approach to the patient with IBS, based on targeting therapy to the predominant symptom.

Figure 8.2 illustrates site and mode of action of classic and new pharmacological therapies in the treatment of IBS. These are based on clinical and/or experimental studies performed in healthy subjects and patients with IBS.

At the end of this section, future applications of newer therapies (e.g. 5-HT$_3$ antagonists, fedotozine, octreotide; 5-HT$_{1A}$ agonists, and 5-HT$_4$ agonists and antagonists) aimed at correcting the underlying mechanisms, are discussed.

Recent reviews, endorsed by the Practice Committee of the American Gastroenterological Association,[73] have outlined the strategies for diagnosis and management of IBS. A greater understanding of sensorimotor pathophysiol-

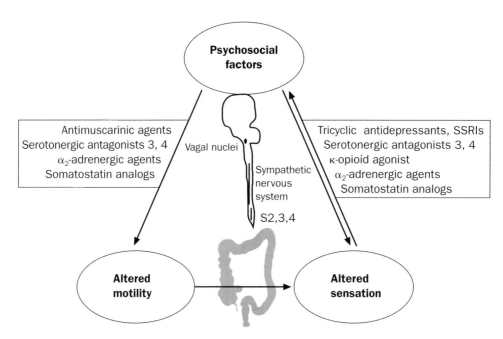

Figure 8.2 Conceptual framework for mechanisms interacting in the development of irritable bowel syndrome, a biopsychosocial disorder involving the brain–gut axis with site and mode of action of classic and new pharmacological therapies in the treatment of IBS. These are based on clinical and/or experimental studies performed in healthy subjects and patients with IBS. Adapted with permission from Camilleri M, Choi M-G. 1997.[72]

ogy, the brain–gut axis, and novel pharmacological agents are reviewed elsewhere,[72] and should lead to improved management of IBS.

Role of fiber in IBS

Fiber accelerates colonic or oro-anal transit in constipation-predominant IBS patients.[113] Based on these and other data, dietary fiber supplements or psyllium products are frequently recommended for patients with constipation-predominant IBS, even though, as a group, these patients do not consume less dietary fiber than control subjects.[114] The mechanisms by which additional fiber may alleviate symptoms in constipation-predominant IBS are not entirely clear. There is evidence that fiber decreases whole-gut transit time; fiber may also decrease intracolonic pressures, thus reducing pain based on the fact that wall tension is one of the factors that contributes to visceral pain.[115–117] Furthermore, fiber reduces bile salt concentrations in the colon, which may indirectly reduce colonic contractile activity.[118] Formal testing, however, failed to show any effect of fiber supplementation on phasic contractile activity in IBS patients.[119] The effects of fiber supplementation on colonic tone, sensation, and compliance in IBS have not been evaluated.

Clinical studies have reported that bran does not provide any benefit over placebo in relief of overall IBS symptoms,[120] and may possibly be worse than a normal diet[121] for some of the symptoms of IBS. The reason for this aggravation of IBS symptoms with fiber is unclear. Patients with IBS may be more sensitive to products of bacterial fermentation of fiber, having a lower threshold to pain from intraluminal distention.[122–124] In two randomized crossover studies of IBS patients receiving increased fiber, the control groups had similar degrees of symptomatic improvement.[119,125] Moreover, symptom relief was not associated with changes in rectosigmoid motility[119] or stool weight,[125] suggesting that improvement was unrelated to the expected actions of fiber.

Although many patients complain of bloating with higher doses of fiber, there is a significant improvement in constipation if sufficient quantities of fiber (20–30 g/day) are consumed.[113,125] In our practice, we add an osmotic laxative to fiber supplementation to avoid excessive bloating if the fiber alone does not increase bowel movements; however, this strategy has not been tested formally.

In conclusion, in contrast to its benefits in treating constipation, the role of fiber for the treatment of abdominal pain and diarrhea associated with IBS remains controversial. The efficacy of fiber in the long term is also questionable, since it resulted in equivocal benefit in a group of 14 patients with IBS followed up to 3 years.[126] Thus, the uncertain benefits reported in several clinical studies have led to a need to formally reappraise the ubiquitous recommendation to increase intake of fiber in IBS.[121]

Smooth muscle relaxants in IBS

Klein[111] appropriately questioned the role of anticholinergic and antispasmodic agents in IBS, chiefly because of poor trial design and statistical analyses with published studies. However, there has been a considerable improvement in the design of more recent trials. There is improved characterization of patient subgroups, exclusion of physiological disturbances (e.g. pelvic floor dyssynergia) that overlap with or complicate IBS and modify response to treatment, and better trial design of appropriately powered studies with definable, clinically-relevant end-points.

Poynard et al.[112] concluded that, as a therapeutic class, smooth muscle relaxants or antispasmodics were significantly better than placebo for global assessment (62% versus 35% placebo improvement) and abdominal pain (64% versus 45% placebo improvement, both significant). Five drugs showed efficacy over placebo in IBS, namely:

1. The antimuscarinic compound cimetropium bromide
2. The quaternary ammonium derivative pinaverium bromide
3. The quatenary ammonium derivative otilinium bromide

4. The peripheral opiate antagonist trimebutine, and
5. the anticholinergic compound mebeverine.

Eight trials with peppermint oil for IBS, including a meta-analysis of five placebo-controlled, double-blind trials, have not established a role for this treatment in IBS.[127] Further well-designed studies and pharmacological approaches are needed. Currently available antispasmodics and anticholinergic agents are best used on an as-needed basis up to twice a day for acute attacks of pain, distention or bloating. Agents such as dicyclomine or mebeverine seem to retain efficacy when used as needed, but become less effective with chronic use. A comparison of mebeverine and alosetron (see text following) showed the latter to be significantly more effective in adequate relief of pain and discomfort in IBS.[128]

Antidiarrheal agents in IBS

Diarrhea-predominant IBS is associated with acceleration of small bowel and proximal colonic transit.[113,129] Loperamide (2–4 mg, up to four times daily), a synthetic opioid, decreases intestinal transit, enhances intestinal water and ion absorption, and increases anal sphincter tone at rest. These physiological actions explain the improvement in diarrhea, urgency, and fecal soiling observed in patients with IBS.[130] The effect on resting and tone[131–135] may help reduce fecal soiling, in particular at night-time. Loperamide does not cross the blood–brain barrier and is therefore preferred over other opiates such as diphenoxylate, codeine, or other narcotics for treating patients with IBS who have predominant diarrhea and/or incontinence. Loperamide is also used to reduce postprandial urgency associated with a prominent colonic response to a meal or as a means of improving control at times of anticipated stress or other colonic stimuli (e.g. exercise, social gatherings, etc.).

Bile acid sequestrian may relieve the choleric effect of bile acids in patients who have idiopathic bile acid malabsorption.[136] Cholestyramine, however, is considered as a second-line treatment in IBS with predominant diarrhea. The rationale is based on the documentation of bile acid malabsorption in patients with functional diarrhea that mimics IBS with diarrhea.[137,138] The simpler, often more acceptable approach in patients who find cholestyramine distasteful or in whom bile acid sequestrates are contraindicated, is to use loperamide as the first intervention for bile acid malabsorption.

Psychotrophic agents

Tricyclic agents (e.g. amitriptyline, imipramine, doxepin) are now frequently used to treat patients with IBS, particularly those with severe or refractory symptoms, impaired daily function, and associated depression or panic attacks. Although their initial use was based on the fact that a high proportion of patients with IBS reported significant depression,[139–141] it is now well-established that antidepressants have neuromodulatory and visceral analgesic properties, that may benefit patients independently of the psychotrophic effects of the drugs.[60,142] Neuromodulatory effects may occur sooner and with lower dosages than those used in the treatment of depression (e.g. 10–25 mg amitriptyline or 50 mg desipramine). Antidepressants must be used on a continual rather than on an as-needed basis, and are therefore usually reserved for patients with protracted symptoms. A 2–3-month trial is usually needed before abandoning this therapeutic approach.

Table 8.1 summarizes placebo-controlled trials of antidepressants in IBS. In two large studies,[143,144] trimipramine decreased abdominal pain, nausea and depression but did not alter stool frequency. The beneficial effect seems to be greater in those with abdominal pain and diarrhea.[139,145] Tricyclic antidepressants do not result in improvement in constipation-predominant IBS, probably reflecting an anticholinergic effect. There is increasing interest in the potential application of SSRIs which tend not to cause constipation and may even induce diarrhea in some patients.[146] Their role is currently the focus of prospective studies. One uncontrolled study supports the efficacy of SSRIs in treating patients with IBS.[60]

Table 8.1 Placebo-controlled psychotrophic drug trials in patients with IBS.*

Tricyclic agent(s)	Comments	Reference no.
Desipramine (150 mg)	No effect on abdominal pain or stool frequency. Constipation-predominant and diarrhea-predominant patients were combined	35
Desipramine (150 mg)	Separated diarrhea-predominant from constipation-predominant patients and controlled for anticholinergic activity. Diarrhea, abdominal pain, and depression, but not constipation, improved more on drug than atropine or placebo	42
Trimipramine (50 mg HS)	Significant decreases in vomiting, sleeplessness, depression, and mucus content of stools	40
Trimipramine (50 mg HS + 10 mg three times daily)	Abdominal pain, nausea, sleeplessness, and depression decreased more on drug than on placebo	41
Nortriptyline (30 mg + fluphenazine (1.5 mg)	Reductions in abdominal pain and diarrhea, but not constipation or bloating	43
Nortriptyline (30 mg + fluphenazine 1.5 mg)	Combination antidepressant/anxiolytic reduced diarrhea and pain	37

* Adapted from American Gastroenterological Association Medical Position Statement: Irritable Bowel Syndrome. *Gastroenterology* 1997; **112:** 2118–2119.

Hypnotherapy and psychotherapy

An exhaustive overview of the available data on the role of hypno- and psychotherapy falls beyond the scope of this chapter. It suffices to say that hypnotherapy or psychotherapy are alternative approaches, in particular to the patient with intermittent but not chronic pain. They are, however, generally less easily available to the practicing physician.[147–149] Factors indicating a favorable response to psychotherapy include:

- Predominant diarrhea and pain
- Association of irritable bowel syndrome with overt psychiatric symptoms
- Intermittent pain exacerbated by stress[149]

The role of psychological treatments is discussed in detail in a recent review.[73]

New treatment options

Pharmaceutical companies have identified agents with visceral analgesic properties, and this has led to a surge in the development of novel drugs for IBS, such as the kappa opioid agonist fedotozine, 5-HT$_3$ and 5-HT$_4$ antagonists specifically aimed at restoring normal visceral sensation, and 5-HT$_4$ agonists with significant colonic prokinetic activity (Table 8.2). Several of these novel approaches are in the process of thorough evaluation in Phase II or Phase III trials, such as the kappa opioid agonist fedotozine.[150] Alosetron, a 5-HT$_3$ antagonist, is effective in relieving pain and normalizing bowel frequency and reducing urgency in non-constipated IBS female patients.[151,152] The 5-HT$_4$ agonists tegaserod[153,154] and prucalopride[155] are currently in Phase III trials for

Table 8.2   Novel IBS pharmacotherapy based on pathophysiology and pharmacodynamics.

Agent(s)	Comment
Alpha$_2$ agonists	Clonidine reduces tone, increases compliance, decreases pain sensation during mechanical stimulation
Anticholinergics	Selective M3 type
Calcium-channel blockers	Reduce rectosigmoid response to distension
Cholecystokinin (CCK) antagonist	Loxiglumide does not inhibit colonic response to food ingestion in humans
Kappa opioid agonist	Peripheral opioid, pain-relieving agent
5-HT$_1$ agonist	Relaxes colonic tone, reduces sensation
5-HT$_3$ antagonist	Reduces gastrocolonic tonic response
	Reduces colonic compliance
	Possible effect on afferents
5-HT$_4$ agonist	Enhances colonic motility and transit
5-HT$_4$ antagonist	Possibly inhibits colonic sensation
Somatostatin analog	Reduces visceral sensation
	Inhibits tonic response, increases phasic response to meal

constipation-predominant IBS. Other research studies are currently exploring the potential of alpha$_2$ adrenergic agonists (clonidine) and 5-HT$_1$ agonists (buspirone).[156,157]

Treatment regimen

Once organic structural or biochemical disorders are excluded, it is useful to actively stress the negative results of these tests and to reassure the patient of the significance of these normal findings. Figure 8.3 provides a management algorithm, detailing a practical approach to the management of patients presenting with IBS. Additional diagnostic tests depend on the predominant symptom in the individual patient and the previous therapeutic trials undertaken. In patients with predominant diarrhea or pain-gas-bloat symptoms, a more detailed dietary history may identify factors that may be aggravating or indeed causing those symptoms. Among those with predomi-

nant diarrhea, lactose, fructose or sorbitol intake may induce this symptom. Therefore, a lactose-hydrogen breath test should be performed, or a lactose-exclusion diet included in the therapeutic trial. If no specific dietary intolerance is identified, diarrhea should be treated symptomatically with antidiarrheal agents such as loperamide. The tricyclic antidepressants, such as desipramine, 50 mg three times daily, or amitriptyline, 10–25 mg twice daily, significantly relieve diarrhea and associated pain. Calcium-channel blockers (e.g. verapamil, 40 mg twice daily) may be used as a secondary treatment.

In patients with IBS with constipation, dietary fiber supplementation (20 g/day) and an osmotic laxative such as a magnesium salt or lactulose are usually efficacious.

Among patients with predominant 'pain-gas-bloat', a plain abdominal radiograph during an acute episode of pain provides some reassurance that there is no mechanical obstruction. Thereafter, a therapeutic trial with a smooth

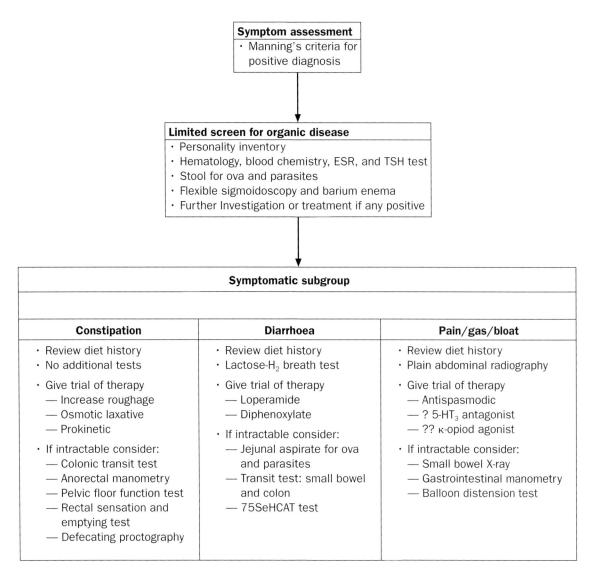

Figure 8.3 Management algorithm detailing a practical approach to the patient presenting with IBS. Reproduced with permission from Coulie B, Camilleri M. *Clin Perspectives Gastroenterol* 1999; **2**: 329–338.

muscle relaxant (as already discussed) is reasonable, although there is no medication that is consistently efficacious. Preliminary data suggest that novel agents such as the 5-HT$_3$ antagonist, alosetron, or the kappa opioid agonist, fedotozine, may be effective but further trials are awaited.

Pharmacology of major new drugs

It is not our intention to discuss in detail the pharmacology of the more traditional drugs used in the treatment of IBS such as smooth muscle-relaxing drugs and antidepressants. We will review alosetron (Lotronex),[158] a 5-HT$_3$

antagonist that appears to be very promising in the treatment of abdominal pain and discomfort and normalizing bowel function in patients with non-constipated IBS, and tegaserod (Zelmac) and prucalopride, 5-HT$_4$ agonists with potential for treating constipation-predominant IBS. The discussion of the latter drugs is more limited since they are somewhat behind alosetron in the drug-development process.

Alosetron

Mode of action

Alosetron is a potent and selective antagonist at the 5-HT$_3$ receptor, which mediates physiological functions in the gastrointestinal tract. 5-HT$_3$ receptors are located on vagal and visceral afferents. Thus, antagonists operating either on vagal afferents or on central receptors in the chemoreceptor trigger zone and vomiting center in the base of the fourth ventricle result in a marked diminution in emesis following chemotherapy and radiotherapy. In the gastrointestinal tract, 5-HT$_3$ receptors appear to be located on postsynaptic enteric neurons and on afferent sensory fibers.[159,160]

In irritable bowel syndrome, hyperactivity of the motor response to meal ingestion, or hypersensitivity to luminal distention result in symptoms that originate in the small bowel and colon. Pharmacodynamic studies of an earlier 5-HT$_3$ antagonist, ondansetron, demonstrated that the antagonist suppressed the reflex activation of colonic motor function in response to food ingestion in health[161] and disease states.[162] The latter reflex is a prominent feature of normal postprandial function but, in certain disease states, it tends to be exaggerated. This manifests as urgency, abdominal cramping, and diarrhea in the early postprandial period in patients with diarrhea-predominant or alternating form of irritable bowel syndrome.

The effects of 5-HT$_3$ antagonists appear to be mediated predominantly by inhibiting visceral afferent responses that either result in direct pain activation or stimulate motor function of the colon. When 5-HT$_3$ antagonists are given intravenously, there is no significant relaxation of colonic tone.[161,162] Orally administered alosetron

(4 mg, twice daily) significantly increased colonic compliance.[163] Conversely, 5-HT$_3$ antagonists such as ondansetron and granisetron inhibit the colonic[161,162,164] and rectal[165] response to meal ingestion. It is still unclear whether the relief of pain from 5-HT$_3$ antagonists results from an inhibition of 5-HT$_3$ receptors on visceral afferents or from inhibition of the postprandial tone, thereby inhibiting the activation of pain-sensitive receptors in the wall of the colon. Delvaux et al.[163] and Thumshirn et al.[166] could not demonstrate significant effects of alosetron on isobaric distention in fasting IBS patients.

Pharmacodynamics

Oral alosetron decreases mouth-to-cecum transit time in healthy male subjects,[167] and 2 mg given twice daily significantly prolonged left-sided colonic transit in IBS relative to placebo.[168] Alosetron did not alter gastric compliance or gastric sensation scores in response to isobaric distensions in healthy subjects; however, in 25 patients with irritable bowel syndrome, compliance of the left side of the colon was increased in response to treatment with alosetron 4 mg twice daily.[163] There was no effect on perception and pain thresholds in response to isobaric distensions but alosetron treatment was associated with higher volume thresholds for first perception and pain; these effects on perception reflect the increased compliance of the colon.

In Phase II studies, 1 mg twice daily alosetron produced a 27% greater increase in the proportion of women reporting adequate relief response than was seen with placebo ($p < 0.05$).[169,170] There was no improvement in pain relief or bowel-related functions relative to placebo in men with irritable bowel syndrome with any dose of alosetron (range 1–8 mg twice daily). Improvement started with the second week of treatment and persisted through Week 12 of the study (Fig. 8.4). In female patients, all doses of alosetron significantly decreased the percentage of days with urgency, hardened stool consistency, and decreased stool frequency compared with placebo.

Two Phase III double-blind, placebo-controlled, parallel-group studies compared placebo and alosetron, 1 mg twice daily, in the

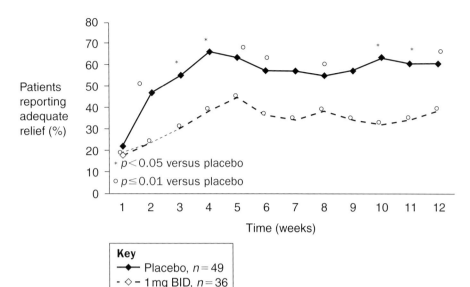

Figure 8.4
Comparison of effect of alosetron 1 mg twice daily and placebo on adequate relief of pain in non-constipated female IBS patients. Reprinted with permission from Camilleri M, et al. 1999.[169]

treatment of female patients with non-constipated irritable bowel syndrome.[152,171] The results of the two trials are essentially similar and confirm the results seen in females in the second Phase II trial.

A recently published report on a Phase III comparison of alosetron with mebeverine, a drug approved for the treatment of irritable bowel syndrome in Europe, also confirmed a higher proportion of adequate relief responders to alosetron than mebeverine during the second and third months of the trial.[172] Compared with mebeverine, the alosetron-treated group of patients also experienced significant decreases in proportions of days with urgency and mean stool frequency, and had firmer stools within 1 week of starting treatment.

Pharmacokinetics
Alosetron has a bioavailability of approximately 60% and a plasma half-life of about 1.5 h. The pharmacokinetics of a single oral dose of alosetron were linear, up to an 8 mg dose. Table 8.3 shows a summary of derived

Table 8.3 Summary of derived pharmacokinetic data following 4 mg oral and intravenous doses of alosetron. Values expressed as mean ± standard deviation (median in parentheses). Reprinted with permission from Camilleri M, Pharmacology and clinical experience with alosetron, *Exp Opin Invest Drugs* 2000; 9: 147–159.

Route of administration	C_{max} (ng/ml)	t_{max} (h)	$t_{1/2}$ (h)	AUC (ngl/ml)
Oral ($n = 16$)	17.2 (14.5–20.4)	1.5 (0.75–3.0)	1.5 (1.4–1.7)	47.8 (38.4–59.6)
Intravenous ($n = 16$)	72.9 (61.9–85.9)	0.25 (0.25)	1.6 (1.5–1.7)	86.8 (74.9–100.7)

* C_{max}, maximum alosetron plasma concentration achieved; T_{max}, times of the sample in which the maximum alosetron concentrations were achieved; $t_{1/2}$, terminal half-life; AUC, area under plasma concentration time curve extrapolated to infinite time.

pharmacokinetic data following 4 mg oral and intravenous doses of alosetron.[158]

Anticipated indications for alosetron

The main indication for alosetron is irritable bowel syndrome in non-constipated female patients; in these patients, alosetron results in adequate relief of pain, reduced urgency to defecate, increase stool consistency, and reduced frequency of bowel movements. The optimal dose is 1 mg twice daily. It will probably be used as an adjunct to loperamide for those with urgency and uncontrollable diarrhea, or to control diarrhea and pain especially if loperamide causes rebound constipation, or when antispasmodics/antidepressants do not provide sufficient pain relief.

Adverse reactions

Over 1200 patients with irritable bowel syndrome have received alosetron for at least 12 weeks during the Phase II and III clinical trials to date. The most common reason for withdrawal of patients from all alosetron trials has been the development of constipation. Constipation is an expected side-effect of 5-HT$_3$ receptor antagonists. Constipation was reported more frequently in patients with alternating irritable bowel syndrome compared to diarrhea-predominant irritable bowel syndrome (44% versus 25% respectively).

The next most common adverse event was headache, ranging from 7–13% with the different dosages, with similar frequency of headaches on placebo. No other drug-related adverse event was reported with a frequency of 5% or greater in the alosetron group.

Drug interactions and contraindications

There are as yet no known drug interactions or specific contraindications. Studies with cytochrome P_{450}-3A4-modifying drugs, such as theophylline, showed no interactions. Animal studies show no harm to the fetus but no adequate well controlled studies in humans. Alosetron and/or metabolites are secreted into breast milk in lactating rats. The safety in breastfeeding women is not known. No pharmacokinetic data in renal or hepatic disease.

Tegaserod

Mode of action

Tegaserod is an amino guanidine-indole with selective and partial 5-HT$_4$ receptor agonist activity.[173,174] 5-HT$_4$ agonists possess gastrointestinal stimulatory effects, partially by facilitation of enteric cholinergic transmission.[175]

Pharmacodynamics

Initial studies evaluating the effects of tegaserod in animals showed stimulatory effects on motor activity through the digestive tract in a variety of species. The peristaltic reflex was stimulated in isolated guinea pig ileum and colon when tegaserod was added.[176] Tegaserod accelerated the gastric emptying of solids in rats and induced Phase II type activity in canine small bowel.[173] Studies by Nguyen *et al.* using 0.03, 0.1, and 0.3 mg/kg of tegaserod in dogs showed acceleration in colonic transit, although the effects on upper gatrointestinal transit were more variable.[177] This dog study did not show the higher doses to be more efficacious than the lowest dose.

Tegaserod, given in doses of 25–100 mg twice daily, accelerated the transit time through the left colon in healthy subjects.[178] Acceleration of left colonic transit was also observed in a model of slow-transit constipation at a dose of 5 mg twice daily.[179] In a Phase 2 trial of 1, 4, 12, and 24 mg for 12 weeks in over 500 patients with constipation-predominant IBS, tegaserod improved the subjective symptoms of IBS, increased stool frequency and decreased abdominal discomfort.[180] The maximum effect was observed with 2 mg and 6 mg twice daily. A dose-dependent increase in stool frequency occurred with diarrhea in some subjects. In constipation-predominant IBS, tegaserod accelerates orocecal transit, and tends to accelerate colonic transit.[153] A more recent study by Lefkowitz *et al.*[154] showed a significant improvement of abdominal discomfort or pain in 799 patients with constipation-predominant IBS. Symptomatic improvement was accompanied by normalization of the frequency of bowel movements.

Pharmacokinetics

Pharmacokinetic parameters of tegaserod are summarized in Table 8.4.[178]

Anticipated indications

The main indications for tegaserod will probably be slow-transit constipation and constipation-predominant IBS. The optimal dose will be between 2 mg and 6 mg twice daily.

Adverse reactions

The most frequent adverse reactions reported with the intake of tegaserod 25–100 mg twice daily are mild to moderate diarrhea, flatulence, and headache.[178] The side-effect profile of lower doses, which are likely to be used clinically, is safer; at a dose of 6 mg twice daily, the prevalence of diarrhea <2%.

Drug interactions and contraindications

There are as yet no known drug interactions or specific contraindications. There is no change in pharmacokinetics in patients with either renal or hepatic disease. The medication is not indicated in pregnant and breastfeeding women.

Prucalopride

Mode of action

Prucalopride is a benzofuran 5-HT$_4$ receptor agonist that has been shown to facilitate colonic neurotransmission.[181] It enhances colonic contractility, including giant migrating contractions, and accelerates the propulsion of stool in dogs.[182] Preclinical, pharmacology, and toxicology studies suggest medication safety, and previous work has demonstrated colokinetic properties in healthy humans.[183,184] In conscious

Table 8.4 Pharmacokinetic parameters of tegaserod after single and twice-daily administration over 2 weeks.[*] Values are presented as mean ± standard deviation (median) in parentheses. Reproduced with permission from Appel *et al.* First pharmacokinetic-pharmacodynamic study in humans with a selective 5-hydroxytryptamine$_4$ receptor agonist. *J Clin Pharmacol* 1997; 37: 229–237.[178] Reprinted by permission of Sage Publications Inc.

Parameter	Value after tegaserod administration		
	25 mg ($n = 8$)	50 mg ($n = 8$)	100 mg ($n = 8$)
Single dose			
t_{max} (h)	1.4 ± 0.4 (1.5)	1.3 ± 0.4 (1.0)	1.7 ± 0.4 (1.8)
C_{max} (ng/ml)	10 ± 4 (10)	16 ± 6 (15)	36 ± 12 (32)
AUC (h ng/ml)	25 ± 12 (22)	39 ± 23 (28)	105 ± 38 (109)
Multiple doses			
$t_{max,ss}$ (h)	1.2 ± 0.3 (1.0)	1.5 ± 0.5 (1.5)	1.8 ± 0.7 (1.8)
$C_{max,ss}$ (ng/ml)	8 ± 3[a] (8)	12 ± 5[a] (12)	38 ± 17 (41)
$AUC_{r,ss}$ (h ng/ml)	26 ± 12 (28)	46 ± 23 (47)	132 ± 50 (127)
R_{ac}	1.2 ± 0.5 (1.2)	1.4 ± 0.6 (1.1)	1.5 ± 0.5 (1.4)

[*] t_{max}, time to reach C_{max} at steady state; C_{max}, maximum plasma concentration; $C_{max,ss}$, maximum plasma concentration at steady state; AUC, area under the plasma concentration-time curve from time zero to infinity; $AUC_{r,ss}$, area under the plasma concentration-time curve over one dosage interval (12 h) at steady state; R_{ac}, accumulation ratio.
[a] Within-dose statistical comparisons, $p < 0.05$.

dogs, intravenous prucalopride induces high-amplitude contractile clusters in the proximal colon.[181] These observations suggest that prucalopride exerts its main propulsive effects via its action in the proximal colon. *In vitro* studies suggest that prucalopride is specific and selective for 5-HT$_4$ receptors in that it is devoid of affinity to muscarinic M$_3$ cholinoceptors, 5-HT$_{2A}$ and 5-HT$_3$ receptors, and cholinesterases.[181]

Pharmacodynamics

In a recent study of 39 patients with functional constipation or constipation-predominant IBS, we showed that prucalopride 2 mg and 4 mg daily accelerated overall gastric emptying and small bowel transit. Prucalopride tended to accelerate overall colonic transit, with significantly faster overall colonic transit and ascending colon emptying with the 4 mg dose.[185]

Several placebo-controlled trials of longer duration have investigated the effects of prucalopride on reported bowel movement frequency in patients with constipation.[155,186,187] Each of these Phase II trials, where prucalopride was given daily for 4 weeks, showed a dose-dependent increase in the number of bowel movements when prucalopride was compared with placebo. Taken together, these findings suggest that prucalopride accelerates colonic transit and improves bowel habit. This agent may play a future role in the management of patients with functional constipation or constipation-predominant IBS. Ongoing Phase III trials of prucalopride are being pursued for the long-term management of patients with constipation.

Pharmacokinetics

The pharmacokinetic parameters of prucalopride are summarized in Table 8.5.

Anticipated indications

As for tegaserod, the main indications for prucalopride will probably be slow-transit constipation and constipation-predominant IBS. The optimal dose will be 2–4 mg daily.

Adverse reactions

The most frequent adverse reactions reported with the intake of prucalopride 0.5–4 mg daily are mild to moderate diarrhea, flatulence, abdominal pain, nausea, and headache.

Drug interactions and contraindications

There are as yet no known drug interactions or specific contraindications. Toxicity studies in experimental animals are ongoing, and the clinical studies are currently on hold.

Table 8.5 Pharmacokinetic parameters in 12 subjects after repeated oral dosing of 2 mg prucalopride succinate.[*] Values are presented as the mean ± standard deviation. Reproduced with permission from *Prucalopride Investigator's Brochure*, 7th edn. Janssen Research Foundation, February 1999, 90.

Parameter*	Value after 2 mg prucalopride
t_{max} (h)	1.7 ± 1.3
C_{max} (ng/ml)	7.5 ± 1.5
$AUC_{0-24 h}$ (ng h/ml)	109 ± 23
Acc ratio	1.9 ± 0.4
$C_{ss,av}$ (ng/ml)	4.5 ± 1.0
$t_{1/2,term}$ (h)	30.5 ± 4.6

[*] t_{max}, time to reach C_{max} at steady state; C_{max}, maximum plasma concentration; $AUC_{0-24 h}$, area under the plasma concentration-time curve from time zero to 24 h; Acc, ratio, $AUC_{0-24 h}$; $C_{ss,av}$, average concentration at steady state; $t_{1/2 term}$, terminal half-life at steady state.

SUMMARY

In general, smooth muscle relaxants are best used sparingly, on an as-needed basis, since their overall efficacy is unclear. The 5-HT$_3$ antagonist, alosetron, results in adequate relief of pain and improvements in bowel function in female, non-constipated IBS patients. Psychotropic agents are important in relieving depression and are of proven benefit for pain and diarrhea in patients with depression associated with IBS. Further trials with selective serotonin re-uptake inhibitors (SSRIs) are awaited.

In summary, current therapies in non-ulcer dyspepsia and IBS are moderately successful. Since the sensorimotor and limbic system disturbances of functional diseases of the gastrointestinal tract are more clearly understood, we should anticipate other pharmacological approaches in the near future, including α_2-adrenergic agents, 5-HT$_{1A}$ and 5-HT$_4$ agents. New therapies are needed to relieve these *syndromes* more effectively, and not just *symptoms*.

REFERENCES

1. Barbara L, Camilleri M, Corinaldesi R, *et al.* Definition and investigation of dyspepsia: consensus of an international ad hoc working party. *Dig Dis Sci* 1989; **34:** 1272–1276.
2. Stanghellini V, Ghidini C, Maccarini MR, Paparo GF, Corinaldesi R, Barbara L. Fasting and postprandial gastrointestinal motility in ulcer and non-ulcer dyspepsia. *Gut* 1992; **33:** 184–190.
3. Greydanus MP, Vassallo M, Camilleri M, Nelson DK, Hanson RB, Thomforde GM. Neurohormonal factors in functional dyspepsia: insights on pathophysiological mechanisms. *Gastroenterology* 1991; **100:** 1311–1318.
4. Waldron B, Cullen PT, Kumar R, *et al.* Evidence for hypomotility in non-ulcer dyspepsia: a prospective multifactorial study. *Gut* 1991; **32:** 246–251.
5. Tack J, Piessevaux H, Coulie B, Caenepeel P, Janssens J. Role if impaired gastric accommodation to a meal in functional dyspepsia. *Gastroenterology* 1998; **115:** 1346–1352.
6. Thumshirn M, Camilleri M, Saslow SB, Williams DE, Burton DD, Hanson RB. Gastric accommodation in non-ulcer dyspepsia and the roles of *Helicobacter pylori* infection and vagal function. *Gut* 1999; **44:** 55–64.
7. Salet GAM, Samsom M, Roelofs JMM, vanBerge Henegouwen GP, Smout AJPM, Akkermans LMA. Responses to gastric distension in functional dyspepsia. *Gut* 1998; **42:** 823–829.
8. Jebbink HJ, Van Berge-Henegouwen GP, Bruijs PP, Akkermans LM, Smout AJ. Gastric myoelectrical activity and gastrointestinal motility in patients with functional dyspepsia. *Eur J Clin Invest* 1995; **25:** 429–437.
9. Agreus L, Svardsudd K, Nyren O, Tibblin G. Irritable bowel syndrome and dyspepsia in the general population: overlap and lack of stability over time. *Gastroenterology* 1995; **109:** 671–680.
10. Kerlin P. Postprandial antral hypomotility in patients with idiopathic nausea and vomiting. *Gut* 1989; **30:** 54–59.
11. Corinaldesi R, Stanghellini V, Raiti C, Rea E, Salgemini R, Barbara L. Effect of chronic administration of cisapride on gastric emptying of a solid meal and on dyspeptic symptoms in patients with idiopathic gastroparesis. *Gut* 1987; **28:** 300–305.
12. Jian R, Ducrot F, Ruskone A, *et al.* Symptomatic, radionuclide and therapeutic assessment of chronic idiopathic dyspepsia: a double-blind placebo-controlled evaluation of cisapride. *Dig Dis Sci* 1989; **34:** 657–664.
13. Wegener M, Borsch G, Schaffstein J, Reuter C, Leverkus F. Frequency of idiopathic gastric stasis and intestinal transit disorders in essential dyspepsia. *J Clin Gastroenterol* 1989; **11:** 163–168.
14. Geldof H, van der Schee EJ, van Blankenstein M, Grashuis JL. Electrogastrophic study of gastric myoelectrical activity in patients with unexplained nausea and vomiting. *Gut* 1986; **27:** 799–808.
15. Quartero AO, de Wit NJ, Lodder AC, Numans ME, Smout AJ, Hoes AW. Disturbed solid-phase gastric emptying in functional dyspepsia: a meta-analysis. *Dig Dis Sci* 1998; **43:** 2028–2033.
16. Scott AM, Kellow JE, Shuter B, *et al.* Intragastric distribution and gastric emptying of solids and liquids in functional dyspepsia: lack of influence of symptom subgroups and *H. pylori*-associated gastritis. *Dig Dis Sci* 1993; **38:** 2247–2254.
17. Troncon LE, Bennett RJ, Ahluwalia NK, Thompson DG. Abnormal intragastric distribu-

tion of food during gastric emptying in functional dyspepsia patients. *Gut* 1994; **35**: 327–332.

18. Crean GP, Holden RJ, Knill-Jones RP, *et al.* A database on dyspepsia. *Gut* 1994; **35**: 191–202.

19. Holtmann G, Goebell H, Jockenhoevel F, Talley NJ. Altered vagal and intestinal mechanosensory function in chronic unexplained dyspepsia. *Gut* 1998; **42**: 501–506.

20. Gilja OH, Hausken T, Wilhelmsen I, Berstad A. Impaired accommodation of proximal stomach to a meal in functional dyspepsia. *Dig Dis Sci* 1996; **41**: 689–696.

21. Lemann M, Dederding JP, Flourie B, Franchisseur C, Rambaud JC, Jian R. Abnormal perception of visceral pain in response to gastric distension in chronic idiopathic dyspepsia: the irritable stomach syndrome. *Dig Dis Sci* 1991; **36**: 1249–1254.

22. Mearin F, Cucala M, Azpiroz F, Malagelada JR. The origin of symptoms on the brain–gut axis in functional dyspepsia. *Gastroenterology* 1991; **101**: 999–1006.

23. Bradette M, Pare P, Douville P, Morin A. Visceral perception in health and functional dyspepsia. Crossover study of gastric distensions with placebo and domperidone. *Dig Dis Sci* 1991; **36**: 52–58.

24. Mertz H, Fullerton S, Naliboff B, Mayer EA. Symptoms and visceral perception in severe functional and organic dyspepsia. *Gut* 1998; **42**: 814–822.

25. Tack J, Piessevaux H, Coulie B, Caenepeel P, Janssens J. Role of visceral hypersensitivity in patients with functional dyspepsia. *Gastroenterology* 1998; **114**: G1232.

26. Tack J, Coulie B, Piessevaux H, Demedts I, Janssens J. Postprandial gastric tone determines the sensitivity to postprandial distention in functional dyspepsia. *Neurogastroenterol Mot* 1998; **10**: 102.

27. Coffin B, Azpiroz F, Guarner F, Malagelada JR. Selective gastric hypersensitivity and reflex hyporeactivity in functional dyspepsia. *Gastroenterology* 1994; **107**: 1345–1351.

28. Notivol R, Coffin B, Azpiroz F, Mearin F, Serra J, Malagelada JR. Gastric tone determines the sensitivity of the stomach to distension. *Gastroenterology* 1995; **108**: 330–336.

29. Dooley CP, Cohen H, Fitzgibbons PL, *et al.* Prevalence of *Helicobacter pylori* infection and histologic gastritis in asymptomatic persons. *N Engl J Med* 1989; **321**: 1562–1566.

30. Bernersen B, Johnson R, Bostad L, Straume B, Sommer AI, Burhol PG. Is *Helicobacter pylori* the cause of dyspepsia? *Br Med J* 1992; **304**: 1276–1279.

31. Heikkinen M, Pikkarained P, Takala J, Rasanen H, Julkunen R. Etiology of dyspepsia: four hundred unselected consecutive patients in general practice. *Scand J Gastroenterol* 1995; **30**: 519–523.

32. Talley NJ. A critique of therapeutic trials in *Helicobacter pylori*-positive functional dyspepsia. *Gastroenterology* 1994; **106**: 1174–1183.

33. Barnett JL, Behler EM, Appelman HD, Elta GH. *Campylobacter pylori* is not associated with gastroparesis. *Dig Dis Sci* 1989; **34**: 1677–1680.

34. Lambert JR. The role of *Helicobacter pylori* in nonulcer dyspepsia: a debate—for. *Gastroenterol Clin North Am* 1993; **22**: 141–151.

35. Talley NJ, Vakil N, Ballard ED, Fennert MB. Absence of benefit of eradicating *Helicobacter pylori* in patients with nonulcer dyspepsia. *N Engl J Med* 1999; **341**: 1106–1111.

36. Blum AL, Talley NJ, O'Morain C, *et al.* Lack of effect of treating *Helicobacter pylori* infection in patients with nonulcer dyspepsia. *N Engl J Med* 1998; **339**: 1875–1881.

37. McColl KEL, Murray LS, El-Omar E, *et al.* Symptomatic benefit from eradicating *Helicobacter pylori* infection in patients with nonulcer dyspepsia. *N Engl J Med* 1998; **339**: 1869–1874.

38. Tucci A, Corinaldesi R, Stanghellini V, *et al.* *Helicobacter pylori* infection and gastric function in patients with chronic idiopathic dyspepsia. *Gastroenterology* 1992; **103**: 768–774.

39. Collen MJ, Loebenberg MJ. Basal gastric acid secretion in nonulcer dyspepsia with or without duodenitis. *Dig Dis Sci* 1989; **34**: 246–250.

40. Nyren O. Secretory abnormalities in functional dyspepsia. *Scand J Gastroenterol Suppl* 1991; **182**: 25–28.

41. Dobrilla G, Comberlato M, Steele A, Vallaperta P. Drug treatment of functional dyspepsia: a meta-analysis of randomized controlled clinical trials. *J Clin Gastroenterol* 1989; **11**: 169–177.

42. Samsom M, Verhagen MAMT, vanBerge Henegouwen GP, Smouth AJPM. Abnormal clearance of exogenous acid and increased acid sensitivity of the proximal duodenum in dyspeptic patients. *Gastroenterology* 1999; **116**: 515–520.

43. Richter JE. Stress and psychologic and environmental factors in functional dyspepsia. *Scand J Gastroenterol Suppl* 1991; **182**: 40–46.

44. Nyren O, Adami HO, Gustavsson S, Loof L. Excess sick-listing in nonulcer dyspepsia. *J Clin Gastroenterol* 1986; **8:** 339–345.

45. Kellner R. Psychosomatic syndromes, somatization and somatoform disorders. *Psychother Psychosom* 1994; **61:** 4–24.

46. Haug TT, Svebak S, Wilhelmsen I, Berstad A, Ursin H. Psychological factors and somatic symptoms in functional dyspepsia: a comparison with duodenal ulcer and healthy controls. *J Psychosom Res* 1994; **38:** 281–291.

47. Ford MJ, Zinsmeister AR, Hanson RB, Camilleri M. Psychosensory modulation of colonic sensation in health: evidence for regional and sensory specificity [Abstract]. *Gastroenterology* 1995; **108(Suppl.):** A600.

48. Bharucha AE, Camilleri M, Ford MJ, O'Connor MK, Hanson RB, Thomforde GM. Hyperventilation alters colonic motor and sensory function: effects and mechanisms in humans. *Gastroenterology* 1996; **111:** 368–377.

49. Bennett EJ, Kellow JE, Cowan H, *et al.* Suppression of anger and gastric emptying in patients with functional dyspepsia. *Scand J Gastroenterol* 1992; **27:** 869–874.

50. Whitehead WE. Behavioral medicine approaches to gastrointestinal disorders. *J Consult Clin Psychol* 1992; **60:** 605–612.

51. Veldhuyzen van Zanten SJO, Cleary C, Talley NJ, *et al.* Drug treatment of functional dyspepsia: a systematic analysis of trial methodology with recommendations for design of future trials. *Am J Gastroenterol* 1996; **91:** 660–671.

52. American Gastroenterological Association medical position statement: evaluation of dyspepsia. *Gastroenterology* 1998; **114:** 579–581.

53. Fisher RS, Parkman HP. Management of nonulcer dyspepsia. *N Engl J Med* 1998; **19:** 1376–1381.

54. Talley NJ, Meineche-Schmidt V, Pare P, *et al.* Efficacy of omeprazole in functional dyspepsia: double-blind, randomized, placebo-controlled trials (the Bond and Opera studies). *Aliment Pharm Ther* 1998; **12:** 1055–1065.

55. Halter F, Miazza B, Brignoli R. Cisapride or cimetidine in the treatment of functional dyspepsia: results of a double-blind, randomized, Swiss multicentre study. *Scand J Gastroenterol* 1994; **29:** 618–623.

56. Jian R, Ducrot F, Ruskone A, *et al.* Symptomatic, radionuclide and therapeutic assessment of chronic idiopathic dyspepsia. A double-blind placebo-controlled evaluation of cisapride. *Dig Dis Sci* 1989; **34:** 657–664.

57. Corinaldesi R, Stanghellini V, Raiti C, Rea E, Salgemini R, Barbara L. Effect of chronic administration of cisapride on gastric emptying of a solid meal and on dyspeptic symptoms in patients with idiopathic gastroparesis. *Gut* 1987; **28:** 300–305.

58. Ghoos YF, Maes BD, Geypens BJ, *et al.* Measurement of gastric emptying rate of solids by means of a carbon-labeled octanoic acid breath test. *Gastroenterology* 1993; **104:** 1640–1647.

59. Choi MG, Camilleri M, Burton DD, Zinsmeister AR, Forstrom LA, Nair KS. [^{13}C]octanoic acid breath test for gastric emptying of solids: accuracy, reproducibility, and comparison with scintigraphy. *Gastroenterology* 1997; **112:** 1155–1162.

60. Clouse RE. Antidepressants for functional gastrointestinal syndromes. *Dig Dis Sci* 1994; **39:** 2352–2363.

61. Gorelick AB, Koshy SS, Hooper FG, Bennett TC, Chey WD, Hasler WL. Differential effects of amitriptyline on perception of somatic and visceral stimulation in healthy humans. *Am J Physiol* 1998; **275:** G460–466.

62. Mertz H, Fass R, Kodner A, Yan-Go F, Fullerton S, Mayer EA. Effect of amitriptyline on symptoms, sleep, and visceral perception in patients with functional dyspepsia. *Am J Gastroenterol* 1998; **93:** 160–165.

63. Thumshirn M, Camilleri M, Choi MG, Zinsmeister AR. Modulation of gastric sensory and motor functions by nitrergic and alpha2-adrenergic agents in humans. *Gastroenterology* 1999; **116:** 573–585.

64. Read NW, Abitbol JL, Bardhan KD, Whorwell PJ, Fraitag B. Efficacy and safety of the peripheral kappa agonist fedotozine versus placebo in the treatment of functional dyspepsia. *Gut* 1997; **41:** 664–668.

65. Zerbib F, Bruley des Varannes S, Oriola RC, McDonald J, Isal JP, Galmiche JP. Alosetron does not affect the visceral perception of gastric distension in healthy subjects. *Aliment Pharm Ther* 1994; **8:** 403–407.

66. Tack J, Coulie B, Wilmer A, Andrioli A, Janssens J. Influence of sumatriptan on gastric fundus tone and on the perception of gastric distention in man. *Gut* 2000; **46:** 468–473.

67. Tack J, Piessevaux H, Coulie B, Fischler B, De

Gucht V, Janssens J. A placebo-controlled trial of buspirone, a fundus-relaxing drug, in functional dyspepsia: effect on symptoms and gastric sensory and motor function. *Gastroenterology* 1999; **116**: A325.

68. Manning AP, Thompson WG, Heaton KW, Morris AF. Towards a positive diagnosis of the irritable bowel. *Br Med J* 1978; **2**: 653–654.

69. Talley NJ, Phillips SF, Melton LJ, *et al.* Diagnostic value of the Manning criteria in irritable bowel syndrome. *Gut* 1990; **31**: 77–81.

70. Thompson WG, Dotevall G, Drossman DA, Heaton KW, Kruis W. Irritable bowel syndrome: guidelines for the diagnosis. *Gastroenterol Int* 1989; **2**: 92–95.

71. Thompson WG, Longstreth GF, Drossman DA, Heaton KW, Irvine EJ, Muller-Lissner SA. Functional bowel disorders and functional abdominal pain. *Gut* 1999; **45 (Suppl II)**: II43–II47.

72. Camilleri M, Choi MG. Review article: irritable bowel syndrome. *Aliment Pharmacol Ther* 1997; **11**: 3–15.

73. Drossman DA, Whitehead WE, Camilleri M. Irritable bowel syndrome: a technical review for practice guideline development. *Gastroenterology* 1997; **112**: 2120–2137.

74. Gwee KA, Leong YL, Graham C, *et al.* The role of psychological and biological factors in postinfective gut dysfunction. *Gut* 1999; **44**: 400–406.

75. Camilleri M, Neri M. Motility and stress. *Dig Dis Sci* 1989; **34**: 1777–1786.

76. Alvarez WC. Ways in which emotion can affect the digestive tract, and help in sizing up the patient. In: *Nervousness, Indigestion and Pain.* Paul B. Hoeber, New York, 1943, 2–21, 83–99.

77. Almy TP, Tulin M. Alterations in man under stress. Experimental production of changes simulating 'irritable colon'. *Gastroenterology* 1947; **8**: 616–626.

78. Chaudhary NA, Truelove SC. Human colonic motility: a comparative study of normal subjects, patients with ulcerative colitis, and patients with the irritable colon syndrome. I. Resting patterns of motility. *Gastroenterology* 1961; **40**: 1–17.

79. Horowitz L, Farrar JT. Intraluminal small intestinal pressure in normal patients and in patients with functional gastrointestinal disorders. *Gastroenterology* 1962; **42**: 455–464.

80. Kellow JE, Phillips SF. Altered small bowel motility in irritable bowel syndrome is correlated with symptoms. *Gastroenterology* 1987; **92**: 1885–1893.

81. Whitehead WE, Engel BT, Schuster MM. Irritable bowel syndrome. Physiological and psychological differences between diarrhea-predominant and constipation-predominant patients. *Dig Dis Sci* 1980; **25**: 404–413.

82. Bazzocchi G, Ellis J, Meyer J, *et al.* Colonic scintigraphy and manometry in constipation, diarrhea, and inflammatory bowel disease. *Gastroenterology* 1988; **94**: 29 [Abstract].

83. Bazzocchi G, Ellis J, Villanueva-Meyer J, *et al.* Postprandial colonic transit and motor activity in chronic constipation. *Gastroenterology* 1990; **98**: 686–693.

84. Cann PA, Read NW, Brown C, Hobson N, Holdsworth CD. Irritable bowel syndrome: relationship of disorders in the transit of a single solid meal to symptom patterns. *Gut* 1983; **24**: 405–411.

85. Vassallo M, Camilleri M, Phillips SF, *et al.* Transit through the proximal colon influences stool weight in irritable bowel syndrome. *Gastroenterology* 1992; **102**: 102–108.

86. Stivland T, Camilleri M, Vassallo M, *et al.* Scintigraphic measurement of regional gut transit in idiopathic constipation. *Gastroenterology* 1991; **101**: 107–115.

87. Talley NJ, Fett SL, Zinsmeister AR. Self-reported abuse and gastrointestinal disease in outpatients: association with irritable bowel-type symptoms. *Am J Gastroenterol* 1995; **90**: 366–371.

88. Ritchie J. Pain from distension of the pelvic colon by inflating a balloon in the irritable bowel syndrome. *Gut* 1973; **14**: 125–132.

89. Prior A, Maxton DG, Whorwell PJ. Anorectal manometry in irritable bowel syndrome: differences between diarrhoea and constipation predominant subjects. *Gut* 1990; **31**: 458–462.

90. Mertz H, Naliboff B, Munakata J, Niazi N, Mayer EA. Altered rectal perception is a biological marker of patients with irritable bowel syndrome. *Gastroenterology* 1995; **109**: 40–52.

91. Cook IJ, van Eeden A, Collins SM. Patients with irritable bowel syndrome have greater pain tolerance than normal subjects. *Gastroenterology* 1987; **93**: 727–733.

92. Mayer EA, Raybould HE. Role of visceral afferent mechanisms in functional bowel disorders. *Gastroenterology* 1990; **99**: 1688–1704.

93. Aggarwal A, Cutts TF, Abell TL, *et al.* Predominant symptoms in irritable bowel syndrome correlate with specific autonomic nervous system abnormalities. *Gastroenterology* 1994; **106:** 945–950.

94. Drossman DA, McKee DC, Sandler RS, *et al.* Psychosocial factors in the irritable bowel syndrome: a multivariate study of patients and nonpatients with irritable bowel syndrome. *Gastroenterology* 1988; **95:** 701–708.

95. Whitehead WE, Bosmajian L, Zonderman A, Costa PT, Schuster MM. Role of psychologic symptoms in irritable bowel syndrome: comparison of community and clinic samples. *Gastroenterology* 1988; **95:** 709–714.

96. Drossman DA, Talley NJ, Leserman J, Olden KW, Barreiro MA. Sexual and physical abuse and gastrointestinal illness. *Ann Intern Med* 1995; **123:** 782–794.

97. Painter NS. Irritable or irritated bowel. *Br Med J* 1972; **2:** 46.

98. McMichael HB, Webb J, Dawson AM. Lactase deficiency in adults: a cause of functional diarrhoea. *Lancet* 1965; **1:** 717–720.

99. Bayless TM, Rosensweig NS. A racial difference in incidence of lactase deficiency: a survey of milk intolerance and lactase deficiency in healthy adult males. *J Am Med Assoc* 1966; **197:** 968–972.

100. Newcomer AD, McGill DB. Irritable bowel syndrome: role of lactase deficiency. *Mayo Clin Proc* 1983; **59:** 339–341.

101. Hyams JS. Sorbitol intolerance: an unappreciated cause of functional gastrointestinal complaints. *Gastroenterology* 1983; **84:** 30–33.

102. Rumessen JJ, Gudmand-Hoyer E. Functional bowel disease: malabsorption and abdominal distress after ingestion of fructose, sorbitol and fructose–sorbitol mixtures. *Gastroenterology* 1988; **95:** 694–700.

103. Spiller RC, Brown ML, Phillips SF. Decreased fluid tolerance, accelerated transit, and abnormal motility of the human colon induced by oleic acid. *Gastroenterology* 1986; **91:** 100–107.

104. Kamath PS, Hoepfner MT, Phillips SF. Short-chain fatty acids stimulate motility of the canine ileum. *Am J Physiol* 1987; **253:** G427–433.

105. Nelis GF, Vermeeren M, Jansen W. Does fructose-sorbitol malabsorption (FSM) play a role in the aetiology of the irritable bowel syndrome? *Gastroenterology* 1990; **98:** A194.

106. Scott RB, Dramant SC, Gall DG. Motility effects of intestinal anaphylaxis in the rat. *Am J Physiol* 1988; **255:** G505–511.

107. Nanda R, James R, Smith H, Dudley CRK, Jewell DP. Food intolerance and the irritable bowel syndrome. *Gut* 1989; **30:** 1098–1104.

108. Oddsson E, Rask-Madsen J, Krag E. A secretory epithelium of the small intestine with increased sensitivity to bile acids in irritable bowel syndrome associated with diarrhoea. *Scand J Gastroenterol* 1978; **13:** 409–416.

109. Merrick MV, Eastwood MA, Ford MJ. Is bile acid malabsorption underdiagnosed? An evaluation of accuracy of diagnosis by measurement of SeHCAT retention. *Br Med J* 1985; **290:** 665–668.

110. Chaudhary NA, Truelove SC. The irritable colon syndrome. A study of the clinical features, predisposing causes, and prognosis in 130 cases. *Quart J Med* 1962; **31:** 307–322.

111. Klein KB. Controlled treatment trials in the irritable bowel syndrome. *Gastroenterology* 1988; **95:** 232–241.

112. Poynard T, Naveau S, Mory B, Chaput JC. Meta-analysis of smooth muscle relaxants in the treatment of irritable bowel syndrome. *Aliment Pharmacol Ther* 1994; **8:** 499–510.

113. Cann PA, Read NW, Holdsworth CD. What is the benefit of coarse wheat bran in patients with irritable bowel syndrome? *Gut* 1984; **25:** 168–173.

114. Jarrett M, Heitkemper MM, Bond EF, Georges J. Comparison of diet composition in women with and without functional bowel disorder. *Gastroenterol Nursing* 1994; **6:** 253.

115. Distrutti E, Azpiroz F, Soldevilla A, Malagelada J-R. Gastric wall tension determines perception of gastric distention. *Gastroenterology* 1999; **116:** 1035–1042.

116. Thumshirn M, Camilleri M, Choi M-G, Zinsmeister AR. Modulation of gastric sensory and motor functions by nitrergic and alpha$_2$-adrenergic agents in humans. *Gastroenterology* 1999; **116:** 573–585.

117. Malcolm A, Phillips SF, Camilleri M, Hanson RP. Pharmacological modulation of rectal tone alters perception of distention in humans. *Am J Gastroenterol* 1997; **92:** 2073–2079.

118. Mueller-Lissner SA. Effect of wheat bran on weight of stool and gastrointestinal transit time: a meta-analysis. *Br Med J* 1988; **296:** 615–617.

119. Cook IJ, Irvine EJ, Campbell D, Shannon S, Reddy SN, Collins SM. Effect of dietary fiber on symptoms and rectosigmoid motility in patients

with irritable bowel syndrome. *Gastroenterology* 1990; **98**: 66–72.

120. Snook J, Shepherd HA. Bran supplementation in the treatment of irritable bowel syndrome. *Aliment Pharmacol Ther* 1994; **8**: 511–514.

121. Francis CY, Whorwell PJ. Bran and irritable bowel syndrome: time for reappraisal. *Lancet* 1994; **344**: 39–40.

122. Whitehead WE, Holtkotter B, Enck P, Hoelzl R, Holmes KD, Anthony J, Shabsin HS, Schuster MM. Tolerance for rectosigmoid distention in irritable bowel syndrome. *Gastroenterology* 1990; **98**: 1187–1192.

123. Haderstorfer B, Psycholgin D, Whitehead WE, Schuster MM. Intestinal gas production from bacterial fermentation of undigested carbohydrate in irritable bowel syndrome. *Am J Gastroenterol* 1989; **84**: 375–378.

124. Lasser RB, Levitt MD. The role of intestinal gas in functional abdominal pain. *N Engl J Med* 1975; **293**: 524–526.

125. Lucey MR, Clark ML, Lowndes J, Dawson AM. Is bran efficacious in irritable bowel syndrome? A double-blind, placebo-controlled crossover study. *Gut* 1987; **28**: 221–225.

126. Hillman LC, Stace NH, Pomare EW. Irritable bowel patients and their long-term response to a high fiber diet. *Am J Gastroenterol* 1984; **79**: 1–7.

127. Pittler MH, Ernst E. Peppermint oil for irritable bowel syndrome: a critical review and meta-analysis. *Am J Gastroenterol* 1998; **93**: 1131–1135.

128. Jones RH, Holtmann G, Rodrigo L, *et al.* Alosetron relieves pain and improves bowel function compared with mebeverine in female nonconstipated irritable bowel syndrome patients. *Aliment Pharmacol Ther* 1999; **13**: 1419–1427.

129. Vassallo MJ, Camilleri M, Phillips SF, Steadman CJ, Hanson RB, Haddad AC. Colonic tone and motility in patients with irritable bowel syndrome. *Mayo Clin Proc* 1992; **67**: 725–731.

130. Cann PA, Read NW, Holdsworth CD, Barends D. Role of loperamide and placebo in management of irritable bowel syndrome. *Dig Dis Sci* 1984; **29**: 239–247.

131. Read M, Read NW, Barber DC, Duthie HL. Effects of loperamide on anal sphincter function in patients complaining of chronic diarrhea with fecal incontinence and urgency. *Dig Dis Sci* 1982; **27**: 807–814.

132. Rattan S, Culver PJ. Influence of loperamide on

the internal anal sphincter in the opossum. *Gastroenterology* 1987; **93**: 121–128.

133. Musial F, Enck P, Kalveram KT, Erckenbrecht JF. The effect of loperamide on anorectal unction in normal healthy men. *J Clin Gastroenterol* 1992; **15**: 321–324.

134. Hallgren T, Fasth S, Delbro DS, Nordgren S, Oresland T, Hulter L. Loperamide improves anal sphincter function and continence after restorative proctocolectomy. *Dig Dis Sci* 1994; **39**: 2612–2618.

135. Sun WM, Read NW, Verlinden M. Effects of loperamide oxide on gastrointestinal transit time and anorectal function in patients with chronic diarrhoea and faecal incontinence. *Scand J Gastroenterol* 1997; **32**: 34–38.

136. Sciarretta G, Fagioli G, Fumo A, *et al.* 75Se HCAT test in the detection of bile acid malabsorption in functional diarrhoea and its correlation with small bowel transit. *Gut* 1987; **28**: 970–975.

137. Thaysen EH, Pedersen L. Idiopathic bile salt catharsis. *Gut* 1976; **17**: 965–970.

138. Luman W, Williams AJ, Merrick MV, Eastwood MA. Idiopathic bile acid malabsorption: long-term outcome. *Eur J Gastroenterol Hepatol* 1995; **7**: 641–645.

139. Heefner JD, Wilder RM, Wilson JD. Irritable colon and depression. *Psychosomatics* 1978; **19**: 540–547.

140. Hislop IG. Psychological significance of the irritable colon syndrome. *Gut* 1971; **12**: 452–457.

141. Lancaster-Smith MJ, Prout BJ, Pinto T, Anderson JA, Schiff AA. Influence of drug treatment on the irritable bowel syndrome and its interaction with psychoneurotic morbidity. *Acta Psychiatr Scand* 1982; **66**: 33–41.

142. Onghena P, Houdenhove BV. Antidepressant-induced analgesia in chronic non-malignant pain: a meta-analysis of 39 placebo-controlled studies. *Pain* 1992; **49**: 205–219.

143. Myren J, Groth H, Larssen SE, Larsen S. The effect of trimipramine in patients with the irritable bowel syndrome. *Scand J Gastroenterol* 1982; **17**: 871–875.

144. Myren J, Lovland B, Larssen S-E, Larsen S. A double-blind study of the effect of trimipramine in patients with the irritable bowel syndrome. *Scand J Gastroenterol* 1984; **19**: 835–843.

145. Greenbaum DS, Mayle JE, Vanegeren LE, *et al.* The effects of desipramine on IBS compared

with atropine and placebo. *Dig Dis Sci* 1987; **32:** 257–266.

146. Gram LF. Fluoxetine. *N Engl J Med* 1994; **20:** 1354–1361.

147. Whorwell PJ, Prior A, Faragher EB. Hypnotherapy in irritable bowel syndrome. *Lancet* 1984; **ii:** 1232–1234.

148. Svedlund J. Psychotherapy in irritable bowel syndrome: a controlled outcome study. *Acta Psychiatr Scand* 1983; **67:** 1–86.

149. Guthrie E, Creed F, Dawson D, Tomerson B. A controlled trial of psychological treatment for the irritable bowel syndrome. *Gastroenterology* 1991; **100:** 450–457.

150. Dapoigny M, Abitbol JL, Fraitag B. Efficacy of peripheral kappa agonist, fedotozine, vs placebo in treatment of irritable bowel syndrome. A multicenter dose-response study. *Dig Dis Sci* 1995; **40:** 2244–2249.

151. Camilleri M, Mayer EA, Drossman DA, *et al.* Improvement in pain and bowel function in female irritable bowel patients with alosetron, a 5-HT$_3$-receptor antagonist. *Aliment Pharmacol Ther* 1999; **13:** 1149–1159.

152. Camilleri M, Northcutt AR, Kong S, Dukes GE, McSorley D, Mangel AW. The efficacy and safety of alosetron in female patients with irritable bowel syndrome: a randomised, placebo-controlled trial. *Lancet* 2000; **355:** 1030–1031.

153. Prather CM, Camilleri M, Zinsmeister AR, McKinzie S, Thomforde G. Tegaserod accelerates orocecal transit in patients with constipation-predominant irritable bowel syndrome. *Gastroenterology* 2000; **118:** 463–468.

154. Lefkowitz M, Shi Y, Schmitt C, Krumholz S, Tanghe J. The 5HT$_4$ partial agonist, tegaserod, improves abdominal discomfort/pain and normalizes altered bowel function in irritable bowel syndrome (IBS). *Am J Gastroenterol* 1999; **94:** 396.

155. Coremans G, Kerstens R, De Pauw M, Stevens M. Effects of a new enterokinetic drug, prucalopride, on symptoms of patients with severe chronic constipation: a double-blind, placebo-controlled pilot study. *Gastroenterology* 1999; **116:** A978.

156. Coulie B, Tack J, Vos R, Janssens J. Influence of the 5-HT$_{1A}$ agonist buspirone on rectal tone and on the perception of rectal distension in man. *Gastroenterology* 1998; **114:** G3046.

157. Viramontes B, Malcolm A, Szarka L, *et al.* Dose-related effects of α_2-adrenergic agent, clonidine,

on human gastrointestinal motor, transit and sensory functions. *Gastroenterology* 2000; **118:** A666 [Abstract].

158. Camilleri M. Pharmacology and clinical experience with alosetron. *Exp Opin Invest Drugs* 2000; **9:** 1–13.

159. Gershon MD. Serotonin: its role and receptors in enteric neurotransmission. *Adv Exper Med Biol* 1991; **294:** 221–230.

160. Gershon MD. Review article: roles played by 5-hydroxytryptamine in the physiology of the bowel. *Aliment Pharm Ther* 1999; **13:** 15–30.

161. von der Ohe MR, Camilleri M, Kvols LK. A 5-HT$_3$ antagonist corrects the postprandial colonic hypertonic response in carcinoid diarrhea. *Gastroenterology* 1994; **106:** 1184–1189.

162. von der Ohe MR, Hanson RB, Camilleri M. Serotonergic mediation of postprandial colonic tonic and phasic responses in humans. *Gut* 1994; **35:** 536–541.

163. Delvaux M, Louvel D, Mamet JP, Campos-Oriola R, Frexinos J. Effect of alosetron on responses to colonic distension in patients with irritable bowel syndrome. *Aliment Pharm Ther* 1998; **12:** 849–855.

164. von der Ohe MR, Camilleri M, Kvols LK, Thomforde GM. Motor dysfunction of the small bowel and colon in patients with the carcinoid syndrome and diarrhea. *N Engl J Med* 1993; **329:** 1073–1078.

165. Prior A, Read NW. Reduction of rectal sensitivity and postprandial motility by granisetron, a 5-HT$_3$ receptor antagonist, in patients with irritable bowel syndrome. *Aliment Pharm Ther* 1993; **7:** 175–180.

166. Thumshirn M, Coulie B, Camilleri M, Burton D, Zinsmeister AR. Evaluation of potential sites of action of alosetron in irritable bowel syndrome. *Neurogastroenterol Motility* 1999; **11:** 295 [Abstract].

167. Houghton LA, Foster J, Whorwell PJ, McDonald JN. Effect of alosetron, a new 5-HT$_3$ antagonist, on gastrointestinal transit in normal healthy volunteers. *Gastroenterology* 1995; **108:** A618 [Abstract].

168. Foster JM, Houghton LA, Whorwell PJ. Alosetron slows colonic transit in patients with irritable bowel syndrome. *Gastroenterology* 1997; **112:** A732 [Abstract].

169. Camilleri M, Mayer EA, Drossman DA, *et al.* Improvement in pain and bowel function in female irritable bowel patients with alosetron, a

5-HT$_3$-receptor antagonist. *Aliment Pharmacol Ther* 1999; **13:** 1149–1159.

170. Bardhan K, Bodemar G, Geldof H, Schutz E, Snell C, Darekar B. A double-blind, placebo-controlled study to evaluate the efficacy of alosetron in the treatment of irritable bowel syndrome. *Gastroenterology* 1996; **110:** A630 [Abstract].

171. Camilleri M, Chey WY, Mayer EA, *et al.* Alosetron in the treatment of pain and bowel function in female, non-constipated, irritable bowel syndrome patients. *Arch Intern Med.* In press.

172. Jones RH, Holtmann G, Rodrigo L, *et al.* Alosetron relieves pain and improves bowel function compared with mebeverine in female nonconstipated irritable bowel syndrome patients. *Aliment Pharm Ther* 1999; **13:** 1419–1427.

173. Pfannkuche HJ, Buhl T, Gamse R, Hoyer D, Mattes H, Buchheit KH. The properties of a new prokinetically active drug, SDZ HTF 919. *Neurogastroenterol Mot* 1995; **7:** 280.

174. Hoyer D, Fehlmann D, Langenegger D, *et al.* High-affinity of SDZ HTF 919 and related molecules for calf and human caudate 5-HT$_4$ receptors. Naunyn-Schmied. *Arch Pharmacol* 1998; **357:** R29.

175. Wiseman LR, Faulds D. Cisapride. An updated review of its pharmacology and therapeutic efficacy as a prokinetic agent in gastrointestinal motility disorders. *Drugs* 1994; **47:** 116–152.

176. Grider J, Foxx-Orenstein AE, Jin JG. 5-Hydroxytryptamine$_4$ receptor agonists initiate the peristaltic reflex in human, rat and guinea pig intestine. *Gastroenterology* 1998; **115:** 370–380.

177. Nguyen A, Camilleri M, Kost LJ, *et al.* SDZ HTF 919 stimulates canine colonic motility and transit *in vivo. J Pharmacol Exper Ther* 1997; **280:** 1270–1276.

178. Appel S, Kumle A, Hubert M, Duvauchelle T. First pharmacokinetic–pharmacodynamic study in humans with a selective 5-hydroxytryptamine$_4$ receptor agonist. *J Clin Pharmacol* 1997; **37:** 229–237.

179. Appel S, Kumle A, Meier R. Clinical pharmacodynamics of SDZ HTF 919, a new 5-HT$_4$ receptor agonist, in a model of slow colonic transit. *Clin Pharmacol Ther* 1997; **62:** 546–555.

180. Langaker KJ, Morris D, Pruitt R, Otten M, Stewart W, Rueegg PC. The partial 5-HT$_4$ agonist (HTF 919) improves symptoms in constipation-predominant irritable bowel syndrome. *Digestion* 1998; **59:** 20.

181. Briejer MR, Meulemans AL, Bosmans J-P, *et al.* *In vitro* pharmacology of the novel enterokinetic R093877. *Gastroenterology* 1997; **112:** A705.

182. Briejer MR, Ghoos E, Eelen J, Schuurkes JAJ. Serotonin 5-HT$_4$ receptors mediate the R093877-induced changes in contractile patterns in the canine colon. *Gastroenterology* 1997; **112:** A705.

183. Emmanuel AV, Kamm MA, Roy AJ, *et al.* Effect of a novel prokinetic drug, R093877, on gastrointestinal transit in healthy volunteers. *Gut* 1998; **42:** 511–516.

184. Bouras EP, Camilleri M, Burton DD, McKinzie S. Selective stimulation of colonic transit by the benzofuran 5-HT$_4$ agonist, prucalopride, in healthy humans. *Gut* 1999; **44:** 682–686.

185. Camilleri M, McKinzie S, Burton D, Thomforde G, Zinsmeister AR, Bouras EP. Prucalopride accelerates small bowel and colonic transit in patients with chronic functional constipation (FC) or constipation-predominant irritable bowel syndrome (C-IBS). *Gastroenterology* 2000; **118:** A845 [Abstract].

186. D'Hooghe B, Guillaume D, Medaer R, *et al.* Treatment of constipation in a multiple sclerosis patients: pilot study with the novel enterokinetic prucalopride. *Neurogastroenterol Mot* 1999; **11:** A256.

187. Miner PB, Nicholas T Jr, Silvers DR, Joslyn A, Woods M. The efficacy and safety of prucalopride in patients with chronic constipation. *Gastroenterology* 1999; **116:** A1043.

9

Gastrointestinal cancer

Justin S Waters, David Cunningham

INTRODUCTION

Cancer of the gastrointestinal tract (GIT) is a major health problem worldwide. Colorectal cancer is the second most common malignancy in men and women in the European Union (EU). The overall incidence of gastrointestinal tract tumours in the EU in 1990 was 68.5 per 100 000 population in men, and 38.3 per 100 000 in women. Mortality rates in that year were 51.1 per 100 000 men, and 26.9 per 100 000 women, reflecting the fact that between two-thirds and three-quarters of patients diagnosed with GIT gastrointestinal tract malignancy ultimately die as a result of their disease, a number exceeding 250 000 patients per year in the EU.[1]

The medical management of gastrointestinal tract cancer has evolved rapidly over recent years. Although traditionally considered to be chemotherapy insensitive, these tumours have proven responsive to several new cytotoxic agents and combination regimens. Adjuvant treatment has become established in colorectal cancer, and neoadjuvant chemotherapy is being investigated in gastric and oesophageal cancer. In the advanced disease setting, palliative chemotherapy has shown survival and quality of life benefits in several tumour types. Combined modality treatment with chemotherapy and radiotherapy exploits the ability of some drugs to sensitize cells to the cytotoxic effects of radiation, while simultaneously delivering a systemic treatment to eradicate microscopic disease outside the radiotherapy field. This approach has been adopted successfully for the treatment of locally advanced tumours of the oesophagus, pancreas, rectum and anus.

The explosion in knowledge resulting from the substantial advances being made in molecular biology has introduced the exciting possibility of targeted tumour therapy. Angiogenesis inhibitors, antibody-based therapy, tumour vaccines, antisense oligonucleotide therapy and gene therapy are some of the fields in which clinical progress is being made.

Pathophysiology

Conventional cytotoxic agents are all designed to target aspects of cell replication, thus exploiting the differential rate of cell division in malignant and normal tissues. This is achieved in several different ways. Several classes of chemotherapeutic drugs target DNA directly, either by intercalation, or by forming cross-linking adducts within or between DNA strands. These lesions have several effects, notably inhibition of DNA replication but also impairment of DNA repair processes, and inhibition of transcription. Examples of drugs with this mechanism of action include the platinum drugs, and mitomycin C.

Topoisomerases are enzymes that alter DNA topology, which is an essential part of the DNA replication process. The topoisomerase forms a complex with the DNA molecule and introduces a single-stranded break, allowing the passage of a second double helix through the break, or rotation of the molecule around the remaining intact strand. The break is then resealed, and the topoisomerase dissociates from the DNA. The anthracyclines and etoposide stabilize the topoisomerase II/DNA complex, thus stimulating DNA cleavage. A similar effect is produced on topoisomerase I by the camptothecins. In the presence of ongoing DNA synthesis, the breaks produced are converted into double-strand breaks, leading to S/G_2 cell cycle arrest, and ultimately to cell death.

Indirect effects on DNA synthesis are produced by the antimetabolite drugs, which have substantial importance in the field of gastrointestinal malignancy. De novo thymidine biosynthesis is required for DNA synthesis, and this pathway is the target of several antimetabolites (Fig. 9.1). 5-Fluorouracil is metabolized by the enzyme phosphoribosyl pyrophosphate transferase to 5-fluorodeoxyuridine monophosphate. This inhibits thymidylate synthase by forming a stable complex with the enzyme and folate. Incorporation of 5-fluorouracil and its metabolites into RNA and DNA also occurs, and may also contribute to its cytotoxicity, although the lack of specificity of its action may be responsible for some of the toxicity seen with this drug. The activity of 5-fluorouracil is enhanced by the co-administration of folinic acid. This increases the cellular pool of N_5N_{10}-methylene tetrahydrofolate, resulting in increased stability of the 5-fluorouracil/ thymidylate synthase/folate complex. Other strategies adopted to enhance the activity of 5-fluorouracil are the co-administration of inhibitors of dihydropyrimidine dehydrogenase, an enzyme involved in the metabolism of 5-fluorouracil, and the use of prodrugs that can be converted into 5-fluorouracil by enzymatic action within the liver or within the tumour itself. These strategies have allowed the development of orally bioavailable drugs. A more

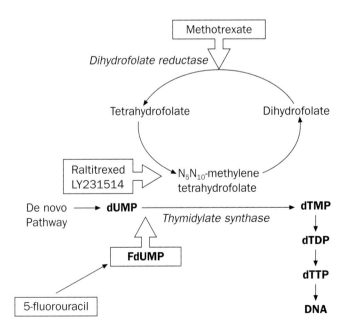

Figure 9.1 Mechanism of action of four antimetabolite cytotoxic drugs. The action of 5-fluorouracil, methotrexate and the two direct thymidylate synthase inhibitors raltitrexed and LY231514 on the nucleotide synthetic pathway is shown.
FdUMP, fluoro deoxyuridine monophosphate;
dUMP, deoxyuridine monophosphate;
dTMP, deoxthymidine monophosphate;
dTDP, deoxthymidine diphosphate;
dTTP, deoxthymidine triphosphate.

specific inhibition of thymidylate synthase has been attempted by the development of folate analogues such as raltitrexed and LY231514. Polyglutamation of these drugs within the cell enhances their affinity for the folate binding site of thymidylate synthase, and prolongs their intracellular half-life.

Methotrexate is another antimetabolite used in the gastrointestinal malignancies. This inhibits the enzyme dihydrofolate reductase, which catalyses the conversion of dihydrofolate to tetrahydrofolate, providing a source of reduced folate for one-carbon transfer reactions. A functional enzyme is therefore required for the maintenance of *de novo* purine and thymidylate biosynthesis, for protein synthesis, and for various methylation pathways. Methotrexate appears also to have direct inhibitory activity on other folate-dependent enzymes including thymidylate synthase, and it is probably a combination of these activities that result in its cytotoxic effects.

A more recently developed antimetabolite drug that is proving very useful, particularly in carcinoma of the pancreas, is gemcitabine. This is a cytidine analogue that is incorporated into DNA in its triphosphate form, after activation by deoxycytidine kinase. This results in chain termination after the addition of one further nucleotide. It also inhibits the activity of several enzymes involved in cytidine metabolism, including ribonucleotide reductase, dCMP deaminase, and CTP synthetase, and is incorporated into RNA, leading to inhibition of RNA synthesis. Cell cycle arrest occurs in the S phase followed by the induction of cell death by apoptosis.

The taxanes are a novel class of drugs that interfere with cell division by interaction with microtubules rather than with DNA or RNA. Paclitaxel and docetaxel bind to β-tubulin, resulting in conformational changes in tubulin dimers, and stabilization of the microtubule, thus inhibiting its function. The precise mechanism by which this leads to cytotoxicity has not yet been fully elucidated. Studies of the taxanes in various systems have demonstrated that exposure of cells to these agents can lead to the induction of apoptosis, possibly involving phosphoregulation pathways. However, cell-cycle arrest without apoptosis has also been observed, suggesting that cell death may result by more than one mechanism. The involvement of several cell-cycle and apoptosis-related genes in this process, including P53 and *bcl-2*, is currently the subject of investigation.

The obvious disadvantage of cytotoxic agents is their propensity to cause significant side-effects, largely as a result of killing normal cells undergoing division, as well as malignant ones. Several strategies are now being developed to target more specifically the tumour cell, drawing on advances in knowledge of the molecular biology of carcinogenesis and metastasis. Most of these approaches are currently in the preclinical or very early clinical stages of development, and are beyond the scope of this chapter to discuss in detail.

THERAPEUTIC APPROACHES AND TREATMENT REGIMENS FOR GASTROINTESTINAL CANCER

Epithelial malignancies

Carcinoma may arise at any site in the gastrointestinal tract, from the oesophagus to the anus. Tumours of the mouth and pharynx are traditionally considered separately from those of the remainder of the gastrointestinal tract, falling under the remit of specialists in head and neck cancer. Tumours arising at different sites present very different problems to the gastrointestinal oncology team, owing to differences in the feasibility of curative surgery and radical radiotherapy. In addition, the natural history of carcinoma arising from different sites is variable, as is the sensitivity of the tumour to cytotoxic drug therapy.

Oesophagus
Carcinoma of the oesophagus is a chemotherapy-sensitive tumour, and such treatment is useful in the palliation of advanced disease. In addition, although surgery remains the

mainstay of therapy for localized disease, the relatively poor outcome of this approach has prompted the investigation of chemotherapy, radiotherapy, and combined chemoradiation as either adjuvant or definitive treatment. Although squamous cell carcinoma has been the most common histological type in the past, distal adenocarcinoma is increasing in frequency, particularly in developed countries.

Chemotherapy for advanced disease

A single randomized trial has been performed comparing palliative chemotherapy with no treatment for advanced oesophageal squamous cell carcinoma.[2] This failed to demonstrate any benefit from chemotherapy, either in survival or in symptom control. Nevertheless, the majority of patients in this trial had previously undergone surgical oesophagectomy, and were included because of lymph node involvement, or incomplete resection of tumour. Extrapolation from the multicentre UK randomized studies in advanced oesophagogastric cancer shows the same benefit from palliative chemotherapy in patients with locally advanced or metastatic adenocarcinoma of the oesophagus as in those with advanced tumours of the oesophageal–gastric junction or stomach, diseases in which a definite palliative benefit has been demonstrated (see p. 197) (Table 9.1; Fig. 9.2).[3,4]

Historically, several cytotoxic drugs have shown single-agent activity in squamous and adenocarcinoma of the oesophagus. These have included bleomycin, 5-fluorouracil, mitomycin C, doxorubicin, methotrexate, cisplatin and paclitaxel. Response rates in single-agent trials have, however, been generally low and response duration very limited. More recently, combination chemotherapy has been used with more success. Cisplatin combined with 5-fluorouracil infusion has been adopted by many authorities as the gold standard but very few randomized studies have been performed to compare different regimens. These drugs show synergism *in vitro*[5] and are both radiosensitizers. Response rates of around 50% have been reported with this combination, although most studies have been of patients with squamous carcinoma and localized or locally advanced disease.[6,7] The addition of epirubicin may provide an advantage in the treatment of adenocarcinoma, as suggested by a randomized study comparing bolus 5-fluorouracil, doxorubicin and high-dose methotrexate (FAMTX) with bolus epirubicin, cisplatin and protracted infusion 5-fluorouracil (ECF).[3,8] This trial included 51 patients with locally advanced or metastatic adenocarcinoma of the oesophagus. Twelve out of 27 (44%) evaluable patients treated with ECF had a response compared with 5 out of 21 (24%) patients treated with FAMTX. The response rate to ECF was confirmed in a second randomized trial in which it was compared with mito-

Table 9.1 Survival by site of primary in a randomized trial of ECF versus FAMTX chemotherapy for locally advanced or metastatic oesophagogastric cancer.

	All patients		Oesophagus		O-G junction		Stomach	
	ECF	FAMTX	ECF	FAMTX	ECF	FAMTX	ECF	FAMTX
Number	126	130	27	24	27	33	72	73
1-year survival	36.5%	21.5%	37.0%	12.5%	33.3%	27.3%	37.5%	21.9%
p value	0.0004		0.032		0.075		0.020	

O–G junction, oesophageal–gastric junction.

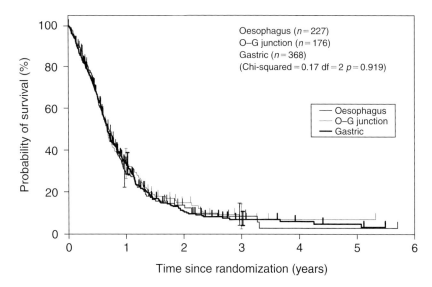

Oesophagus ($n=227$)
O–G junction ($n=176$)
Gastric ($n=368$)
(Chi-squared $=0.17$ df $=2$ $p=0.919$)

— Oesophagus
— O–G junction
— Gastric

Figure 9.2 Actuarial survival curves for patients treated in the multicentre UK randomized trials of ECF versus FAMTX and ECF versus MCF according to site of primary tumour. O–G junction, oesophagogastric junction.

mycin C, cisplatin and protracted infusion 5-fluorouracil.[4] However, the ECF regimen has not been compared with 5-fluorouracil and cisplatin alone in a randomized study. Combinations of paclitaxel and cisplatin have also shown promise in Phase II studies with reported response rates of 40–50%, and a median survival of 7 months.[9,10]

Combined modality treatment (1): chemoradiation
Concurrent radiotherapy and cisplatin and 5-fluorouracil chemotherapy produced a survival advantage over radiotherapy alone for locally advanced carcinoma of the oesophagus. Response rates were reported as 73% in the combined modality group and 60% in the radiotherapy alone group. Median survival was also significantly improved (12.5 versus 8.9 months; $p = 0.009$).[11] Similar results were seen with a combination of 5-fluorouracil, mitomycin C and radiotherapy in an Eastern Cooperative Oncology Group study (median survival 14.9 versus 9.0 months; $p = 0.03$).[12]

Combined modality treatment (2): adjuvant or neoadjuvant chemotherapy
Evidence regarding postoperative chemotherapy is minimal. A randomized trial of two cycles of postoperative cisplatin and vindesine versus surgery alone showed no significant difference in survival between the two arms.[13] A subsequent study used cisplatin and 5-fluorouracil for the chemotherapy arm.[14] Although there was an effect on 5-year disease-free survival, no overall survival benefit was observed with combination treatment (surgery, 51%; surgery plus chemotherapy, 61%; $p = 0.3$). A randomized trial of pre- and postoperative cisplatin and 5-fluorouracil versus surgery alone demonstrated no benefit from the addition of chemotherapy; however, very few patients actually received the full course of chemotherapy allocated in this study.[15] At present, neoadjuvant or postoperative chemotherapy for patients with operable oesophageal cancer must be considered investigational, and the results of ongoing studies including the Medical Research Council's OEO2 trial are awaited.

Combined modality treatment (3): neoadjuvant chemoradiation
Five randomized trials compared chemoradiation and surgery with surgery alone for operable carcinoma of the oesophagus (Table 9.2).[16–20] These have used a variety of chemoradiation regimens, and have studied adenocarcinoma,

Table 9.2 Randomized trials of preoperative chemoradiation in operable oesophageal cancer.[a]

Trial	Treatment arms	No. of patients	Histology and stage	No. of complete resections/no. of operations	Pathological complete remission rate	Survival (median unless otherwise stated)
Nygaard[16]	Cisplatin/bleomycin	50	Squamous carcinoma, Stage I–II	NR	NR	8 months
	Radiotherapy	48				11 months
	Cisplatin/Bleomycin/RT	47				9 months
	Surgery alone	41				8 months
Le Prise[17]	Cisplatin/5-FU/RT	41	Squamous carcinoma, Stage I–II	35/35	10%	10 months
	Surgery alone	45		38/42	—	10.5 months
Bosset[18]	Cisplatin/RT	143	Squamous carcinoma, Stage I–II	112/138	21%	18.6 months
	Surgery alone	139		94/137*	—	18.6 months
Walsh[19]	Cisplatin/5-FU/RT	58	Adeno carcinoma, Stage I–III	NR	25%	16 months
	Surgery alone	55			—	11 months*
Urba[20]	Cisplatin/Vinblastine/ 5-fluorouracil/RT	50	Squamous and adeno carcinoma, Stage I–II	NR	28%	32% at 3 years
	Surgery alone	50		NR	—	15% at 3 years*

[a]NR, not reported; *, statistically significant difference between arms.

squamous carcinoma, or both. Two studies have shown a survival benefit for the combined modality arm. These both used schedules in which chemotherapy and radiation were administered concurrently, and the chemotherapy incorporated cisplatin and 5-fluorouracil. A recent Phase II trial using preoperative paclitaxel, carboplatin, 5-fluorouracil and radiotherapy reported a pathological complete response rate of 54%, and a median survival of 24 months among 73 patients.[21] These results will require substantiation in a randomized trial but appear very promising.

Stomach and oesophagogastric junction

Adenocarcinoma of the stomach is sensitive to combination chemotherapy. There is evidence that tumours of the oesophagogastric junction should be considered as part of the same disease spectrum, both in terms of clinical behaviour,[4] and molecular and cellular origin.[22] Several randomized trials have demonstrated a survival and quality-of-life benefit of palliative chemotherapy for advanced disease, and this is now considered standard treatment for patients who are sufficiently fit. Nevertheless, median survival with optimal treatment remains less than 1 year, owing to the fairly rapid emergence of chemoresistance. Surgery remains the standard of care for localized disease but there is ongoing investigation of adjuvant and neoadjuvant chemotherapy. The latter is also of possible value in downstaging locally advanced tumours initially unsuitable for operation.

Palliative chemotherapy

Three randomized studies have shown a statistically significant improvement in survival following treatment with combination chemotherapy compared with supportive care alone.[23–25] This provides compelling evidence for the use of chemotherapy but the optimal regimen remains controversial. There is a large body of evidence from randomized trials comparing different regimens in this disease. Improved response rates and progression-free survival have been demonstrated with the addition of cisplatin to single-agent 5-fluoro-

uracil, although no survival advantage was obtained.[26] This combination remains popular in Europe but there is evidence that the addition of an anthracycline results in increased activity.[27] The combination of protracted venous infusion 5-fluorouracil, cisplatin and epirubicin (ECF) has produced among the highest response rates seen in a Phase II trial,[28] and has also demonstrated improved response rates (46% versus 21%; $p < 0.001$) and survival (8.7 versus 6.1 months; $p < 0.001$) compared with FAMTX in a randomized study.[3,8] Substitution of epirubicin with mitomycin C in this regimen did not improve outcome despite an increased dose of 5-fluorouracil, and resulted in poorer quality of life.[4] A Phase II study of an intensive weekly regimen of bolus 5-fluorouracil, cisplatin, epirubicin, and leucovorin (supported with glutathione to reduce cisplatin-associated neurotoxicity and G-CSF to limit leucopenia) produced a response rate of 62%, and a median survival of 11 months. Toxicity was moderate but was mainly haematological and was reasonably well-tolerated.[29] This regimen has not yet undergone Phase III testing.

New agents with activity in gastric cancer have been evaluated in combination regimens in Phase II studies. For example, paclitaxel, cisplatin and 5-fluorouracil produced an overall response rate of 51%, with a median survival of 6 months among 41 patients.[30] Toxicity predominantly consisted of myelosuppression. A combination of cisplatin and irinotecan was studied in 29 chemotherapy-naïve, and 15 previously treated patients. The overall response rate was 48%, and was 59% in the chemotherapy naïve group. Median survival was 9 months in the entire patient group.[31] Docetaxel, oxaliplatin and the oral fluoropyrimidines are also undergoing evaluation in this disease. The different mechanism of action and spectrum of resistance to these drugs introduces the possibility of second-line chemotherapy for patients remaining sufficiently fit after failure of conventional first-line treatment.

Adjuvant chemotherapy

As yet there is no definitive evidence to support the use of postoperative adjuvant chemotherapy following resection of gastric cancer. Clinical trials addressing this question date back 25 years, and the earlier studies used chemotherapy regimens that would no longer be considered optimal. A meta-analysis conducted in 1993 failed to show a benefit of adjuvant chemotherapy over surgery alone (odds ratio 0.88; 95% confidence interval (CI) 0.78–1.08).[32] This was criticized for the exclusion of two positive studies, however, the inclusion of which resulted in a statistically significant benefit for adjuvant chemotherapy.[33] A recent updated meta-analysis, including 13 trials conducted in non-Asian patients, produced an odds ratio for death of 0.8 (95% CI 0.66–0.97) in the treated group, corresponding to a relative risk of death of 0.94 (95% CI 0.89–1.00). There was a trend to greater benefit in trials in which a greater proportion of patients had node-positive disease.[34] The substantially higher response rates observed with modern combination chemotherapy regimens may translate into a more substantial survival advantage when these are used in the adjuvant setting.

Neoadjuvant chemotherapy

The possible efficacy of neoadjuvant chemotherapy for gastric cancer has been suggested by the observation of long-term survival in a minority of patients with locally advanced disease. This usually results from downstaging of the disease by 'palliative' chemotherapy, which then allows surgical removal of the primary tumour. In our trial of ECF versus FAMTX, complete surgical resection was rendered possible in 10 out of the 43 patients with locally advanced disease who were treated with ECF. Three of these had a pathological complete response to chemotherapy.[8] Furthermore, in a series of 30 patients with Stage IIIA, IIIB, or IV gastric cancer treated with etoposide, doxorubicin and cisplatin, multivariate analysis showed that complete clinical response to chemotherapy ($n = 8$; $p < 0.01$) and complete tumour resection ($n = 24$; $p < 0.01$) were the major independent predictors of long-term survival.[35] At present, however, randomized evidence for improvement in survival following neoadjuvant chemotherapy for

resectable disease is lacking. Two reported studies have been negative, one using preoperative FAMTX,[36] and the other using pre- and postoperative cisplatin, etoposide and 5-fluorouracil.[37] The latter trial showed a significantly improved operability rate for the chemotherapy-treated patients but the difference in median survival did not reach statistical significance (3.58 versus 2.48 years; $p = 0.114$).

Chemoradiation for localized disease

Radiation therapy has not played a major role in the treatment of localized gastric cancer, owing to the poor radiotherapy tolerance of the normal gastric mucosa. Nevertheless, the use of paclitaxel as a radiosensitizing agent has been evaluated in this disease, since it appears to have a degree of selectivity for the tumour cells. The mechanism of radiosensitization appears to relate to the synchronization of cells at G_2/M, and to involve P53-independent initiation of apoptosis.[38] In a Phase II trial, a response rate of 56% was observed with a combination of weekly paclitaxel and concurrent radiotherapy to 45 Gy. However, 47% of patients had Grade III/IV toxicity, including oesophagitis, gastritis, nausea and anorexia, and four patients required total parenteral nutritional support. At present, this approach remains investigational.

Pancreas

Adenocarcinoma of the pancreas has one of the poorest outcomes of any tumour type, with a 5-year survival of only 2–5%, and a median survival for advanced disease of 3–5 months. Only about 20% of patients present with potentially resectable disease, and the median survival following complete resection remains poor at 11–12 months. At present, palliative chemotherapy is not universally accepted by the oncology community but there is evidence for both survival and quality-of-life benefit over supportive care alone from randomized trials. Survival was approximately doubled in the chemotherapy arm to between 6 and 11 months.[39–41] One difficulty is that many patients presenting with pancreatic cancer have a poor performance status, have suffered significant weight loss, and may have obstructive jaundice, all of which limit the tolerance of cytotoxic chemotherapy. Thus the results of clinical trials that exclude such patients should be interpreted with caution when extrapolating to a general population.

Palliative chemotherapy

The optimal palliative treatment regimen for this disease is not established. Very few randomized trials have been conducted to compare different regimens, and differences in patient inclusion and response assessment criteria make interpretation of the many small Phase II studies very difficult. Single-agent activity has generally been limited. 5-Fluorouracil is used widely, but response rates have been under 20% in most series, and median survival has rarely been longer than 6 months.[42] Mitomycin C produced similar activity in a single Phase II trial,[43] but has subsequently only been evaluated in combination with other agents. Similarly, cisplatin has limited activity.[44] Gemcitabine, a novel cytidine analogue has been used extensively in this disease. Response rates in two Phase II studies were 14% and 6.3%, with a median survival of 5.6 months and 6.3 months, respectively. The drug was well-tolerated with low rates of grade III/IV toxicity.[45,46] A subsequent randomized trial compared gemcitabine with 5-fluorouracil.[47] A significantly superior outcome was obtained with gemcitabine in this study for traditional measures such as objective response rate (5.4% versus 0%; $p = 0.077$), median time to tumour progression (3.2 versus 1.0 months; $p = 0.0002$), and median survival (5.65 versus 4.41 months; $p = 0.0025$). In addition, the investigators assessed 'clinical benefit', a composite measure including improvement in pain, reduced analgesic requirements, weight gain, and improvement in performance status. This was also significantly greater in the gemcitabine-treated patients (23.8% versus 4.8%; $p = 0.0022$). This trial has been criticized for the use of a suboptimal 5-fluorouracil regimen of 600 mg/m² infused over 30 min once a week in the control arm.

A great variety of combination chemotherapy regimens have been assessed in Phase II studies. However, few have been compared with single-agent treatment in randomized trials, and there is no convincing evidence for an advantage of multi-agent therapy. As in the other upper gastrointestinal malignancies, combinations of cisplatin and 5-fluorouracil have been popular, and have produced response rates of up to 26%, and a median survival of up to 7 months.[42] A recently reported randomized trial demonstrated a small but significant improvement in response rate (12% versus 0%; $p < 0.01$) and 6-month progression-free survival (38% versus 28%; $p = 0.01$) for a combination of 5-day 5-fluorouracil infusion plus cisplatin compared with 5-day bolus 5-fluorouracil alone. There was no significant overall survival advantage, however, and the combination regimen produced greater toxicity.[48] The ECF regimen has also been evaluated in pancreatic cancer, and appeared active, with response rates of between 17% and 27%; however, median survival duration was only 6–8.5 months. Toxicity was substantially greater than that produced by single-agent therapy.[49–51] Combinations of cisplatin and gemcitabine have also been disappointing in Phase II studies, without substantially extending survival.[52,53] A regimen of 5-fluorouracil infusion, leucovorin, mitomycin C, and dipyridamole produced a response rate of 41%, and a median survival duration of 15 months among 46 patients of good performance status with locally advanced disease.[54] A second trial, however, using the same regimen produced a disappointing median survival of 4.4 months, suggesting that patient selection may have played a part in producing the earlier highly favourable results.[55] At present, further randomized trials are required to define the place of combination chemotherapy in the treatment of advanced pancreatic cancer, and single-agent 5-fluorouracil or gemcitabine remain appropriate control arms for such studies.

Chemoradiation

The poor outcome of surgery for localized disease has prompted the evaluation of chemoradiation in this setting. Postoperative adjuvant chemotherapy[56] or chemoradiation[57] have been reported to produce improved median survival over surgery alone; however, these trials were hampered by poor recruitment, largely because of the long recovery time following pancreato-duodenectomy. Preoperative chemoradiation has been evaluated in several Phase II studies. This appears to reduce the rate of local relapse but has little impact on overall survival because of the development of metastatic disease at a high frequency.[58,59] Chemoradiation has also been used for locally advanced disease not amenable to surgical resection. This has been shown to improve median survival to 10 months compared with 6 months for radiotherapy alone.[60] However, a comparison of 5-fluorouracil-based chemoradiation with 5-fluorouracil chemotherapy alone did not show a significant survival difference between the two arms, questioning the importance of local control in determining survival.[61] Chemoradiation regimens have commonly incorporated 5-fluorouracil, delivered as a bolus or an infusion, together with radiotherapy. The addition of cisplatin appears to increase toxicity without any substantial gains in efficacy. Newer alternatives to 5-fluorouracil with radiosensitizing activity include paclitaxel and gemcitabine. Phase I and II trials have demonstrated the feasibility of combining these agents with radiotherapy in the treatment of localized pancreatic cancer.[62,63] At present, however, their efficacy does not appear superior to 5-fluorouracil.

Biliary tract

Cancers of the biliary tract, including carcinoma of the gall bladder and cholangiocarcinoma, are rare, and few clinical trials have addressed their management. Patients frequently present with advanced disease that is not amenable to surgical resection, and the prognosis is poor, with a median survival of less than 6 months. Palliative chemotherapy may have a role, as suggested by a trial comparing 5-fluorouracil, leucovorin and etoposide with best supportive care alone. This demonstrated improved survival (6 versus 2.5 months; $p < 0.01$) and quality of life in the chemotherapy arm.[40] This trial included both biliary and pancreatic cancer patients (a feature of many studies of this disease) but the benefits of treatment were seen in both tumour types. 5-Fluorouracil is the most commonly used single agent, with response rates of about 10–20%. Combination of cisplatin and 5-fluorouracil increased the response rate to 32%,[64] and further addition of epirubicin (the ECF regimen) produced a 40% response rate and a 40% 1-year survival.[65] An interesting agent in this disease is alpha-interferon. A regimen combining a 5-day infusion of 5-fluorouracil with alpha-interferon on Days 1, 3 and 5, repeated every 2 weeks produced a response rate of 39%, and a median survival of 1 year among 19 patients.[66]

Adjuvant chemotherapy or chemoradiation has also been investigated in several small Phase II studies but there is no definitive evidence for a survival benefit over surgery alone. Randomized trials of the most active regimens in advanced disease, such as ECF, are ongoing.

Liver

Hepatocellular carcinoma is a common disease worldwide but its incidence in Europe and the USA is low. Systemic chemotherapy has proved largely ineffective in inducing tumour remissions, or in prolonging survival of patients with inoperable disease. In contrast, a variety of regional therapies have been used successfully to reduce the mass of tumours confined to the liver; however, the impact of such treatment on survival is not established. Liver tumours derive the majority of their blood supply from the hepatic artery, whereas normal liver parenchyma is supplied mostly by the portal vein. This provides the rationale for two strategies:

1. Intrahepatic arterial chemotherapy, and
2. Selective hepatic artery embolization.

Intrahepatic arterial (IHA) chemotherapy with single-agent cisplatin, has produced response rates of between 40 and 55%.[67] The addition of an embolization agent such as lipiodol, gelfoam, starch microspheres, or arterial ligation to IHA chemotherapy with cisplatin or doxorubicin or both, has also been evaluated extensively in Phase II trials, producing response rates of above 50%. A randomized trial of IHA cisplatin and doxorubicin with or without lipiodol produced a greater response rate in the chemo-embolization group (57% versus 44%) but there was no difference in survival between the two arms.[68] A meta-analysis of all therapeutic modalities that have been evaluated in two or more randomized trials found no evidence of survival benefit at 1 year resulting from systemic treatment with doxorubicin or 5-fluorouracil, from percutaneous ethanol injection, or from intrahepatic arterial chemotherapy. A marginal benefit could not be excluded from systemic interferon, or from tamoxifen but there was insufficient data to clearly demonstrate the efficacy of either of these modalities.[69] A subsequently reported large prospective randomized trial comparing tamoxifen with best supportive care, including 496 patients, showed no difference in progression-free or overall survival between the two arms.[70] These results effectively rule out any possible benefit from this approach.

Drug therapy may have an adjuvant role in the management of operable hepatocellular carcinoma, although there is conflicting evidence from randomized studies. Two trials have reported negative results, one using postoperative adjuvant epirubicin plus chemoembolization with iodized oil and cisplatin,[71] and the second using a combination of IHA epirubicin, intravenous epirubicin and oral carmofur.[72] In contrast, positive results have been reported for adjuvant IHA doxorubicin and lipiodol,[73] for a complex pre- and postoperative regimen of tumour-targeted IHA therapy containing a cocktail of lipiodol, urographin, mitomycin C, carboplatin, epirubicin, leucovorin, 5-fluorouracil, γ-interferon, and interleukin-2,[74] and for a single postoperative IHA dose of ^{131}I-labelled lipiodol.[75]

Small intestine
Adenocarcinoma of the small intestine is an extremely rare disease, and there is little pub-lished data regarding the role of chemotherapy in its management. We have reported a series of eight patients treated with infusional 5-fluoro-uracil-based regimens for locally advanced or metastatic disease between 1990 and 1995 at our institution.[76] Five patients received the ECF regimen, one received protracted venous infusion (PVI) 5-fluorouracil plus mitomycin C, and the remaining two received PVI 5-fluorouracil alone. There were one complete and two partial responses, for an overall response rate of 37%, and the median survival was 13 months. The four symptomatic patients all improved on chemotherapy. Other anecdotal reports of responses to fluoropyrimidine-based treatment support the results of this series. Neoadjuvant chemoradiation has also proven efficacious in this disease, four out of five patients with duodenal adenocarcinoma achieving pathological complete remissions following treatment with concurrent radiotherapy, 5-fluorouracil infusion and mitomycin C.[77]

Colon and rectum
Palliative chemotherapy for advanced disease
Chemotherapy has been shown to produce a survival advantage and palliative benefits to patients with advanced colorectal cancer compared with supportive care alone.[78,79] Furthermore, early treatment produces a better outcome compared with treatment initiated at the time of symptom onset.[80] Leucovorin-modulated bolus 5-fluorouracil has been considered the standard treatment and remains the most commonly used regimen but is associated with significant toxicity, notably mucositis, diarrhoea and leucopenia. Infusional delivery of 5-fluorouracil has been shown to result in less toxicity and at least equivalent efficacy, and is now widely accepted as standard therapy.[81–83] Several different infusional regimens are used, including protracted venous infusion, biweekly 48 h infusion plus leucovorin (de Gramont regimen), and weekly 24 h infusion (AIO regimen). Single-agent raltitrexed, a direct thymidylate synthase inhibitor, has produced similar survival to leucovorin-modulated 5-fluorouracil bolus in two out of three randomized trials. In

the third study, survival was slightly inferior with raltitrexed.[84] Raltitrexed has a more convenient administration schedule of a 3-weekly bolus injection and has a different spectrum of toxicity compared with 5-fluorouracil. Oral fluoropyrimidines also have a potential role. Capecitabine, is converted to 5-fluorouracil by the tumour-associated angiogenesis factor thymidine phosphorylase, thus reducing exposure of normal tissues to the active metabolite. Two separate Phase III randomized trials showed improved response rates with capecitabine compared with bolus 5-fluorouracil/leucovorin, although statistically equivalent progression-free survival was observed.[85,86] Oral UFT (a combination of ftorafur (1-(2-tetrahydrofuryl)-5-fluorouracil) and uracil at a molar ratio of 1:4) plus oral leucovorin also produced a similar response rate and median survival compared with bolus 5-fluorouracil/leucovorin.[87]

Combination chemotherapy has also been investigated in this setting. The addition of bolus mitomycin C to protracted venous infusion 5-fluorouracil resulted in an improved response rate and median failure-free survival, and marginally improved actuarial overall survival.[88] Similarly, the addition of oxaliplatin to the de Gramont schedule of infusional 5-fluorouracil significantly prolonged the median progression-free survival, and treatment with oxaliplatin was found to be a significant prognostic factor for overall survival on multivariate analysis.[89] Two recently reported randomized trials have demonstrated a progression-free survival advantage for the addition of irinotecan to standard 5-fluorouracil/leucovorin regimens, with a significant overall survival benefit in one study.[90,91]

Second-line chemotherapy following 5-fluorouracil failure is becoming more widely adopted. Several Phase II studies have demonstrated tumour responses to infusional 5-fluorouracil regimens following failure of 5-fluorouracil bolus.[92–94] The addition of oxaliplatin to 5-fluorouracil infusion may further improve response rates.[95] Two recent studies have demonstrated that irinotecan produces a survival advantage in this setting compared with supportive care (2.8 months)[96] or 5-fluorouracil infusion (2.3 months),[97] with improved quality of life. These results provide a sound basis for the use of second-line chemotherapy in selected patients.

Patients with isolated liver metastases should be considered for surgical resection, with curative potential; however, in many patients surgery is not technically feasible. An alternative approach is intrahepatic arterial chemotherapy. Floxuridine (5-fluoro-2'deoxyuridine; FUDR) has superior pharmacokinetics compared with 5-fluorouracil by this route, and is the preferred agent.[98] A meta-analysis of trials comparing IHA chemotherapy with supportive care or systemic chemotherapy demonstrated a significantly improved response rate in the IHA group, although no significant survival advantage.[99]

Adjuvant chemotherapy for colon cancer

There is now an established role for systemic adjuvant 5-fluorouracil-based chemotherapy in Dukes C colon cancer following curative resection, having been shown to reduce the risk of recurrence by 19–40% and of death by 16–33%.[100–103] The benefit of adjuvant chemotherapy for patients with Duke's B colon cancer is less clear. An analysis of four NSABP studies has shown that the relative benefit is similar to that seen in Duke's C disease but that the absolute improvement in survival is small because of the relatively good prognosis of this group.[104] Similar findings were reported by the Netherlands Adjuvant Colorectal Cancer Project in a trial of 5-fluorouracil and levamisole versus surgery alone.[105] An analysis performed by the IMPACT B2 Investigators of five separate trials showed only a 2% absolute improvement in survival from 80% to 82% produced by 6 or 12 months adjuvant therapy with 5-fluorouracil and leucovorin.[106] It appears that this population of patients encompasses some with a very low risk of recurrence, and others in whom this risk is substantial, with several prognostic factors now well-defined. It remains to be established whether any individual factors can be used to select patients for adjuvant chemotherapy. Enrolment of these patients into prospective trials should be encouraged.

Adjuvant therapy for rectal cancer

Adjuvant chemotherapy was shown to be effective for Duke's B and C rectal cancer in the National Surgical Adjuvant Breast and Bowel Project (NSABP) R-01 study. A 5-year survival advantage for chemotherapy (methyl-CCNU, vincristine and bolus 5-fluorouracil [MOF]) over surgery alone was demonstrated (53% versus 43%; $p = 0.05$).[107] Other studies have investigated the role of combined chemoradiation. In a four-arm trial, the Gastrointestinal Tumour Study Group (GITSG) showed a statistically significant survival advantage for chemoradiation over surgery ($p = 0.005$); postoperative chemotherapy or radiotherapy alone were not superior to surgery in this trial.[108] The North Central Cancer Treatment Group (NCCTG) compared postoperative radiotherapy with chemoradiation, consisting of methyl-CCNU and bolus 5-fluorouracil administered both before, during (5-fluorouracil only), and after the course of radiotherapy.[109] With a follow-up of 7 years, the recurrence rate was reduced by 34% ($p = 0.0016$), and the death rate by 29% ($p = 0.025$) in the combination arm. Following the publication of these results, the National Cancer Institute Consensus Conference concluded in 1990 that combined modality therapy should be considered the standard postoperative adjuvant treatment for stage T_3 and/or node-positive rectal cancer.[110] The NSABP R-02 study confirmed the benefit of the addition of radiotherapy to adjuvant chemotherapy in reducing local recurrence rates, although there was no additional survival advantage.[111] Further trials have attempted to define the optimal chemoradiation regimen. The NCCTG showed an advantage for infusional 5-fluorouracil over bolus 5-fluorouracil in combination with radiotherapy.[112] The addition of methyl-CCNU to 5-fluorouracil conferred no advantage. Preoperative chemoradiation is also being investigated. The NSABP R-03 trial compares preoperative with postoperative chemoradiation. An early analysis following the randomization of 116 patients was reported to show a higher rate of sphincter-preserving operations and evidence for tumour downstaging in the preoperative group.[113]

New approaches to adjuvant therapy of colorectal cancer

Following the demonstration of activity in advanced disease, there is considerable interest in the use of irinotecan and oxaliplatin in the adjuvant setting for colon and rectal cancer. The very high response rates observed with combinations of either of these agents and fluoropyrimidines make these an attractive choice for further evaluation. Randomized trials will clearly be required to establish the optimal regimen. Monoclonal antibody therapy has also been investigated as adjuvant therapy for Duke's C colorectal cancer. A randomized trial compared surgery alone with murine monoclonal antibody 17-1A given at a dose of 500 mg infused over 1 h on postoperative Day 15, followed by four further doses of 100 mg at monthly intervals.[114] With a median follow-up of 7 years, there was a reduction in recurrence rate in the treatment arm of 23% ($p < 0.04$) and a reduction in mortality of 32% ($p < 0.01$). Thus the survival advantage seen in this study was of the same order as that produced by standard 5-fluorouracil plus leucovorin chemotherapy, and the associated toxicity was negligible.

Anus

Squamous carcinoma of the anus is sensitive to chemotherapy and radiotherapy. If surgery is selected as the primary treatment modality, most patients require abdominoperineal resection and consequently need a permanent colostomy. For this reason, chemoradiation is widely accepted to be the optimal primary therapy, with surgery reserved for those patients not achieving an adequate response, or for those suffering local relapse. A large randomized trial conducted by the UK Co-ordinating Committee on Cancer Research (UKCCCR) demonstrated improved response rates and local tumour control, and a reduced risk of death from anal cancer, following treatment with 5-fluorouracil and mitomycin C together with radiotherapy, compared with radiotherapy alone.[115] In this study, 5-fluorouracil was given as a continuous infusion for 4 days at the beginning and end of radiotherapy (dosage 45 Gy), with a single bolus dose of mitomycin C on Day 1. A very similar, although smaller study conducted by the European Organisation for the Research and Treatment of Cancer (EORTC) supported these results.[116] The importance of mitomycin C in this type of regimen was shown in an Intergroup randomized trial comparing radiotherapy plus 5-fluorouracil, with a combination of radiotherapy, 5-fluorouracil and mitomycin C.[117] Cisplatin has also been evaluated together with 5-fluorouracil and radiotherapy on the basis of the known efficacy of this combination in squamous carcinomas at other sites. Response rates and toxicity are comparable with those of the 5-fluorouracil/mitomycin C chemoradiation regimens, but local control may be improved,[118] however, randomized studies will be required to establish the superior regimen.

Chemotherapy probably also has a role in the management of locally advanced and metastatic disease, although there are no large Phase II studies in the literature, let alone randomized trials. In addition to 5-fluorouracil, mitomycin C and cisplatin, other agents with activity include carboplatin and doxorubicin.

Primary lymphoma of the gastrointestinal tract

The gastrointestinal tract is the most common site of origin of extranodal lymphomas. Non-Hodgkin's lymphoma (NHL) accounts for approximately 3–10% of all gastric neoplasms, and 20% of small intestinal cancers but for less than 1% of all large bowel malignancies. Other relatively rare sites of origin include the oesophagus, the pancreas and the liver. All histological subtypes are represented but there is a greater proportion of histologically aggressive NHL than is seen with nodal lymphomas.

The specific management of gastrointestinal tract NHL depends on the histological classification, site and stage of the disease. In the past, surgery has played a major role in the management of localized aggressive gastric lymphoma but the morbidity and mortality associated with gastrectomy have led to alternative approaches

being advocated. A randomized trial has shown that combination chemotherapy is equally effective as gastrectomy followed by chemotherapy for Stage IE and IIE disease.[119] The risk of bleeding or perforation during chemotherapy was very low in this study. High complete-response rates of 90% and a 5-year actuarial survival of 82% following chemotherapy, and in some cases consolidation radiotherapy, were reported recently in a similar cohort of patients.[120] Advanced gastrointestinal tract NHL is also treated optimally with combination chemotherapy, producing a similar outcome to nodal NHL of similar histology and International Prognostic Index.[121]

Coeliac disease is a known risk factor for the development of T-cell lymphomas, the so-called enteropathy associated T-cell lymphoma (EATCL). The relative risk of developing EATCL in this group ranges from about 17 to 80 times that of the normal population, depending on adherence to a gluten-free diet.[122] Treatment usually includes surgical resection followed by chemotherapy and/or radiotherapy for localized disease, and combination chemotherapy alone for advanced-stage disease. The prognosis is extremely poor, however, with a median survival of less than 6 months and a 5 year survival of only 9.5% in the largest reported series.[123]

Gastric MALT lymphoma has only relatively recently been recognized as a distinct entity,[124] and its management is somewhat controversial. The overall prognosis appears excellent, and the observation that eradication of *Helicobacter pylori* leads to regression of lymphoma in a proportion of cases has brought the role of aggressive treatment modalities such as surgery and chemotherapy into question.[125] However, the natural history of this disease is not yet completely understood, and the use of cytotoxic chemotherapy undoubtedly has a part to play—particularly in patients failing to respond to antibiotics.

Neuroendocrine tumours

The neuroendocrine tumours include carcinoid tumours and enteropancreatic endocrine tumours, including gastrinomas, insulinomas, vasoactive intestinal peptide (VIP)omas, glucagonomas, somatostatinomas, and growth releasing factor (GRF)omas, all of which arise from the amine precursor uptake and decarboxylation (APUD) system. They are rare, with incidence rates of 1–2 per 100 000 population per year, although post-mortem studies suggest a higher incidence, reflecting the fact that up to three-quarters of these tumours remain asymptomatic and are undetected in life. The principles of management of these tumours are two-fold. Firstly to control the symptoms resulting from the production of bioactive amines and polypeptides and, secondly, to prevent tumour growth and metastasis. Surgical resection remains the priority as this represents the only curative therapy, and benign and malignant primary tumours cannot be distinguished reliably on histopathological grounds. Only a minority of symptomatic tumours present, however, with completely resectable disease and systemic therapy is often required.

Long-acting somatostatin analogues have become the drugs of choice for the symptomatic treatment of the carcinoid syndrome, insulinoma, VIPoma, glucagonoma, and GRFoma, and may also have cytostatic activity via an action on tumour somatostatin receptors.[126] There is extensive experience with octreotide (given 50 μg twice daily by subcutaneous injection, increased according to response to 200 μg three times daily, higher doses exceptionally required), which reduces symptoms, and decreases 5-hydroxyindolacetic acid (5-HIAA) levels in a high proportion of carcinoid patients.[127] Patients with neuroendocrine tumours who are adequately controlled on subcutaneous octreotide may be switched to a long-acting depot preparation given by deep intramuscular injection (into the gluteal muscle), initially 20 mg every 4 weeks for 3 months, adjusted according to response; a maximum of 30 mg is given every 4 weeks. The newer agent,

lanreotide, available in a slow-release formulation allowing twice-monthly administration, had comparable efficacy in a Phase II study.[128] Alpha-interferon also has efficacy in reducing the symptoms of the carcinoid syndrome and other neuroendocrine syndromes, either as single-agent treatment,[129] or in combination with octreotide.[130] In a trial of alpha-interferon treatment after resection of primary mid-gut carcinoids, and hepatic artery embolization of liver metastases, 39% of patients showed an objective response after 1 year. Those patients who continued alpha-interferon treatment had a significantly improved 5-year survival compared with those who stopped after 1 year.[131] Other complications of the carcinoid syndrome, such as bronchoconstriction and cardiac failure, are treated symptomatically with bronchodilators and diuretics, respectively. Occasionally, tricuspid valve replacement is indicated for severe incompetence. Symptoms of the Zollinger-Ellison syndrome are effectively treated with the proton-pump inhibitors, omeprazole or lansoprazole, in the majority of patients; total gastrectomy is rarely required to control gastric acid hypersecretion.

Tumour growth can often be contained with the use of somatostatin analogues and alpha-interferon, as alluded to previously. If these relatively non-toxic measures are unsuccessful, other approaches include the use of high-dose radiolabelled metaiodobenzylguanidine (MIBG)[132] or octreotide.[133,134] Chemotherapy is usually reserved for progressive hepatic or systemic metastatic disease. Pancreatic endocrine tumours (PET) are relatively more sensitive to chemotherapy than are carcinoids. The standard regimen for well-differentiated PETs is streptozotocin and doxorubicin, which has shown greater activity than streptozotocin plus 5-fluorouracil or single-agent chlorozotocin in a randomized trial.[135] Poorly differentiated PETs appear responsive to a combination of etoposide and cisplatin.[136] Conversely, carcinoid tumours respond no better to combination chemotherapy than to single-agent 5-fluorouracil, streptozotocin or doxorubicin. The relative lack of toxicity of 5-fluorouracil makes this the agent of choice. Embolization or chemoembolization of hepatic metastases has also been successful in inducing objective and symptomatic responses in patients with carcinoids and PETs.[137] The timing of such therapy will be determined by the contribution of the hepatic disease to the overall clinical situation, since it is associated with substantial toxicity.

Chemoprevention of gastrointestinal cancer

The relatively poor outcome of cancers of the gastrointestinal tract has driven the search for agents that modulate the process of carcinogenesis, and hence may have utility in cancer prevention. By far the greatest experience is in colorectal cancer, a disease in which there is a well-developed hypothesis of cancer development, a recognized high-risk population in which pilot studies can be carried out, and several surrogate endpoints such as adenoma recurrence that precede the development of malignancy. Epidemiological studies have suggested several dietary factors that may reduce the incidence of colorectal cancer, including high fibre,[138] calcium,[139] and the antioxidant vitamins: folic acid,[140] vitamin C,[141] tocopherol (vitamin E)[142] and retinoids.[143] Case-control studies have also suggested that non-steroidal anti-inflammatory drugs (NSAIDs) may have a role in colon cancer prevention.[144] At present few randomized trials have been completed to assess the effect of intervention with these agents on colon cancer development. Most studies either completed or underway have enrolled patients with a previous adenoma, or either familial adenomatous polyposis or hereditary non-polyposis colon cancer, and the primary endpoint is polyp recurrence. A small but statistically significant reduction in risk of adenoma recurrence was observed in patients receiving a daily dose of 3 g calcium carbonate for 4 years, compared with placebo-treated controls.[145] An earlier report from the same group failed to show a benefit from β-carotene, or from vitamins C and E.[146] Ongoing randomized studies are evaluating, among others, the role of aspirin, sulindac and folate in this setting.[147]

PHARMACOLOGY OF MAJOR DRUGS

The use of cytotoxic drugs for the treatment of malignant disease should, in general, be confined to specialists in oncology. All of these drugs have a narrow therapeutic index, and side-effects are expected at the doses required for therapeutic efficacy. Dose reduction or delay is often required to allow recovery from toxicity. There is relatively little experience of their use in pregnancy, and this should generally be considered an absolute contraindication. Similarly, gametogenesis is likely to be disrupted, and all patients receiving cytotoxic treatment should therefore take adequate contraceptive precautions. Many of these drugs have the potential to cause reversible or permanent infertility. Details of the pharmacology, indications, commonly encountered toxicity, drug interactions and contraindications for the drugs in routine clinical use in gastrointestinal cancer are given in the text following.

Fluoropyrimidines

The fluoropyrimidines are antimetabolite drugs that inhibit DNA synthesis by several mechanisms including inhibition of thymidylate synthase, and mis-incorporation into DNA. They also inhibit RNA synthesis by mis-incorporation into RNA.

Fluorouracil (5-FU)
This drug has unreliable oral availability, and is usually administered by intravenous injection or infusion. The plasma elimination half-life is about 16 min, and is dose-dependent. Following a single i.v. dose, 15% is excreted unchanged in the urine, and the remainder is metabolized in the liver. It is converted to 5-fluorodeoxyuridine monophosphate (FdUMP) by the enzyme phosphoribosyl pyrophosphate transferase. FdUMP forms a stable complex with thymidylate synthase and folate, thus inhibiting the enzyme. Toxicity comprises myelosuppression, mucositis, diarrhoea, palmar-plantar erythema and, rarely, a cerebellar syndrome.

Indications

Palliative treatment of all epithelial gastrointestinal malignancies and adjuvant treatment of colorectal cancer are indications for treatment.

Drug interactions

Biochemical modulation of the action of 5-fluorouracil is produced by leucovorin and methotrexate. Metronidazole, allopurinol and cimetidine inhibit the metabolism of 5-fluorouracil.

Cautions and contraindications

Caution is advised in treating patients with a history of heart disease, since 5-fluorouracil can induce coronary artery spasm. Caution is required in patients with impaired renal or hepatic function.

Uracil ftorafur (UFT)

This drug is a combination of ftorafur (1-(2-tetrahydrofuryl)-5-fluorouracil) and uracil at a molar ratio of 1:4. Ftorafur is reliably absorbed from the gastrointestinal tract, and is converted into 5-fluorouracil in the liver. The addition of uracil inhibits the degradation of 5-fluorouracil to 2-fluoro-β-alanine. Blood levels of 5-fluorouracil peak 30 min after an oral dose of UFT, and subsequently decline gradually. Toxicity is similar to that produced by 5-fluorouracil, with the addition of nausea and vomiting, and hyperbilirubinaemia. This drug is not yet in routine clinical use in the UK but is the subject of investigation for the palliative treatment of colorectal cancer.

Capecitabine

This drug is absorbed unchanged from the gastrointestinal tract. It is primarily metabolized in the liver by the enzyme carboxylesterase to 5′-deoxy-5-fluorocytidine (5′-DFCR), which is then converted to 5′-deoxy-5-fluorouracil (5′-DFUR) by cytidine deaminase, principally located in the liver and in tumour tissue. The final conversion to 5-fluorouracil is catalysed by the enzyme pyrimidine nucleoside phosphorylase, which is present at higher levels in tumour than in normal tissue. After oral administration, peak plasma levels of capecitabine and its two main metabolites, 5′-DFCR and 5′-DFUR, are reached within 30–90 min, after which concentrations decline exponentially with a half life of about 30–60 min. Plasma levels of 5-fluorouracil are approximately 30 times lower than those produced by an intravenous bolus of 5-fluorouracil.

Indications

This drug is not yet in routine clinical use in the UK but is the subject of investigation for the palliative treatment of colorectal cancer.

Cautions and contraindications

Diarrhoea and palmar-plantar erythema are the most common toxic effects encountered with this drug.

Direct thymidylate synthase inhibitors

Raltitrexed

Direct inhibition of thymidylate synthase is produced by the folate analogue raltitrexed. This is administered intravenously, and is transported into the cell by the reduced folate carrier. Within the cell, raltitrexed undergoes polyglutamation by the enzyme folyl polyglutamate synthetase. Polyglutamated forms have increased potency for thymidylate synthase, and are retained within the cell, prolonging the inhibitory activity. Plasma levels of raltitrexed after i.v. injection decline rapidly in an initial phase, with a β half-life of 90–120 min, followed by a slow elimination phase, with a terminal half-life of about 8 days. Approximately 40–50% of the drug is excreted in the urine.

Indications

This drug is used for the palliative treatment of advanced colorectal cancer.

Drug interactions

Leucovorin and folic acid may interfere with its action. Other interactions are not known.

Cautions and contraindications

Toxicity associated with this drug includes myelosuppression, nausea and vomiting, diarrhoea, asthenia, reversible increases in transaminases, and skin rash. Severe diarrhoea associated with neutropenia may be life-threatening.

Severe renal impairment (creatinine clearance <25 ml/min) is a contraindication to its use. A 50% dose reduction is required for moderate renal impairment (creatinine clearance 25–65 ml/min). Caution should be exercised in hepatic impairment.

Platinum analogues

This group of drugs inhibits DNA synthesis by producing intra- and inter-strand cross-linking adducts within the DNA molecule.

Cisplatin

Cisplatin is administered intravenously by infusion over 6–8 h. It is cleared initially rapidly from the plasma but this slows subsequently owing to covalent binding to serum proteins. The majority of drug is eliminated via the kidneys; 15–25% within the first 4 h, and 20–80% within 24 h. The remainder represents drug bound to tissues or plasma proteins. Toxic effects of cisplatin are common, and include nephrotoxicity, ototoxicity, myelosuppression, peripheral neuropathy, nausea and vomiting, hypomagnesemia, and occasionally anaphylaxis.

Indications

In combination regimens, cisplatin is indicated for the palliative treatment of upper gastrointestinal cancers. It is also used in chemoradiation regimens together with 5-fluorouracil.

Drug interactions

Antihypertensive therapy with frusemide, hydralazine, diazoxide and propranolol has been reported to exacerbate nephrotoxicity. Cisplatin forms a black precipitate with aluminium.

Cautions and contraindications

Cisplatin is contraindicated in renal impairment and in patients with hearing impairment. Both creatinine clearance and audiometry should be monitored during treatment. In addition, cisplatin is contraindicated in patients with a history of allergy to this drug. Cisplatin must be given with pre- and postadministration hydration with mannitol-induced diuresis to prevent renal toxicity, together with magnesium and potassium supplementation.

Carboplatin

Carboplatin is administered as a 1-h i.v. infusion. Plasma clearance is biphasic with an α half-life of 90 min and a β half-life of 6 h. Extensive binding to plasma proteins occurs, and elimination is mainly in the urine, with recovery of approximately 65% of administered drug within the first 24 h. Toxicity comprises predominantly myelosuppression and nausea and vomiting. Less commonly, nephrotoxicity, ototoxicity, and peripheral neuropathy occur. These are more frequent in patients who have previously experienced these toxicities with cisplatin.

Indications

Carboplatin has not demonstrated equivalent activity to cisplatin in upper gastrointestinal tumours, and should not be used routinely in this setting; however, in the presence of a contraindication to the use of cisplatin, its substitution with carboplatin may be considered.

Drug interactions

Concurrent therapy with nephrotoxic drugs should be avoided. Carboplatin forms a black precipitate with aluminium.

Cautions and contraindications

This drug is contraindicated in patients with severe renal impairment (EDTA clearance <20 ml/min) or those with a previous history of allergy to platinum-containing drugs.

Oxaliplatin

Oxaliplatin is a diaminocyclohexane platinum

compound administered as a 2-h i.v. infusion. The pharmacokinetics of this compound are less well characterized than for the older platinum analogues; however, it appears to produce dose-proportionate plasma levels over a wide dose range and is excreted mainly in the urine. Toxicity with this drug is primarily neurological, and comprises acute paraesthesias and dysaesthesias (sometimes cold-related) that usually resolve over the course of a few hours or days, and cumulative sensory neuropathy that appears to be at least partly reversible on discontinuation of the drug. Other toxicities include myelosuppression, nausea and vomiting, and diarrhoea (particularly when given in combination with 5-fluorouracil).

Indications

In combination with 5-fluorouracil, oxaliplatin is indicated for the palliative treatment of colorectal cancer.

Drug interactions

No drug interactions are known.

Cautions and contraindications

Oxaliplatin is contraindicated in patients with a previous history of allergy to platinum-containing drugs. Caution should be exercised in patients with pre-existent peripheral neuropathy.

Anthracyclines

The anthracyclines inhibit DNA synthesis at least in part by interaction with topoisomerase II.

Doxorubicin (Adriamycin)

This drug is administered as an i.v. bolus. Its elimination from the plasma follows a triphasic pharmacokinetic pattern, with half-lives of 12 min, 3.3 h and 29.6 h, respectively. It is bound by tissues extensively. It is metabolized in the liver, and approximately 50% is excreted in the bile. Only 5% is excreted in the urine. Toxic effects include myelosuppression, nausea

and vomiting, mucositis, alopecia, and cumulative cardiac toxicity (the risk of cardiac failure increases greatly once cumulative doses above $450 \, mg/m^2$ have been reached). It is also a vesicant drug and causes local tissue necrosis if extravasation occurs during administration.

Indications

Doxorubicin is indicated for the palliative treatment of upper gastrointestinal tumours, for neuroendocrine tumours and for primary gastrointestinal lymphomas.

Drug interactions

No drug interactions are known.

Cautions and contraindications

Cardiac toxicity should be monitored with regular assessment of left ventricular ejection fraction once cumulative doses approach or exceed $400 \, mg/m^2$. A dose reduction is required in hepatic impairment, and doxorubicin should be used with caution in this situation.

Epirubicin

This drug has similar pharmacokinetics as doxorubicin, although it is metabolized in addition by glucuronidation, which is thought to account for a slightly more favourable toxicity profile. Toxicity is, however, qualitatively similar to that produced by doxorubicin, including the risk of cardiotoxicity with high cumulative doses ($900–1000 \, mg/m^2$).

Indications

Epirubicin is indicated for the palliative treatment of upper gastrointestinal tumours.

Drug interactions

None are known.

Cautions and contraindications

Cardiac toxicity should be monitored with regular assessment of left ventricular ejection fraction once cumulative doses approach or exceed $900 \, mg/m^2$. A dose reduction is required in hepatic impairment, and epirubicin should be used with caution in this situation.

Mitomycin C

This drug is activated within the cell to an alkylating agent, and forms a complex with DNA. In addition it inhibits the biosynthesis of DNA, and may also inhibit RNA and protein synthesis. Following intravenous injection, mitomycin is rapidly cleared from the plasma by metabolism in the liver and other tissues. The half-life is inversely proportional to dose owing to saturation of metabolic pathways. Approximately 10% is excreted unchanged in the urine. Toxicity comprises predominantly thrombocytopenia and leucopenia. Nausea and vomiting occur occasionally but are rarely severe. With cumulative doses approaching $40\,\text{mg}/\text{m}^2$, a microangiopathic haemolytic anaemia has been reported, and is frequently fatal. Diffuse pulmonary infiltration is also encountered rarely. Extravasation during administration produces local tissue necrosis.

Indications
Mitomycin C is indicated for the palliative treatment of upper and lower gastrointestinal tract tumours, usually in combination with other cytotoxic agents.

Drug interactions
Microsomal enzyme inducers such as barbiturates or liver enzyme inducers such as cimetidine may alter the activity of mitomycin C by an effect on host and tumour metabolism.

Cautions and contraindications
Mitomycin C is contraindicated in patients with platelet counts less than $75 \times 10^9/\text{l}$, in patients with coagulation disorders, or in patients with moderate or severe renal impairment. In addition it is contraindicated in patients who have experienced previous hypersensitivity reactions to this drug. Owing to the risk of microangiopathic haemolytic anaemia, we would recommend limiting the cumulative dose of mitomycin C to $28\,\text{mg}/\text{m}^2$ or 56 mg total. In addition, screening of a blood film for red cell fragmentation is recommended prior to each dose, with discontinuation of this drug if red cell fragments are present.

Taxanes

The taxanes inhibit cell division by stabilization of microtubules.

Paclitaxel (Taxol)
This drug is administered as an i.v. infusion. It appears to be extensively protein bound, and is cleared primarily by hepatic metabolism, and excretion in the bile, with approximately 10% being excreted unchanged in the urine. Toxicity comprises myelosuppression, hypersensitivity reactions, including dyspnoea, hypotension, angioedema, and generalized urticaria, cardiac conduction abnormalities, peripheral neuropathy, arthralgia or myalgia, alopecia and nausea and vomiting. Cellulitis may result from extravasation.

Indications
Paclitaxel is not in current routine use for gastrointestinal malignancy but is the subject of ongoing study in the treatment of upper gastrointestinal tract cancers, particularly as a radiosensitizer.

Drug interactions
Administration after cisplatin increases haematological toxicity. Ketoconazole may inhibit the metabolism of paclitaxel.

Cautions and contraindications
Premedication with corticosteroids, antihistamines and H_2-receptor antagonists is recommended to prevent hypersensitivity reactions. Previous severe hypersensitivity reactions to paclitaxel are a contraindication to its use. Caution should be exercised in patients with hepatic impairment; paclitaxel should probably not be used in patients with severe hepatic impairment.

Docetaxel (Taxotere)
This drug is administered as a short i.v. infusion. It is highly bound to plasma protein, and exhibits dose-independent pharmacokinetics consistent with a three-compartment model, with half-lives for the α, β, and γ phases of

4 min, 36 min and 11.1 h, respectively. Excretion is primarily via the bile, after cytochrome P$_{450}$-mediated oxidative metabolism, with approximately 6% of the dose excreted unchanged in the urine. Toxicity includes myelosuppression (particularly neutropenia), hypersensitivity reactions, fluid retention, cutaneous reactions including erythema of the extremities followed by desquamation, peripheral neuropathy, nausea and vomiting, diarrhoea, stomatitis, alopecia, arthralgia, myalgia, and asthenia.

Indications

Docetaxel is not currently indicated for the treatment of gastrointestinal tract malignancy, but is under investigation for the treatment of upper gastrointestinal tumours.

Drug interactions

No formal studies have been conducted but there is potential for interaction with drugs that induce or inhibit or are metabolized by cytochrome P$_{450}$-3A (e.g. cyclosporin, terfenadine, ketoconazole, and erythromycin).

Cautions and contraindications

Premedication with corticosteroids, antihistamines and H$_2$-receptor antagonists is recommended to prevent hypersensitivity reactions. Previous severe hypersensitivity reactions to docetaxel are a contraindication to its use. Caution should be exercised in patients with hepatic impairment, and a dose reduction instituted; docetaxel should probably not be used in patients with severe hepatic impairment.

Irinotecan

Irinotecan (CPT-11, Campto) is a semi-synthetic camptothecin that inhibits DNA replication via an interaction with topoisomerase I. It is metabolized by carboxylesterase in most tissues to SN-38, which is more active in binding to topoisomerase I than the parent compound. It is administered as a short i.v. infusion over 30–90 min. It displays dose-independent tripha-

sic pharmacokinetics, with half-lives for the three phases of 12 min, 2.5 h and 14.2 h, respectively. Irinotecan is approximately 65% protein bound but SN-38 is 95% protein bound. Approximately 20% of irinotecan and 0.25% of SN-38 is excreted in the urine in the first 24 h. Toxicity of irinotecan includes diarrhoea, which may be severe and prolonged, myelosuppression, nausea and vomiting, acute cholinergic syndrome (early diarrhoea, abdominal pain, rhinitis, conjunctivitis, hypotension, vasodilation, sweating, chills, malaise, dizziness, visual disturbances, myosis, lachrymation, and increased salivation, occurring within 24 h of administration), elevation of hepatic transaminases, alkaline phosphatase or bilirubin, asthenia, and alopecia.

Indications

Irinotecan is indicated for the palliative treatment of 5-fluorouracil-refractory colorectal cancer. It is also being investigated in combination with 5-fluorouracil for the first-line palliative treatment of colorectal cancer.

Drug interactions

There have been no formal studies to assess possible drug interactions. Interaction with neuromuscular blocking agents cannot be ruled out; drugs with anticholinesterase activity may prolong the neuromuscular blocking effects of suxamethonium, and the neuromuscular blockade of non-depolarizing drugs may be antagonized. Loperamide should not be given prophylactically.

Cautions and contraindications

Patients should be warned of the potential for severe delayed diarrhoea and supplied with loperamide and broad-spectrum oral antibiotics (e.g. ciprofloxacin). Loperamide must be commenced immediately a liquid stool occurs, and the patient should drink large volumes of fluids containing electrolytes. Loperamide should be continued at high dosage (2 mg every 2 h) until 12 h after the last liquid stool. If the diarrhoea persists for longer than 24 h, the patient should be asked to contact the hospital and to commence antibiotics. Loperamide should not be continued for longer than 48 h. If the diarrhoea persists at this point, or if it is associated with fever or vomiting at any point, the patient should be admitted to hospital for supportive measures. Patients who experience the acute cholinergic syndrome should receive treatment with atropine (0.25 mg subcutaneously), and this should be given prior to subsequent courses. Irinotecan should be used with caution in patients with mild renal or hepatic impairment, and is not recommended for patients with moderate or severe renal or hepatic impairment. Irinotecan is contraindicated in patients of WHO performance status >2, in patients with chronic inflammatory bowel disease or bowel obstruction, and in patients with a history of severe hypersensitivity reactions with this drug.

REFERENCES

1. World Health Organisation, International Agency for Research on Cancer, European Commission. *Survival of Cancer Patients in Europe: The Eurocare Study.* IARC Scientific Publications, Lyon, 1995, 132.

2. Levard H, Pouliquen X, Hay JM, *et al.* 5-Fluorouracil and cisplatin as palliative treatment of advanced oesophageal squamous cell carcinoma. A multicentre randomised controlled trial. The French Associations for Surgical Research. *Eur J Surg* 1998; **164:** 849–857.

3. Webb A, Cunningham D, Scarffe JH, *et al.* Randomized trial comparing epirubicin, cisplatin, and fluorouracil versus fluorouracil, doxorubicin, and methotrexate in advanced esophagogastric cancer, *J Clin Oncol* 1997; **15:** 261–267.

4. Ross P, Cunningham D, Scarffe H, *et al.* Results of a randomised trial comparing ECF with MCF in advanced oesophagogastric cancer [Abstract]. *Proc Am Soc Clin Oncol* 1999; **18:** 272a.

5. Etienne MC, Bernard S, Fischel JL, *et al.* Dose reduction without loss of efficacy for 5-fluorouracil and cisplatin combined with folinic acid. *In vitro* study on human head and neck carcinoma cell lines. *Br J Cancer* 1991; **63:** 372–377.

6. Ajani JA, Ryan B, Rich TA, *et al.* Prolonged chemotherapy for localised squamous carcinoma of the oesophagus, *Eur J Cancer* 1992; **28A:** 880–884.

7. Mercke C, Albertsson M, Hambraeus G, *et al.* Cisplatin and 5-FU combined with radiotherapy and surgery in the treatment of squamous cell carcinoma of the esophagus. Palliative effects and tumor response. *Acta Oncol* 1991; **30:** 617–622.

8. Waters JS, Norman A, Cunningham D, *et al.* Long-term survival after epirubicin, cisplatin and fluorouracil for gastric cancer: results of a randomized trial. *Br J Cancer* 1999; **80:** 269–272.

9. Petrasch S, Welt A, Reinacher A, Graeven U, Konig M, Schmiegel W. Chemotherapy with cisplatin and paclitaxel in patients with locally advanced, recurrent or metastatic oesophageal cancer. *Br J Cancer* 1998; **78:** 511–514.

10. Kelsen D, Ginsberg R, Bains M, *et al.* A phase II trial of paclitaxel and cisplatin in patients with locally advanced metastatic esophageal cancer: a preliminary report. *Semin Oncol* 1997; **24 (6 Suppl. 19):** 77–81.

11. Herskovic A, Martz K, Al Sarraf M, *et al.* Combined chemotherapy and radiotherapy compared with radiotherapy alone in patients with cancer of the esophagus. *N Engl J Med* 1992; **326:** 1593–1598.

12. Sischy B, Ryan L, Haller D, *et al.* Interim report of Est 1282 Phase III protocol for the evaluation of combined modalities in the treatment of patients with carcinoma of the esophagus, Stage I and II [Abstract]. *Proc Am Soc Clin Oncol* 1990; **9:** A407.

13. Ando N, Iizuka T, Kakegawa T, *et al.* A randomized trial of surgery with and without chemotherapy for localized squamous carcinoma of the thoracic esophagus: the Japan Clinical Oncology Group Study. *J Thorac Cardiovasc Surg* 1997; **114:** 205–209.

14. Ando N, Iizuka T, Ide H, *et al.* A randomised trial of surgery alone v surgery plus postoperative chemotherapy with cisplatin and 5-fluorouracil for localized squamous carcinoma of the thoracic esophagus: the Japan Clinical Oncology Group Study (JCOG 9204). *Proc Am Soc Clin Oncol* 1999; **18:** 269a.

15. Kelsen DP, Ginsberg R, Pajak TF, *et al.* Chemotherapy followed by surgery compared with surgery alone for localized esophageal cancer. *N Engl J Med* 1998; **339:** 1979–1984.

16. Nygaard K, Hagen S, Hansen HS, *et al.* Pre-operative radiotherapy prolongs survival in operable esophageal carcinoma: a randomized, multicenter study of pre-operative radiotherapy and chemotherapy. The second Scandinavian trial in esophageal cancer. *World J Surg* 1992; **16:** 1104–1109.

17. Le Prise E, Etienne PL, Meunier B, *et al.* A randomized study of chemotherapy, radiation therapy, and surgery versus surgery for localized squamous cell carcinoma of the esophagus. *Cancer* 1994; **73:** 1779–1784.

18. Bosset JF, Gignoux M, Triboulet JP, *et al.* Chemoradiotherapy followed by surgery compared with surgery alone in squamous-cell cancer of the esophagus. *N Engl J Med* 1997; **337:** 161–167.

19. Walsh TN, Noonan N, Hollywood D, Kelly A, Keeling N, Hennessy TP. A comparison of multimodal therapy and surgery for esophageal adenocarcinoma. *N Engl J Med* 1996; **335:** 462–467.

20. Urba S, Orringer A, Turrisi R, Whyte R, Iannettoni M, Forastiere A. A randomised trial comparing surgery to preoperative chemoradiation plus surgery in patients with resectable esophageal cancer: updated analysis [Abstract]. *Proc Am Soc Clin Oncol* 1997; **16:** 983.

21. Gray JR, Meluch AA, Kalman L, *et al.* Neoadjuvant paclitaxel/carboplatin/5-FU/radiation therapy for localised esophageal cancer: update of a Minnie Pearl Cancer Research Network Phase II trial. *Proc Am Soc Clin Oncol* 1999; **18:** 271a.

22. Gleeson CM, Sloan JM, McManus DT, *et al.* Comparison of p53 and DNA content abnormalities in adenocarcinoma of the oesophagus and gastric cardia. *Br J Cancer* 1998; **77:** 277–286.

23. Pyrhonen S, Kuitunen T, Nyandoto P, Kouri M. Randomised comparison of fluorouracil, epi-doxorubicin and methotrexate (FEMTX) plus supportive care with supportive care alone in patients with non-resectable gastric cancer. *Br J Cancer* 1995; **71:** 587–591.

24. Glimelius B, Ekstrom K, Hoffman K, *et al.* Randomized comparison between chemotherapy plus best supportive care with best supportive care in advanced gastric cancer. *Ann Oncol* 1997; **8:** 163–168.

25. Murad AM, Santiago FF, Petroianu A, Rocha PR, Rodrigues MA, Rausch M. Modified therapy with 5-fluorouracil, doxorubicin, and methotrexate in advanced gastric cancer. *Cancer* 1993; **72:** 37–41.

26. Kim NK, Park YS, Heo DS, *et al.* A phase III randomized study of 5-fluorouracil and cisplatin versus 5-fluorouracil, doxorubicin, and mitomycin C versus 5-fluorouracil alone in the treatment of advanced gastric cancer. *Cancer* 1993; **71:** 3813–3818.

27. Kyoto Research Group for Chemotherapy of Gastric Cancer (KRGCGC). A randomized, comparative study of combination chemotherapies in advanced gastric cancer: 5-fluorouracil and cisplatin (FP) versus 5-fluorouracil, cisplatin, and 4'-epirubicin (FPEPIR). *Anticancer Res* 1992; **12:** 1983–1988.

28. Findlay M, Cunningham D, Norman A, *et al.* A phase II study in advanced gastro-esophageal cancer using epirubicin and cisplatin in combination with continuous infusion 5-fluorouracil (ECF). *Ann Oncol* 1994; **5:** 609–616.

29. Cascinu S, Labianca R, Alessandroni P, *et al.* Intensive weekly chemotherapy for advanced gastric cancer using fluorouracil, cisplatin, epi-doxorubicin, 6S-leucovorin, glutathione, and fil-grastim: a report from the Italian Group for the Study of Digestive Tract Cancer. *J Clin Oncol* 1997; **15:** 3313–3319.

30. Kim YH, Shin SW, Kim BS, *et al.* Paclitaxel, 5-fluorouracil, and cisplatin combination chemotherapy for the treatment of advanced gastric carcinoma. *Cancer* 1999; **85:** 295–301.

31. Boku N, Ohtsu A, Shimada Y, *et al.* Phase II study of a combination of irinotecan and cisplatin against metastatic gastric cancer. *J Clin Oncol* 1999; **17:** 319–323.

32. Hermans J, Bonenkamp JJ, Boon MC, *et al.* Adjuvant therapy after curative resection for gastric cancer: meta-analysis of randomized trials. *J Clin Oncol* 1993; **11:** 1441–1447.

33. Pignon JP, Ducreux M, Rougier P. Meta-analysis of adjuvant chemotherapy in gastric cancer: a critical reappraisal [Letter]. *J Clin Oncol* 1994; **12:** 877–878.

34. Earle CC, Maroun JA. Adjuvant chemotherapy after curative resection for gastric cancer: revisiting a meta-analysis of randomised trials. *Proc Am Soc Clin Oncol* 1998; **17:** 263a.

35. Fink U, Schuhmacher C, Stein HJ, *et al.* Preoperative chemotherapy for stage III–IV gastric carcinoma: feasibility, response and outcome after complete resection. *Br J Surg* 1995; **82:** 1248–1252.

36. Songun I, Keizer HJ, Hermans J, *et al.* Chemotherapy for operable gastric cancer: results of the Dutch randomised FAMTX trial. *Eur J Cancer* 1999; **35**: 558–562.

37. Kang YK, Choi DW, Im YH, *et al.* A phase III randomized comparison of neoadjuvant chemotherapy followed by surgery versus surgery for locally advanced stomach cancer [Abstract]. *Proc Am Soc Clin Oncol* 1996; **15**: A503.

38. Saito Y, Milross CG, Hittelman WN, *et al.* Effect of radiation and paclitaxel on p53 expression in murine tumors sensitive or resistant to apoptosis induction. *Int J Radiat Oncol Biol Phys* 1997; **38**: 623–631.

39. Mallinson CN, Rake MO, Cocking JB, *et al.* Chemotherapy in pancreatic cancer: results of a controlled, prospective, randomised, multicentre trial. *Br Med J* 1980; **281**: 1589–1591.

40. Glimelius B, Hoffman K, Sjoden PO, *et al.* Chemotherapy improves survival and quality of life in advanced pancreatic and biliary cancer. *Ann Oncol* 1996; **7**: 593–600.

41. Palmer KR, Kerr M, Knowles G, Cull A, Carter DC, Leonard RC. Chemotherapy prolongs survival in inoperable pancreatic carcinoma, *Br J Surg* 1994; **81**: 882–885.

42. Kollmannsberger C, Peters HD, Fink U. Chemotherapy in advanced pancreatic adenocarcinoma. *Cancer Treat Rev* 1998; **24**: 133–156.

43. Carter SK, Comis RL. The integration of chemotherapy into a combined modality approach for cancer treatment. VI. Pancreatic adenocarcinoma. *Cancer Treat Rev* 1975; **2**: 193–214.

44. Wils JA, Kok T, Wagener DJ, Selleslags J, Duez N. Activity of cisplatin in adenocarcinoma of the pancreas. *Eur J Cancer* 1993; **2**: 203–204.

45. Casper ES, Green MR, Kelsen DP, *et al.* Phase II trial of gemcitabine (2,2'-difluorodeoxycytidine) in patients with adenocarcinoma of the pancreas. *Invest New Drugs* 1994; **12**: 29–34.

46. Carmichael J, Fink U, Russell RC, *et al.* Phase II study of gemcitabine in patients with advanced pancreatic cancer. *Br J Cancer* 1996; **73**: 101–105.

47. Burris HA, 3rd, Moore MJ, Andersen J, *et al.* Improvements in survival and clinical benefit with gemcitabine as first-line therapy for patients with advanced pancreas cancer: a randomized trial. *J Clin Oncol* 1997; **15**: 2403–2413.

48. Rougier P, Ducreux M, Douillard JF, *et al.* Efficacy of 5-FU and cisplatin compared to bolus 5-FU in advanced pancreatic carcinoma: a randomised trial from the French Anticancer Centers Digestive Group [Abstract]. *Proc Am Soc Clin Oncol* 1999; **18**: 274a.

49. Underhill CR, Highley MS, Parnis FX, *et al.* Epirubicin, cisplatin and infusional 5-FU—an active regimen in pancreatic carcinoma [Abstract]. *Proc Am Soc Clin Oncol* 1996; **15**: 203.

50. Munzone E, Nole F, de Braud F, *et al.* ECF (epirubicin, cisplatin, fluorouracil) in pancreatic carcinoma (PC): a promising approach [Abstract]. *Proc Am Soc Clin Oncol* 1997; **16**: A1062.

51. Evans TR, Lofts FJ, Mansi JL, Glees JP, Dalgleish AG, Knight MJ. A phase II study of continuous-infusion 5-fluorouracil with cisplatin and epirubicin in inoperable pancreatic cancer. *Br J Cancer* 1996; **73**: 1260–1264.

52. Heinemann V, Wilke H, Possinger K, *et al.* Gemcitabine and cisplatin in the treatment of advanced pancreatic cancer. Final results of a phase II study [Abstract]. *Proc Am Soc Clin Oncol* 1999; **18**: 274a.

53. Philip PA, Zalupski M, Vaitkevicius VK, Arlauskas P, Shields A. Phase II study of gemcitabine and cisplatin in advanced or metastatic pancreatic cancer [Abstract]. *Proc Am Soc Clin Oncol* 1999; **18**: 274a.

54. Isacoff WH, Botnick L, Rose C, *et al.* Treatment of patients (pts) with locally advanced pancreatic carcinoma with continuous infusion (CI), 5-fluorouracil (5-FU), calcium leucovorin (LV), mitomycin-C (Mito-C), and dipyridamole (D) [Abstract]. *Proc Am Soc Clin Oncol* 1993; **12**: A692.

55. Burch PA, Ghosh C, Schroeder G, Woodhouse C, Windschitl H, Tschetter L. A phase II evaluation of continuous infusion 5-FU, leucovorin, mitomycin C, and oral dipyridamole in advanced measurable pancreatic cancer: a NCCTG trial [Abstract]. *Proc Am Soc Clin Oncol* 1996; **15**: 211.

56. Bakkevold KE, Arnesjo B, Dahl O, Kambestad B. Adjuvant combination chemotherapy (AMF) following radical resection of carcinoma of the pancreas and papilla of Vater—results of a controlled, prospective, randomised multicentre study. *Eur J Cancer* 1993; **5**: 698–703.

57. Kalser MH, Ellenberg SS. Pancreatic cancer. Adjuvant combined radiation and chemotherapy following curative resection. *Arch Surg* 1985; **120**: 899–903.

58. Staley CA, Lee JE, Cleary KR, *et al.* Preoperative chemoradiation, pancreaticoduodenectomy, and intraoperative radiation therapy for adenocarcinoma of the pancreatic head. *Am J Surg* 1996; **171:** 118–124.

59. Hoffman JP, Lipsitz S, Pisansky T, Weese JL, Solin L, Benson AB, 3rd. Phase II trial of preoperative radiation therapy and chemotherapy for patients with localized, resectable adenocarcinoma of the pancreas: an Eastern Cooperative Oncology Group Study. *J Clin Oncol* 1998; **16:** 317–323.

60. Moertel CG, Frytak S, Hahn RG, *et al.* Therapy of locally unresectable pancreatic carcinoma: a randomized comparison of high dose (6000 rads) radiation alone, moderate dose radiation (4000 rads + 5-fluorouracil), and high-dose radiation + 5-fluorouracil. The Gastrointestinal Tumor Study Group. *Cancer* 1981; **48:** 1705–1710.

61. Klaassen DJ, MacIntyre JM, Catton GE, Engstrom PF, Moertel CG. Treatment of locally unresectable cancer of the stomach and pancreas: a randomized comparison of 5-fluorouracil alone with radiation plus concurrent and maintenance 5-fluorouracil. An Eastern Cooperative Oncology Group study. *J Clin Oncol* 1985; **3:** 373–378.

62. Safran H, Akerman P, Cioffi W, *et al.* Paclitaxel and concurrent radiation therapy for locally advanced adenocarcinomas of the pancreas, stomach, and gastroesophageal junction. *Semin Radiat Oncol* 1999; **9:** 53–57.

63. McGinn CJ, Shureiqi I, Robertson JM, *et al.* A phase I trial of radiation dose-escalation with full dose gemcitabine in patients with pancreatic cancer [Abstract]. *Proc Am Soc Clin Oncol* 1999; **18:** 274a.

64. Rougier P, Fandi A, Ducreux M, *et al.* Demonstrated efficiency of 5-fluorouracil (5FU) continuous infusion (CI) and cisplatin (P) in patients with advanced biliary tract carcinoma [Abstract]. *Proc Am Soc Clin Oncol* 1995; **14:** A498.

65. Ellis PA, Norman A, Hill A, *et al.* Epirubicin, cisplatin and infusional 5-fluorouracil (5-FU) (ECF) in hepatobiliary tumours [Abstract]. *Eur J Cancer* 1995; **31a:** 1594–1598.

66. Patt YZ, Jones DV, Jr., Hoque A, *et al.* Phase II trial of intravenous fluorouracil and subcutaneous interferon alfa-2b for biliary tract cancer. *J Clin Oncol* 1996; **14:** 2311–2315.

67. Carr BI. Escalating cisplatin doses by hepatic artery infusion (HAI) for advanced-stage hepatocellular carcinoma (HCC) [Abstract]. *Anti Cancer Treatment, Sixth International Congress,* Paris, France, February 6–9, 1996, Abstract 133.

68. Carr BI, Orons P, Zajko A, Sammon J, Bron K, Baron R. Prolonged survival with chemotherapy alone for hepatocellular carcinoma (HCC) with intra-arterial chemotherapy [Abstract]. *Proc Am Soc Clin Oncol* 1994; **13:** A606.

69. Mathurin P, Rixe O, Carbonell N, *et al.* Review article: overview of medical treatments in unresectable hepatocellular carcinoma—an impossible meta-analysis? *Aliment Pharmacol Ther* 1998; **12:** 111–126.

70. Gallo C, Daniele B, Gaeta GB, Perrone F, Pignata S. Tamoxifen in treatment of hepatocellular carcinoma: a randomised controlled trial. *Lancet* 1998; **352:** 17–20.

71. Lai EC, Lo CM, Fan ST, Liu CL, Wong J. Postoperative adjuvant chemotherapy after curative resection of hepatocellular carcinoma: a randomized controlled trial. *Arch Surg* 1998; **133:** 183–188.

72. Ono T, Nagasue N, Kohno H, *et al.* Adjuvant chemotherapy with epirubicin and carmofur after radical resection of hepatocellular carcinoma: a prospective randomized study. *Semin Oncol* 1997; **24 (2 Suppl. 6):** 18–25.

73. Asahara T, Itamoto T, Katayama K, *et al.* Adjuvant hepatic arterial infusion chemotherapy after radical hepatectomy for hepatocellular carcinoma: results of long-term follow-up. *Hepato Gastroenterol* 1999; **46:** 1042–1048.

74. Lygidakis NJ, Pothoulakis J, Konstantinidou AE, Spanos H. Hepatocellular carcinoma: surgical resection versus surgical resection combined with pre- and post-operative locoregional immunotherapy-chemotherapy. A prospective randomized study. *Anticancer Res* 1995; **15:** 543–550.

75. Lau WY, Leung TWT, Ho SKW, *et al.* Adjuvant intra-arterial iodine-131-labelled lipiodol for resectable hepatocellular carcinoma: a prospective randomised trial. *Lancet* 1999; **353:** 797–801.

76. Crawley C, Ross P, Norman A, Hill A, Cunningham D. The Royal Marsden experience of a small bowel adenocarcinoma treated with protracted venous infusion 5-fluorouracil. *Br J Cancer* 1998; **78:** 508–510.

77. Yeung RS, Weese JL, Hoffman JP, *et al.* Neoadjuvant chemoradiation in pancreatic and

duodenal carcinoma. A Phase II Study. *Cancer* 1993; **72:** 2124–2133.

78. Scheithauer W, Rosen H, Kornek GV, Sebesta C, Depisch D. Randomised comparison of combination chemotherapy plus supportive care with supportive care alone in patients with metastatic colorectal cancer. *Br Med J* 1993; **306:** 752–755.

79. Allen Mersh TG, Earlam S, Fordy C, Abrams K, Houghton J. Quality of life and survival with continuous hepatic-artery floxuridine infusion for colorectal liver metastases. *Lancet* 1994; **344:** 1255–1260.

80. Expectancy or primary chemotherapy in patients with advanced asymptomatic colorectal cancer: a randomized trial. Nordic Gastrointestinal Tumor Adjuvant Therapy Group. *J Clin Oncol* 1992; **10:** 904–911.

81. Leichman CG, Fleming TR, Muggia FM, *et al.* Phase II study of fluorouracil and its modulation in advanced colorectal cancer: a Southwest Oncology Group study. *J Clin Oncol* 1995; **13:** 1303–1311.

82. de Gramont A, Bosset JF, Milan C, *et al.* Randomized trial comparing monthly low-dose leucovorin and fluorouracil bolus with bimonthly high-dose leucovorin and fluorouracil bolus plus continuous infusion for advanced colorectal cancer: a French intergroup study. *J Clin Oncol* 1997; **15:** 808–815.

83. Meta-analysis Group In Cancer. Efficacy of intravenous continuous infusion of fluorouracil compared with bolus administration in advanced colorectal cancer. *J Clin Oncol* 1998; **16:** 301–308.

84. Cunningham D. Mature results from three large controlled studies with raltitrexed ('Tomudex'). *Br J Cancer* 1998; **77 (Suppl. 2):** 15–21.

85. Twelves C, Harper P, Van Cutsem E, *et al.* A phase III trial (SO 14796) of Xeloda (capecitabine) in previously untreated advanced/metastatic colorectal cancer [Abstract]. *Proc Am Soc Clin Oncol* 1999; **18:** 263a.

86. Cox JV, Pazdur R, Thibault A, *et al.* A phase III trial (SO 14695) of Xeloda (capecitabine) in previously untreated advanced/metastatic colorectal cancer [Abstract]. *Proc Am Soc Clin Oncol* 1999; **18:** 265a.

87. Pazdur R, Douillard J-Y, Skillings JR, *et al.* Multicentre phase III study of UFT in combination with leucovorin in patients with metastatic

colorectal cancer [Abstract]. *Proc Am Soc Clin Oncol* 1999; **18:** 263a.

88. Ross P, Norman A, Cunningham D, *et al.* A prospective randomised trial of protracted venous infusion 5-fluorouracil with or without mitomycin C in advanced colorectal cancer. *Ann Oncol* 1997; **8:** 995–1001.

89. de Gramont A, Figer A, Seymour M, *et al.* A randomised trial of leucovorin and 5-fluorouracil with or without oxaliplatin in advanced colorectal cancer. *Proc Am Soc Clin Oncol* 1998; **17:** 257a.

90. Doillard J-Y, Cunningham D, Roth AD, *et al.* A randomised phase III trial comparing irinotecan + 5FU/folinic acid to the same schedule of 5FU/FA in patients with metastatic colorectal cancer as front-line chemotherapy [Abstract]. *Proc Am Soc Clin Oncol* 1999; **18:** 233a.

91. Saltz LB, Locker PK, Pirotta N, Elfring GL, Miller LL. Weekly irinotecan, leucovorin, and fluorouracil is superior to daily x 5 LV/FU in patients with previously untreated metastatic colorectal cancer [Abstract]. *Proc Am Soc Clin Oncol* 1999; **18:** 233a.

92. Jager E, Klein O, Wachter B, Muller B, Braun U, Knuth A. Second-line treatment with high-dose 5-fluorouracil and folinic acid in advanced colorectal cancer refractory to standard dose 5-fluorouracil treatment. *Oncology* 1995; **52:** 470–473.

93. Nobile MT, Chiara S, Barzacchi MC, *et al.* Pretreated advanced colorectal cancer: phase II study with high-dose 24 hours 5-fluorouracil infusion plus l-leucovorin [Abstract]. *Proc Am Soc Clin Oncol* 1998; **17:** 275a.

94. Thirion P, Cunningham D, Findlay M, *et al.* Pooled analysis of phase II trials with low-dose 5-fluorouracil continuous infusion as a second-line chemotherapy in advanced colorectal cancer [Abstract]. *Proc Am Soc Clin Oncol* 1998; **17:** 272a.

95. de Gramont A, Vignoud J, Tournigand C, *et al.* Oxaliplatin with high-dose leucovorin and 5-fluorouracil 48-hour continuous infusion in pretreated metastatic colorectal cancer. *Eur J Cancer* 1997; **33:** 214–219.

96. Cunningham D, Pyrhonen S, James RD, *et al.* Randomised trial of irinotecan plus supportive care versus supportive care alone after fluorouracil failure for patients with metastatic colorectal cancer. *Lancet* 1998; **352:** 1413–1418.

97. Rougier P, Van Cutsem E, Bajetta E, *et al.*

Randomised trial of irinotecan versus fluoro-uracil by continuous infusion after fluorouracil failure in patients with metastatic colorectal cancer. *Lancet* 1998; **352**: 1407–1412.

98. Ensminger WD, Gyves JW. Regional chemotherapy of neoplastic diseases. *Pharmacol Ther* 1983; **21**: 277–293.

99. Meta-Analysis Group in Cancer. Reappraisal of hepatic arterial infusion in the treatment of non-resectable liver metastases from colorectal cancer. *J Natl Cancer Inst* 1996; **88**: 252–258.

100. Wolmark N, Fisher B, Rockette H, *et al.* Postoperative adjuvant chemotherapy or BCG for colon cancer: results from NSABP protocol C-01. *J Natl Cancer Inst* 1988; **80**: 30–36.

101. Moertel CG, Fleming TR, Macdonald JS, *et al.* Levamisole and fluorouracil for adjuvant ther-apy of resected colon carcinoma. *N Engl J Med* 1990; **322**: 352–358.

102. International Multicentre Pooled Analysis of Colon Cancer Trials (IMPACT) investigators. Efficacy of adjuvant fluorouracil and folinic acid in colon cancer. *Lancet* 1995; **345**: 939–944.

103. O'Connell MJ, Mailliard JA, Kahn MJ, *et al.* Controlled trial of fluorouracil and low-dose leucovorin given for 6 months as postoperative adjuvant therapy for colon cancer. *J Clin Oncol* 1997; **15**: 246–250.

104. Mamounas E, Wieand S, Wolmark N, *et al.* Comparative efficacy of adjuvant chemother-apy in patients with Dukes' B versus Dukes' C colon cancer: results from four National Surgical Adjuvant Breast and Bowel Project adjuvant studies (C-01, C-02, C-03, and C-04). *J Clin Oncol* 1999; **17**: 1349–1355.

105. Zoetmulder FAN, Taal BG, Van Tinteren H. Adjuvant 5FU plus levamisole improves sur-vival in stage II and III colonic cancer, but not in rectal cancer. Interim analysis of the Netherlands Adjuvant Colorectal Cancer Project (NACCP) [Abstract]. *Proc Am Soc Clin Oncol* 1999; **18**: 266a.

106. International Multicentre Pooled Analysis of B2 Colon Cancer Trials (IMPACT B2) Investigators. Efficacy of adjuvant fluorouracil and folinic acid in B2 colon cancer. *J Clin Oncol* 1999; **17**: 1356–1363.

107. Fisher B, Wolmark N, Rockette H, *et al.* Postoperative adjuvant chemotherapy or radia-tion therapy for rectal cancer: results from NSABP protocol R-01. *J Natl Cancer Inst* 1988; **80**: 21–29.

108. Douglas HO, Moertel CG, Mayer RJ, *et al.*, Survival after postoperative combination treat-ment of rectal cancer. *New Engl J Med* 1986; **315**: 1294–1295.

109. Krook JE, Moertel CG, Gunderson LL, *et al.* Effective surgical adjuvant therapy for high-risk rectal carcinoma. *N Engl J Med* 1991; **324**: 709–715.

110. National Institutes of Health Consensus Conference: adjuvant therapy for patients with colon and rectal cancer. *J Am Med Assoc* 1990; **264**: 1444–1450.

111. Rockette H, Deutsch M, Petrelli N, *et al.* Effect of postoperative radiation therapy (RTX) when used with adjuvant chemotherapy in Dukes' B and C rectal cancer: results from NSABP R-02 [Abstract]. *Proc Am Soc Clin Oncol* 1994; **13**: A560.

112. O'Connell MJ, Martenson JA, Wieand HS, *et al.* Improving adjuvant therapy for rectal cancer by combining protracted-infusion fluorouracil with radiation therapy after curative surgery. *N Engl J Med* 1994; **331**: 502–507.

113. Hyams DM, Mamounas EP, Petrelli N, *et al.* A clinical trial to evaluate the worth of preopera-tive multimodality therapy in patients with operable carcinoma of the rectum: a progress report of National Surgical Breast and Bowel Project Protocol R-03. *Dis Colon Rectum* 1997; **40**: 131–139.

114. Riethmuller G, Holz E, Schlimok G, *et al.* Monoclonal antibody therapy for resected Dukes' C colorectal cancer: seven-year outcome of a multicenter randomized trial. *J Clin Oncol* 1998; **16**: 1788–1794.

115. Arnott SJ, Cunningham D, Gallagher J, *et al.* Epidermoid anal cancer: results from the UKC-CCR randomised trial of radiotherapy alone versus radiotherapy, 5-fluorouracil, and mito-mycin. *Lancet* 1996; **348**: 1049–1054.

116. Bartelink H, Roelofsen F, Eschwege F, *et al.* Concomitant radiotherapy and chemotherapy is superior to radiotherapy alone in the treat-ment of locally advanced anal cancer: results of a phase III randomized trial of the European Organization for Research and Treatment of Cancer Radiotherapy and Gastrointestinal Cooperative Groups. *J Clin Oncol* 1997; **15**: 2040–2049.

117. Flam M, John M, Pajak TF, *et al.* Role of mito-mycin in combination with fluorouracil and radiotherapy, and of salvage chemoradiation in

the definitive nonsurgical treatment of epidermoid carcinoma of the anal canal: results of a phase III randomized intergroup study. *J Clin Oncol* 1996; **14:** 2527–2539.

118. Doci R, Zucali R, La Monica G, *et al.* Primary chemoradiation therapy with fluorouracil and cisplatin for cancer of the anus: results in 35 consecutive patients. *J Clin Oncol* 1996; **14:** 3121–3125.

119. Aviles A, Diaz Maqueo JC, De la Torre A, *et al.* Is surgery necessary in the treatment of primary gastric non-Hodgkin lymphoma? *Leuk Lymphoma* 1991; **5:** 365–369.

120. Ferreri AJ, Cordio S, Ponzoni M, Villa E. Non-surgical treatment with primary chemotherapy, with or without radiation therapy, of stage I-II high-grade gastric lymphoma. *Leuk Lymphoma* 1999; **33:** 531–541.

121. Tondini C, Giardini R, Bozzetti F, *et al.* Combined modality treatment for primary gastrointestinal non-Hodgkin's lymphoma: the Milan Cancer Institute experience. *Ann Oncol* 1993; **4:** 831–837.

122. Holmes GK, Prior P, Lane MR, Pope D, Allan RN. Malignancy in coeliac disease-effect of a gluten free diet. *Gut* 1989; **30:** 333–338.

123. Swinson CM, Slavin G, Coles EC, Booth CC. Coeliac disease and malignancy. *Lancet* 1983; **1:** 111–115.

124. Isaacson PG, Spencer J, Wright DH. Classifying primary gut lymphomas [Letter]. *Lancet* 1988; **2:** 1148–1149.

125. Wotherspoon AC, Doglioni C, Diss TC, *et al.* Regression of primary low-grade B-cell gastric lymphoma of mucosa-associated lymphoid tissue type after eradication of *Helicobacter pylori.* *Lancet* 1993; **342:** 575–577.

126. Saltz L, Trochanowski B, Buckley M, *et al.* Octreotide as an antineoplastic agent in the treatment of functional and nonfunctional neuroendocrine tumors. *Cancer* 1993; **72:** 244–248.

127. Kvols LK, Moertel CG, O'Connell MJ, Schutt AJ, Rubin J, Hahn RG. Treatment of the malignant carcinoid syndrome. Evaluation of a long-acting somatostatin analogue. *N Engl J Med* 1986; **315:** 663–666.

128. Ruszniewski P, Ducreux M, Chayvialle JA, *et al.* Treatment of the carcinoid syndrome with the long-acting somatostatin analogue lanreotide: a prospective study in 39 patients. *Gut* 1996; **39:** 279–283.

129. Oberg K. Chemotherapy and biotherapy in neuroendocrine tumors. *Curr Opin Oncol* 1993; **5:** 110–120.

130. Oberg K, Eriksson B, Janson ET. The clinical use of interferons in the management of neuroendocrine gastroenteropancreatic tumors. *Ann NY Acad Sci* 1994; **733:** 471–478.

131. Jacobsen MB, Hanssen LE, Kolmannskog F, Schrumpf E, Vatn MH, Bergan A. Interferon-alpha 2b, with or without prior hepatic artery embolization: clinical response and survival in mid-gut carcinoid patients. The Norwegian carcinoid study. *Scand J Gastroenterol* 1995; **30:** 789–796.

132. Taal BG, Hoefnagel CA, Valdes Olmos RA, Boot H, Beijnen JH. Palliative effect of metaiodobenzylguanidine in metastatic carcinoid tumors. *J Clin Oncol* 1996; **14:** 1829–1838.

133. Otte A, Mueller Brand J, Dellas S, Nitzsche EU, Herrmann R, Maecke HR. Yttrium-90-labelled somatostatin-analogue for cancer treatment [Letter]. *Lancet* 1998; **351:** 417–418.

134. Janson ET, Eriksson B, Oberg K, *et al.* Tumour-targeting therapy with a radioactive somatostatin analogue in neuroendocrine tumours. *Clin Physiol* 1998; **18:** 281–282.

135. Moertel CG, Lefkopoulo M, Lipsitz S, Hahn RG, Klaassen D. Streptozocin-doxorubicin, streptozocin-fluorouracil or chlorozotocin in the treatment of advanced islet-cell carcinoma. *N Engl J Med* 1992; **326:** 519–523.

136. Moertel CG, Kvols LK, O'Connell MJ, Rubin J. Treatment of neuroendocrine carcinomas with combined etoposide and cisplatin. Evidence of major therapeutic activity in the anaplastic variants of these neoplasms. *Cancer* 1991; **68:** 227–232.

137. Venook AP. Embolization and chemoembolization therapy for neuroendocrine tumors. *Curr Opin Oncol* 1999; **11:** 38–41.

138. Howe GR, Benito E, Castelleto R, *et al.* Dietary intake of fiber and decreased risk of cancers of the colon and rectum: evidence from the combined analysis of 13 case-control studies. *J Natl Cancer Inst* 1992; **84:** 1887–1896.

139. Newmark HL, Lipkin M. Calcium, vitamin D, and colon cancer. *Cancer Res* 1992; **52 (7 Suppl.):** 2067s-2070s.

140. Giovannucci E, Stampfer MJ, Colditz GA, *et al.* Multivitamin use, folate, and colon cancer in women in the Nurses' Health Study. *Ann Intern Med* 1998; **129:** 517–524.

141. Block G. Epidemiologic evidence regarding

vitamin C and cancer. *Am J Clin Nutr* 1991; **54 (6 Suppl.):** 1310s–1314s.

142. Slattery ML, Edwards SL, Anderson K, Caan B. Vitamin E and colon cancer: is there an association? *Nutr Cancer* 1998; **30:** 201–206.

143. La Vecchia C, Braga C, Negri E, *et al.* Intake of selected micronutrients and risk of colorectal cancer. *Int J Cancer* 1997; **73:** 525–530.

144. Muscat JE, Stellman SD, Wynder EL. Nonsteroidal anti-inflammatory drugs and colorectal cancer. *Cancer* 1994; **74:** 1847–1854.

145. Baron JA, Beach M, Mandel JS, *et al.* Calcium supplements for the prevention of colorectal adenomas. Calcium Polyp Prevention Study Group. *N Engl J Med* 1999; **340:** 101–107.

146. Greenberg ER, Baron JA, Tosteson TD, *et al.* A clinical trial of antioxidant vitamins to prevent colorectal adenoma. Polyp Prevention Study Group. *N Engl J Med* 1994; **331:** 141–147.

147. Montoya RG, Wargovich MJ. Chemoprevention of gastrointestinal cancer. *Cancer Metast Rev* 1997; **16:** 405–419.

10

Pancreatitis and pancreatic insufficiency

Stefan Kahl, Peter Malfertheiner

ACUTE PANCREATITIS

Acute pancreatitis is an acute painful abdominal disease of sudden onset that ranges from a mild and self-limited illness to a severe progressive life-threatening condition. The ratio of mild to severe acute pancreatitis is approximately five to one. Patients with severe acute pancreatitis develop systemic complications resulting from either the systemic inflammatory response syndrome (SIRS) or to sepsis, which may lead to multi-organ failure (MOF).

The death rate in severe acute pancreatitis, despite important progress in clinical management, is still 10–20%.[1–7]

Pathophysiology of acute pancreatitis

The initial events of acute pancreatitis are still incompletely elucidated (Fig. 10.1). Basic knowledge, which is still evolving, is derived from animal experiments.[8] Acinar cells of the pancreas are extremely active in the synthesis of digestive enzymes, which are delivered as inactive proenzymes into the duodenal lumen where they are activated by enterokinases. In acute pancreatitis, acinar cell injury leads to co-localization of digestive enzyme zymogens and lysosomes and, in this way, lysosomal hydrolase cathepsin-B

activates trypsinogen to trypsin within the cell compartment. This intracellular digestive enzyme activation produces a local inflammatory process that may extend to a generalized phenomenon, with release of cytokines and tissue damaging factors including the platelet aggregating factor (PAF). This series of events results in systemic inflammatory response syndrome (SIRS), which may progress into individual or multiple organ failure (MOF).

Therapy of acute pancreatitis

The prognostic assessment of the severity of acute pancreatitis into 'mild' and 'severe' has important implications for management.[9] Single biochemical markers such as C-reactive protein and multi-factorial scoring systems (Glasgow criteria and APACHE II scoring system) are well-validated and used widely for prognosis of acute pancreatitis.[10–12]

There is still no specific therapy for patients with acute pancreatitis despite efforts to introduce novel drugs with antagonistic effects on some of the established pathways of the disease. Only in patients with severe acute biliary pancreatitis has early endoscopic retrograde cholangiography (ERC) combined with papillotomy proven to be of significant clinical benefit.[13–15]

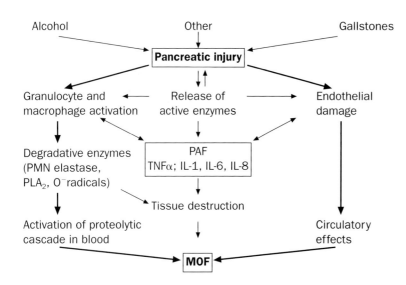

Figure 10.1 Pathophysiology of acute pancreatitis. PMN, polymorphonuclear neutrophil; PLA_2, phospholipase A_2; PAF, platelet activating factor; TNFα, tissue necrosing factor alpha; IL, interleukin; MOF, multiorgan failure

Supportive therapy is mandatory first-line therapy. This consists of adequate volume replacement (3–9 l with appropriate electrolytes) regulated on the central venous pressure, analgesics, and prophylactic antibiotics when there is pancreatic necrosis. Standard therapy in acute pancreatitis is as follows:

- Effective medical therapy
  — Volume replacement and hydration
  — Analgesics for pain relief
  — Correction of electrolyte abnormalities and diabetes mellitus
- Effective therapy in predicted severe cases
  — Antibiotics
  — Parenteral or jejunal feeding

Severe cases should be treated depending on complications, in the setting of high-dependency or intensive care units.

Several drugs aimed at interrupting the acute inflammatory pathway, such as antiproteolytic drugs, aprotinin[16] or gabexate mesilate,[7] or inhibitors of pancreatic secretion,[17,18] have failed to reduce both morbidity and mortality. New therapies designed to antagonize local pancreatic inflammation and to prevent SIRS have also failed as yet.

Gabexate mesilate is a synthetic broad-spectrum antiprotease; it has a low molecular weight and is able to penetrate the pancreatic parenchyma and interstitium. It is the most promising drug developed in the last decade. While a large multicentre study failed to show a significant benefit[7] another study, in which the drug was given very early in the course of the disease, reported a reduction of pancreatic damage.[19] This is often impracticable in routine clinical practice and the use of gabexate mesilate is therefore limited to the prevention of ERCP-induced acute pancreatitis.

Lexipafant, a potent antagonist of platelet activating factor (PAF), was also a new promising candidate. It was probably effective in experimentally-induced pancreatitis in rats, and an initial pilot study in humans showed reduced pancreatic and extrapancreatic inflammation, as well as a reduction in organ complications.[20] However, in a recent large multicentre study, a beneficial effect was not confirmed.[21]

Antibiotics

The majority of deaths in acute pancreatitis relate to septic complications. These complications are usually seen around the 10th to 14th day after onset of the disease. Patients with necrotizing pancreatitis are at greatest risk of secondary infection and death. This risk increases with the degree of pancreatic necrosis.

Current advice is that patients with a severe attack of acute pancreatitis should undergo contrast-enhanced (dynamic) computed tomography (CT) between 3 and 10 days after admission for the assessment of the degree of pancreatic necrosis and surrounding peripancreatic and intra-abdominal fluid collections.[22]

The acute-phase protein, C-reactive protein (CRP), accurately indicates the presence of pancreatic necrosis in up to 90% patients providing the validated level of over 120 mg/l is used.[23] There is an impressive time-dependent increase in infection rates of pancreatic necrosis with the duration of the disease.[24] Most of these infections are caused by *Escherichia coli*, *Pseudomonas* spp., *Staphylococcus aureus*, or *Klebsiella* spp.[25] The benefit of early prophylactic antibiotic therapy (within 48 h) in patients with necrotizing pancreatitis to prevent septic complications is now well-established.[26] The antibiotics must penetrate into pancreatic tissue and cover the full bacterial spectrum.[27] Imipenem and cephalosporins have good tissue penetration and high antibactericidal efficacy.[28–30]

In a direct comparison of pefloxacin (400 mg, twice daily for 14 days) and imipenem (500 mg, three times daily for 14 days) imipenem proved significantly more effective in prevention of the infection and extrapancreatic infections than pefloxacin.[28]

Recent evidence indicates that fungal infection may follow antibiotic treatment, although this may occur even in patients who have not received prior treatment.

If infection of pancreatic necrosis is suspected, CT-guided percutaneous aspiration has proven to be a safe and accurate method of distinguishing sterile from infected necrosis. In cases of infected pancreatic necrosis, the currently accepted practice is to perform early surgical debridement.[31,32] Further studies are needed to evaluate the benefit of non-surgical approaches in infected pancreatic necrosis.

Enteral and parenteral nutrition

Total parenteral nutrition via central venous catheter is recommended for patients with predicted severe acute pancreatitis and in cases with a protracted illness. In mild acute pancreatitis, total parenteral nutrition is unnecessary. In severe cases of acute pancreatitis, parenteral nutrition should be started within the first 72 h after the onset of the illness but there is no definite evidence that total parenteral nutrition improves outcome.[33,34] Recent studies have shown an improvement in clinical outcome of patients with acute pancreatitis if they received enteral nutrition by a nasojejunal tube compared with patients on parenteral nutrition.[34–40]

The concept behind early enteral nutrition is that luminal nutrients will protect the gut from mucosal injury. Without luminal nutrition, within a few hours after the onset of acute pancreatitis intestinal permeability to toxins or bacteria is increased. Endogenous cytokines stimulated by endotoxins and bacterial products from the paralysed gut will enter the systemic circulation and may damage a variety of distant organ systems and lead to SIRS, to sepsis, MOF and death.[41]

It has been shown, that enteral nutrition is safe, that it controls the acute-phase response, decreases disease severity and improves clinical outcome in patients with severe acute pancreatitis.[36,39,40] A large randomized clinical trial for final proof of the enteral feeding concept as a substitute for the parenteral route is essential. The current management options for patients with acute pancreatitis are summarized in Table 10.1.

ERCP induced acute pancreatitis

Depending on how this entity is defined, some degree of post-ERCP pancreatitis or elevated pancreatic enzymes may occur in up to 40% of patients undergoing this procedure.[42,43] Clinically acute post-ERCP pancreatitis appears in 1–3% of patients.[44,45]

The pathophysiology of post-ERCP pancreatitis remains unknown, although the following

Table 10.1 Therapeutic approaches in acute pancreatitis.

	Indication	Therapies	Drugs	Dosage/24 h	Application
All patients	· Dehydration	· Volume replacement	· Intravenous fluids water, glucose and amino acids	3–9 l	Intravenous; according to the central venous pressure and balanced
	· Pain	· Analgesics			
	— Mild		· Acetaminophen	2–3 × 1000 mg	Oral, if not possible tramadol intravenously
			· Tramadol	3–4 × 100 mg	
	— Moderate to severe		· Buprenorphin	6–8 × 0.3 mg max 9 µg/kg Bodyweight/dosage	Intravenous
	· Elevated blood glucose, diabetes mellitus	· Correction of blood glucose level	Insulin	· According to blood glucose	Continuous intravenous infusion
	· Electrolyte abnormalities				
	· Severe hypocalcemia	· Correction of serum calcium level	Administration of calcium	· According to serum calcium level	Intravenous
Predicted severe cases	· Nutritional support	· Parenteral nutrition	Water, glucose and amino acids	Balanced	Intravenous
	· Prevention of infected pancreatic necrosis and septic complications	· Antibiotics	Meropenem Imipenem	3 × 500 mg 3 × 500 mg	Intravenous
	· Nutritional support and prevention of septic complications*	· Enteral (jejunal) feeding	Nutrients via a nasojejunal tube	Balanced	Enteral

* Further studies are needed.

have been proposed as risk factors:

- Increased intrapancreatic pressure caused by retrograde injection of contrast medium, with consequent damage of acinar cells
- A toxic component of injected contrast agents
- Insufficient drainage of injected contrast media and pancreatic juice owing to oedema of the papilla as a consequence of mechanical and thermal injury resulting from manipulations during endoscopy

The ideal solution to prevent post-ERCP pancreatitis would be to provide effective prophylaxis prior to the procedure, probably with a pharmacological agent. Several groups have investigated somatostatin or its long-acting cyclic analogue octreotide. One group found octreotide to be effective in the prevention of post-ERCP pancreatitis[46] but others could not confirm this benefit.[43,47–49] Summarizing all data neither somatostatin nor octreotide can prevent ERCP-induced pancreatitis. Pre-treatment with corticosteroid has been reported to decrease the incidence of post-ERCP pancreatitis,[50] but others have been unable to reproduce these results, and thus cannot be recommended.[51]

Despite initial optimism that non-ionic contrast media would reduce the risk of post-ERCP pancreatitis, a prospective multicentre trial did not show any statistical significance between ionic and non-ionic contrast media.[52]

A significant reduction in the incidence of post-ERCP pancreatitis was shown in a multicentre study from Italy using gabexate mesilate;[19] however gabexate is expensive and as recommended in this study, a 12-h preprocedure infusion is required. This will restrict the use of this drug in routine clinical practice.

A large prospective study analysing the risk factors associated with complications of endoscopic sphinctrotomy identified low-dose anticoagulation to be an independent factor that reduced the risk of post-procedure acute pancreatitis.[53] Again this intervention needs further prospective studies before it can be recommended widely. Data on prevention of post-ERCP pancreatitis is summarized in Table 10.2.

CHRONIC PANCREATITIS

Chronic pancreatitis is a dynamic process in which a progressive destruction of pancreatic parenchyma caused by inflammation, necrosis, and consequent biosynthesis of fibrotic tissue occurs. This necrosis–fibrosis sequence is considered to be a central event in the evolution of chronic pancreatitis.[56–58] Fibrosis leads to a complete change of gland architecture, which is followed by impairment of function. The main features of chronic pancreatitis are:

- Pain
- Loss of exocrine and endocrine pancreatic function

Pain

Pain is the leading symptom in chronic pancreatitis, and presents in a heterogeneous pattern, ranging from a few relapses per year to continuous pain.[59] Two mechanisms are commonly suggested for the generation of pain in the absence of local complications: (1) ductal and (2) intraparenchymal hypertension or inflammatory changes of pancreatic parenchyma with involvement of pancreatic nerves.[59,60]

Analgesic therapy

Pain in chronic pancreatitis poses significant problems for treatment. The first step in pain management consists of the complete avoidance of alcohol. Total abstinence from alcohol as the only measure achieves pain relief in up to 50% of patients, but this effect appears restricted to those with mild to moderate disease.[61–63] Prior to using analgesics, any complication that may be responsible for pain (e.g. pseudocysts, compression of adjacent visceral structures) needs to be excluded. Analgesic drug-treatment should begin with non-narcotic agents (e.g. paracetamol, non-steroidal anti-inflammatory drugs—NSAIDs) but opioid analgesics are often required. Type and doses of analgesic drugs required vary between patients. Treatment should be adopted to individual

Table 10.2 Different approaches for prevention of post-ERCP pancreatitis.

Agent	Data for use	Data against use	Recommendation
Non-ionic contrast medium	Barkin et al. 1991[54]	Johnson et al. 1995[52]	Not recommended
Somatostatin/octreotide	Poon et al. 1999[55]	Arcidiocono et al. 1994,[43] Tulassay et al. 1998,[47] Haber 2000,[48] Binmoeller et al. 1992[49]	Not recommended
Gabexate	Cavallini et al. 1996[19]		Possibly recommended in special cases: 12 h pre-procedure infusion is required; further prospective studies are needed
Anticoagulation	Rabenstein et al. 2000[53]		Presently not recommended; possibly recommended in special cases; further prospective studies are needed
Corticosteroids	Weiner et al. 1995[50]	De Palma and Catazano 1999[51]	Not recommended

needs, with the lowest drug doses necessary to control pain. If a NSAID is used, it should be combined with a proton-pump inhibitor. Analgesic drugs should be increased stepwise according to WHO recommendations.[64]

Co-existing depression may lower the visceral pain threshold in individual patients. In this case, an antidepressant can be useful. Additional to the effect on the depression, antidepressants have an effect on pain and potentiate the effect of opiates.

EXOCRINE INSUFFICIENCY

Exocrine pancreatic insufficiency includes decreased activity of amylase, lipase, and trypsin which results in maldigestion of carbohydrates, fat, and protein.

The clinical picture of pancreatic exocrine insufficiency is dominated by steatorrhoea because of reduced lipase activity; this is due to increased pancreatic output, and also to irreversible inactivation below pH 4.0 and by proteases. Patients with chronic pancreatitis do not have steatorrhoea until maximum stimulated lipase output is below 10% of normal. The indication for pancreatic enzyme replacement is severe exocrine insufficiency accompanied by progressive weight loss and/or complaints associated with steatorrhoea. The amount of lipase activity that abolishes steatorrhoea in achlorhydric patients is approximately 30 000 IU.[65] However, in patients with chronic pancreatitis who may have normal or even increased gastric acid output and decreased pancreatic bicarbonate secretion, this amount is insufficient because of acid inactivation of lipase. This acidic loss can be overcome either by increasing the dose of lipase activity (up to a dose of 50 000–75 000 IU) or by protecting the lipase from inactivation. Protection against acidic inactivation is best achieved by using proton pump inhibitors in a standard dose, or by using enteric-coated mini-dose-unit preparations. A combination of both approaches may be necessary since, in some cases in which there is a simultaneous decrease in bicarbonate secretion, the optimal pH for enzyme activity in the duodenum is only achieved after acid suppression.

The required dose of lipase activity for a main meal ranges from 25 000–75 000 IU lipase and for between meal snacks from 5000–25 000 IU lipase. Consequently, one–three capsules during main meals will usually suffice. Individual patients may require lower or higher doses.

In contrast to earlier treatment recommendations, fat intake should not be restricted. Restrictions of fat intake may seriously compromise caloric intake and lead to loss of body weight.

ENDOCRINE INSUFFICIENCY: DIABETES MELLITUS

Endocrine pancreatic insufficiency (impaired glucose utlization or diabetes mellitus) is a frequent complication in chronic pancreatitis. In acute pancreatitis, temporary hyperglycaemia can be observed in about 50% of patients, while persisting diabetes may affect 1–15%.[66] In chronic pancreatitis, about 60% of patients are reported to have diabetes, 30% of whom will be insulin-dependent.[67] Endocrine pancreatic insufficiency in patients with chronic pancreatitis occurs with the progressive atrophy of the gland. In the majority of cases, the time between diagnosis and onset of pancreatic diabetes ranges from 7–15 years.[68]

During the initial phase of endocrine insufficiency in chronic pancreatitis, dietary restrictions sometimes combined with oral hypoglycaemic agents may be sufficient. Most patients with overt diabetes mellitus will need to be treated with insulin eventually. This is often difficult and associated with a high rate of hypoglycaemic episodes because of the associated lack of regulatory hormones such as glucagon, impaired food assimilation (owing to exocrine pancreatic insufficiency, see earlier text) and poor adherence to dietary regimens. Therapy for chronic pancreatitis is outlined in Table 10.3.

Table 10.3 Therapy of chronic pancreatitis.

Indication	Drugs	Dosage	Problems
· **Pain** (stepwise therapy according to WHO scheme)			
— Mild	Acetaminophen	2–3 × 1000 mg	May be accompanied by spasmolytic agents (N-butylscopolaminumbromid; 3–4 × 10–20 mg/day) or by antidepressants
	Tramadol	3–4 × 100–200 mg	
— Moderate to severe	Buprenorphin	6–8 × 0.3 mg max 9 μg/kg bodyweight/ dosage	
— Severe	Additional interventional therapy: coeliac ganglion block with 25 ml 50% alcohol on each side		
· **Exocrine insufficiency**			
— Without steatorrhoea and without weight loss	No therapy needed		
— With steatorrhoea and/or weight loss	Pancreatin (combination of porcine lipase, amylase and proteases (e.g. Creon™))	3 × 50 000 IU during main meals, 25 000 IU during snacks	Lipase is sometimes inactivated by low pH, add proton pump inhibitor (e.g. omeprazole) in standard dosage, see below
— Protection of oral administered enzyme preparation against acidic inactivation	Proton pump inhibitors	Standard dosage two times daily perorally	
· **Endocrine insufficiency**			
— Impaired glucose utilization	Dietary procedures with restricted oral glucose intake		
— Diabetes mellitus	Insulin	Individual amounts of insulin needed	Oral antidiabetics only sufficient in the early phase of diabetes mellitus.

PSEUDOCYSTS

Pancreatic pseudocysts are fluid collections of pancreatic secretions or transudates without an epithelial lining, resulting from pancreatic inflammation or pancreatic damage.

Acute pseudocysts may develop as a consequence of acute pancreatic inflammation and may contain fluid and necrotic debris. Chronic pseudocysts develop by rupture of a side branch of the pancreatic duct allowing the escape of pancreatic secretions to the surrounding tissue. Peripancreatic fluid collections are found in up to 50% of patients following severe acute pancreatitis. More than one-half regress spontaneously; those persisting beyond 4 weeks and enclosed by a defined wall of fibrous tissue are termed pseudocysts.[69]

Up to one-half (40–50%) of pseudocysts are present for less than 6–12 weeks. Small pseudocysts often disappear spontaneously, whereas larger ones require interventional therapy or surgery.[70]

Complication rates of treated and untreated cysts are similar, so only symptomatic pseudocysts should be treated. Up to now there are no adequate clinical trials to decide whether surgery, internal endoscopic drainage, external drainage, drug therapy or combination of different modalities is the method of choice for treatment of pseudocysts.

Enlarging pseudocysts usually have a connection to the pancreatic duct system, even if not detectable using ERCP. Therefore inhibition of pancreatic secretion should lead to a decrease in pseudocyst size.

Somatostatin has a profound inhibitory effect on the pancreatic secretion, this has been used in the treatment of pseudocysts.[71]

When symptomatic pancreatic pseudocysts are treated non-surgically, a combination of drainage procedures in addition to the inhibition of pancreatic secretion with the somatostatin analogue, octreotide (100–200 µg three times per day subcutaneously) is recommended.

The administration of the long-acting somatostatin analogue, octreotide (500–200 µg s.c. three times daily) has been used success-fully to reduce the duration of catheter drainage and to avoid recurrent cyst formation after treatment.[72,73] Total inhibition of pancreatic exocrine secretion must be accompanied by pancreatic enzyme supplements (containing 50 000 IU or more of lipase activity/standard meal).

PANCREATIC FISTULA

Pancreatic fistulae result from either rupture of a pancreatic duct or from external drainage of a pseudocyst or abscess. They may close spontaneously. Somatostatin is extremely effective in decreasing output of the fistula and expediting closure. The mechanism of action is the same as for pseudocysts. The dosage is 100–200 µg three times per day or octreotide in depot formulation (10–30 mg/monthly for 3 months). Inhibition of pancreatic exocrine secretion must be accompanied by oral enzyme supplementation (at least approx. 50 000 IU of lipase, during meals).

PHARMACOLOGY OF DRUGS

Imipenem with cilastin

Imipenem is partially inactivated in the kidney by dehydropeptidase and is therefore administered with cilastin, a specific enzyme inhibitor, which blocks its renal metabolism. Antibacterial activity includes Gram-positive and Gram-negative bacteria and anaerobes.

Indications
Imipenem with cilastin is used in the prevention of pancreatic infection in patients with acute severe pancreatitis and pancreatic necrosis involving more than 30% of the pancreas on contrast-enhanced CT scan.

Dynamics/kinetics
The half-life of both imipenem and cilastin is 60 min; 70% of both drugs are excreted by the kidney.

Adverse reactions
Adverse reactions include nausea, vomiting, diarrhoea and local reactions at injection site (erythema, pain and induration, and thrombophlebitis). Rarely, allergic reactions, seizures, toxic epidermal necrolysis, pseudomembranous colitis, neutropenia and agranulocytosis, eosinophillia, thrombocytopenia, anaemia, positive Coombs' test, increased liver enzymes, increase in serum creatinine and blood urea, and abnormal urinalysis occur.

Drug interactions
Beta-lactam antibiotics and probenecid may increase toxicity.

Precautions and contraindications
Imipenem appears in breast milk and crosses the placenta and should be avoided in pregnant and breastfeeding patients. The dose and frequency of drug administration should be reduced in patients with renal impairment (see data sheet). Imipenem/cilastin is contraindicated in patients with previous drug hypersensitivity.

Somatostatin

See Chapter 13, p. 303.

Octreotide

See Chapter 13, p. 303.

REFERENCES

1. Karimgani I, Porter KA, Langevin ER, Banks PA. Prognostic factors in sterile pancreatic necrosis. *Gastroenterology* 1992; **103**: 1636–1640.
2. Beger HG, Büchler MW, Bittner R, Nevalainen TJ, Roschere R. Necrosectomy and postoperative local lavage in necrotizing pancreatitis. *Br J Surg* 1988; **75**: 207–221.
3. Sarr M, Nagomey D, Johnson CD, Farnell M. Acute necrotizing pancreatitis: management by planned, staged pancreatic necrosectomy/debridement and delayed primary wound closure over drains. *Br J Surg* 1991; **78**: 576–581.
4. Rattner DW, Legermate DA, Lee MJ, Warshaw AL. Early surgical debridement of symptomatic pancreatic necrosis is beneficial irrespective of infection. *Am J Surg* 1992; **163**: 105–110.
5. Steinberg WM, Schlesselmann SE. Treatment of acute pancreatitis. Comparison of animal and human studies. *Gastroenterology* 1987; **93**: 1420–1427.
6. Leese T, Holliday M, Watkins M, Neoptolemos JP, Hall C, Attard A. A multicentre controlled clinical trial of high-volume fresh frozen plasma therapy in prognostically severe acute pancreatitis. *Ann R Coll Surg Engl* 1991; **73**: 207–214.
7. Büchler MW, Malfertheiner P, Uhl W, *et al.* Gabexate mesilate in human acute pancreatitis. *Gastroenterology* 1993; **104**: 1165–1170.
8. Lerch MM, Saluja A, Dawra R, Ramarao P, Saluja M, Steer ML. Acute necrotizing pancreatitis in the opossum; earliest morphologic changes involve acinar cells. *Gastroenterology* 1992; **103**: 205–213.
9. Glazer G, Mann DV. United Kingdom guidelines for the management of acute pancreatitis. *Gut* 1998; **42 (Suppl. 2):** S1–S13.
10. Knaus WA, Draper EA, Wagner DP, Zimmermann JE. APACHE-I: a severity of disease classification system. *Crit Care Med* 1985; **13**: 818–829.
11. Ranson JHC, Rifkind KM, Roses DF, Fink SD, Eng K, Spencer FC. Prognostic signs and the role of operative management in acute pancreatitis. *Surg Gynecol Obstet* 1974; **139**: 69–81.
12. Imrie CM, Benjamin IS, Ferguson JC, *et al.* A single-centre double-blind trial of Trasylol therapy in primary acute pancreatitis. *Br J Surg* 1978; **65(5):** 337–341.
13. Fan ST, Lai CS, Mok FPT, Lo CM, Rheng SS, Wong J. Early treatment of acute biliary pancreatitis by endoscopic papillotomy. *N Engl J Med* 1993; **325**: 228–232.
14. Neoptolemos JP, London NJ, James D, Carr-Locke DL, Bailey IA, Fossard DP. Controlled trial of urgent endoscopic retrograde cholangiopancreaticography and endoscopic sphincterotomy versus conservative treatment for acute pancreatitis due to gallstones. *Lancet* 1988; **ii:** 979–983.
15. Nowak A, Marek TA, Nowakowska DE, Rybicka J, Kaczor R. Biliary pancreatitis needs endo-

scopic retrograde cholangiopancreatography with endoscopic sphincterotomy for cure. *Endoscopy* 1998; **30(9):** A256–A259.

16. Niederau C, Schulz HU. Current conservative treatment of acute pancreatitis: evidence from animal and human studies. *Hepato-gastroenterology* 1993; **40:** 538–549.

17. Binder M, Uhl W, Friess H, Malfertheiner P, Büchler MW. Octreotide in the treatment of acute pancreatitis: results of an unicenter prospective trial with three different octreotide dosages. *Digestion* 1994; **55 (Suppl. 1):** 20–23.

18. Uhl W, Büchler MW, Malfertheiner P, Beger HG, Adler G, Gaus W. A randomised, double-blind, multicentre trial of octreotide in moderate to severe acute pancreatitis. *Gut* 1999; **45(1):** 97–104.

19. Cavallini G, Titobello A, Frulloni L, Masci E, Mariana A, Di Francesco V. Gabexate for the prevention of pancreatic damage related to endoscopic retrograde cholangiopancreatography. Gabexate in digestive endoscopy—Italian Group. *N Engl J Med* 1996; **335(13):** 919–923.

20. McKay CJ, Curran F, Sharples C, Baxter JN, Imrie CM. Prospective placebo-controlled randomized trial of lexipafant in predicted severe acute pancreatitis. *Br J Surg* 1997; **84:** 1239–1243.

21. Johnson CD, Kingsnorth AN, Imrie CW, *et al.* Double blind, randomised, placebo controlled study of a platelet activating factor antagonist, lexipafant, in the treatment and prevention of organ failure in predicted severe acute pancreatitis, *Gut* 2001; **48:** 62–69.

22. Balthazar EJ, Robinson DL, Megibow AJ, Ransom JHC. Acute pancreatitis: value of CT in establishing prognosis. *Radiology* 1990; **174(2):** 331–336.

23. Büchler MW, Malfertheiner P, Schoetensack C, Uhl W, Bergner M. Sensitivity of antiproteases, complement factors and C-reactive protein in detecting pancreatic necrosis. Results of a prospective clinical study. *Int J Pancreatol* 1986; **3–4(1):** 227–235.

24. Beger HG, Bittner R, Block S, Büchler MW. Bacterial contamination of pancreatic necrosis. *Gastroenterology* 1986; **91:** 433–438.

25. Banks PA, Gerzof SG, Langevin ER, Silverman SG, Sica GT, Hughes MD. CT-guided aspiration of suspected pancreatic infection. Bacteriology and clinical outcome. *Pancreas* 1995; **18:** 265–270.

26. Kramer KM, Levy H. Prophylactic antibiotics for severe acute pancreatitis: the beginning of an era. *Pharmacotherapy* 1999; **19(5):** 592–602.

27. Büchler MW, Malfertheiner P, Friess H, *et al.* Human pancreatic tissue concentration of bactericidal antibiotics. *Gatroenterology* 1992; **103(6):** 1902–1908.

28. Bassi C, Falconi M, Talamini G, *et al.* Controlled trial of pefloxacin versus imipenem in severe acute pancreatitis. *Gastroenterology* 1998; **115(6):** 1513–1517.

29. Pederzoli P, Bassi C, Vesentini S, Campedelli A. A randomized multicenter clinical trial of antibiotic prophylaxis of septic complications in acute necrotizing pancreatitis with imipenem. *Surg Gynecol Obstet* 1993; **176(5):** 480–483.

30. Saino V, Kemppainen E, Puolakkainen P. Early antibiotic treatment in acute necrotizing pancreatitis. *Lancet* 1995; **346:** 663–667.

31. Rau B, Uni W, Büchler MW, Beger HG. Surgical treatment of infected necrosis. *World J Surg* 1997; **21:** 155–161.

32. Banks PA. Practice guidelines in acute pancreatitis. *Am J Gastroenterol* 1997; **92:** 377–386.

33. Pisters PWT, Ranson JHC. Nutritional support for acute pancreatitis. *Surg Gynecol Obstet* 1992; **175:** 275–284.

34. Sitzmann JV, Steiborn PA, Zinner MJ, *et al.* Total parenteral nutrition and alternate energy substrates in treatment of severe acute pancreatitis. *Surg Gynecol Obstet* 1989; **168:** 311–317.

35. Kalfarentzos F, Karafios DD, Karatzas TM, *et al.* Total parenteral nutrition in severe acute pancreatitis. *J Am Coll Nutr* 1991; **10:** 156–162.

36. Kalfarentzos F, Kehagias J, Mead N, Kokkinis K, Gogos CA. Enteral nutrition is superior to parenteral nutrition in severe acute pancreatitis: results of a randomized prospective trial. *Br J Surg* 1997; **84(12):** 1665–1669.

37. Kotani J, Usami M, Nomura H, *et al.* Enteral nutrition prevents bacterial translocation but does not improve survival during acute pancreatitis. *Arch Surg* 1999; **134(3):** 287–292.

38. McClave SA, Greene LM, Snider HL, *et al.* Comparison of the safety of early enteral vs parenteral nutrition in mild acute pancreatitis. *J Parenter Enteral Nutr* 1997; **21(1):** 14–20.

39. Nakad A, Piessevaux H, Margot JC, *et al.* Is early enteral nutrition in acute pancreatitis dangerous? About 20 patients fed by an endoscopically placed nasogastrojejunal tube. *Pancreas* 1998; **17(2):** 187–193.

40. Windsor ACJ, Kanwar S, Li AGK, *et al.* Compared with parenteral nutrition, enteral feeding attenuates the acute-phase response and

improves disease severity in acute pancreatitis. *Gut* 1998; **42**: 431–435.

41. Gardiner KR, Kirk SJ, Rowlands BJ. Novel substrates to maintain gut integrity. *Nutr Res Rev* 1995; **8**: 43–66.

42. Sherman S, Lehman G. ERCP and endoscopic sphincterotomy-induced pancreatitis. *Pancreas* 1991; 350–367.

43. Arcidiacono R, Gambitta P, Rossi A, Grosso C, Bini M, Zanasi G. The use of a long-acting somatostatin analogue (octreotide) for prophylaxis of acute pancreatitis after endoscopic sphincterotomy. *Endoscopy* 1994; **26(9)**: 715–718.

44. Bilbao MK, Dotter CT, Lee TG, Kanton RM. Complications of endoscopic retrograde cholangiopancreatography (ERCP)—a study of 10,000 cases. *Gastroenterology* 1976; **70(3)**: 314–320.

45. Cotton PB, Lenman G, Vennes J, *et al.* Endoscopic sphincterotomy complications and their management: an attempt at consensus. *Gastrointest Endosc* 1991; **37(3)**: 383–393.

46. Poon RTP, Yeung C, Lo CM, Yuen WK, Liu CL, Fan ST. Prophylactic effect of somatostatin on post-ERCP pancreatitis: a randomized controlled trial. *Gastrointest Endosc* 1999; **49(5)**: 593–598.

47. Tulassay Z, Dobronte Z, Pronai L, Zagoni T, Juhasz L. Octreotide in the prevention of pancreatic injury associated with endoscopic cholangiopancreatography. *Aliment Pharmacol Ther* 1998; **12(11)**: 1109–1112.

48. Haber GB. Prevention of post-ERCP pancreatitis [editorial comment]. *Gastrointest Endosc* 2000; **51(1)**: 100–103.

49. Binmoeller KF, Harris AG, Dumas R, Grimaldi C, Delmont JP. Does somatostatin analogue octreotide protect against ERCP induced pancreatitis? *Gut* 1992; **33(8)**: 1129–1133.

50. Weiner GR, Geenen JE, Hogan WJ, Catalano ME. Use of corticosteroids in the prevention of post-ERCP pancreatitis. *Gatrointest Endosc* 1995; **42(6)**: 579–583.

51. De Palma GD, Catanzano C. Use of corticosteroids in the prevention of post-ERCP pancreatitis results of a controlled prospective study. *Am J Gastroenterol* 1999; **94(4)**: 982–985.

52. Johnson GK, Geenen JE, Bedford RA, *et al.* A comparison of nonionic versus ionic contrast media: results of a prospective, multicenter study. Midwest Pancreaticobiliary Study Group. *Gastrointest Endosc* 1995; **42(4)**: 312–316.

53. Rabenstein T, Schneider HT, Bulling D, *et al.* Analysis of the risk factors associated with endo-

scopic sphincterotomy techniques: preliminary results of a prospective study, with emphasis on the reduced risk of acute pancreatitis with low-dose anticoagulation treatment. *Endoscopy* 2000; **32(1)**: 10–19.

54. Barkin JS, Casal GL, Reiner DK, Goldberg RI, Phillips RS, Kaplan S. A comparative study of contrast agents for endoscopic retrograde pancreatography. *Am J Gastroenterol* 1991; **86(10)**: 1437–1441.

55. Poon RT, Yeung C, Lo CM, Yuen WK, Liu CL, Fan ST. Prophylactic effect of somatostatin on post-ERCP pancreatitis: a randomized controlled trial [see comments]. *Gastrointest Endosc* 1999; **49(5)**: 593–598.

56. Ammann RW, Heitz PU, Klöppel G. The 'two-hit' pathogenetic concept of chronic pancreatitis. *Int J Pancreatol* 1999; **25(3)**: 251.

57. Klöppel G, Maillet B. Chronic pancreatitis: evolution of the disease. *Hepatogastroenterology* 1991; **38**: 408–412.

58. Klöppel G, Maillet B. The morphological basis for the evolution of acute pancreatitis into chronic pancreatitis. *Virchows Arch A Pathol Anat Histol* 1992; **420**: 1–4.

59. Malfertheiner P, Mayer D, Büchler MW, Dominguez-Munoz JE, Schiefer B, Ditschuneit H. Treatment of pain in chronic pancreatitis by inhibition of pancreatic secretion with octreotide. *Gut* 1995; **36**: 450–454.

60. Malfertheiner P, Dominguez-Munoz JE, Büchler MW. Chronic pancreatitis: management of pain. *Digestion* 1994; **55(Suppl. 1)**: 29–34.

61. Little JM. Alcohol abuse and chronic pancreatitis. *Surgery* 1987; **101**: 357–360.

62. Hayakawa T, Kondo T, Shibata T, Sugimoto Y, Katigawa M. Chronic alcoholism and evolution of pain in chronic pancreatitis. *Dig Dis Sci* 1989; **34**: 33–38.

63. Bockmann DE, Büchler MW, Malfertheiner P, Beger HG. Analysis of nerves in chronic pancreatitis. *Gastroenterology* 1988; **94**: 1459–1469.

64. World Health Organization. *Cancer Pain Relief and Palliative Care: Report on a WHO Expert Committee,* World Health Organization, Geneva, 1990.

65. DiMagno EP. Controversies in the treatment of exocrine pancreatic insufficiency. *Dig Dis Sci* 1982; **27**: 481–484.

66. Klöppel G, Bommer G, Commandeur G, Heitz PH. The endocrine pancreas in chronic pancreatitis. *Virchows Arch A Pathol Anat Histol* 1978; **337**: 157–174.

67. McKiddie MT, Burchanan KD, McBain GC, Bell G. The insulin response to glucose in patients with pancreatic disease. *Postgrad Med J* 1969; **45(529):** 726–728.

68. Ammann RW, Akovbientz A, Largiader F, Schuler G. Course and outcome of chronic pancreatitis. Longitudinal study of a mixed medical-surgical series of 245 patients. *Gastroenterology* 1984; **82:** 820–826.

69. Bradley ELI, Clements JL, Gonzalez AC. The natural history of pancreatic pseudocysts: a unified concept of management. *Am J Surg* 1979; **137:** 135–141.

70. Yeo CJ, Bastidas JA, Lynch-Nyhan A, Fishman EK, Zinner MJ, Cameron JL. The natural history of pancreatic pseudocysts documented by computed tomography. *Surg Gynecol Obstet* 1990; **170:** 411–417.

71. Gulio L, Barbara L. Treatment of pancreatic pseudocysts with octreotide. *Lancet* 1991; **338:** 540–541.

72. Barkin JS, Reiner DK, Deutch E. Sandostatin for control of catheter drainage of pancreatic pseudocyst. *Pancreas* 1991; **6:** 245–248.

73. D'Agostino HB, van Sonnenberg E, Sanchez RB, Goodacre BW, Viliaveiran RG, Lyche K. Treatment of pancreatic pseudocysts with percutaneous drainage and octreotide. *Radiology* 1993; **187:** 685–688.

11

Viral hepatitis

Eleanor Barnes, George Webster, Geoffrey M Dusheiko

INTRODUCTION

Approximately 450 million people worldwide have persistent hepatitis B and C virus infection, many of whom live in developing countries. The treatment of hepatitis B virus infection (HBV), stimulated by the successful treatment of human immunodeficiency virus (HIV) with nucleoside analogues, is entering a new and potentially exciting phase, but remains challenging. It is likely that the coming decade will see the successful treatment of HBV with combinations of nucleoside analogues and immunomodulatory therapies. Unfortunately, as with human immunodeficiency virus infection, it is likely that these drugs will not be affordable in developing countries where they are needed most, unless expanded access programmes are developed. An effective vaccine for HBV has been available since 1982 and universal vaccination programmes have been implemented in more than 100 countries (but excluding the UK). These programmes have reduced the transmission rate of HBV. Universal vaccination of newborns worldwide remains a major therapeutic and economic challenge.

Up to 2% of the world population may be infected with hepatitis C virus (HCV). End stage hepatitis C disease is a leading indication for liver transplantation in Europe and the USA. Relatively effective treatment with alpha-interferon (α-IFN) and ribavirin is now available for those infected but this treatment is difficult to administer, expensive, and the side-effects may be considerable. There is currently no vaccine against HCV infection, which has an inherent ability to mutate and evade immune surveillance and usually leads to persistent infection. Many research groups are currently attempting to elucidate the mechanism of viral persistence in HCV infection with a view to vaccine development and improved treatment.

Hepatitis A virus (HAV) does not cause chronic infection but is a significant cause of acute hepatitis and occasionally of fulminant liver failure in adults. A vaccine is available for at risk groups. Likewise, hepatitis E may lead to fulminant hepatitis but does not cause chronic hepatitis. Hepatitis D can cause co-infection or superinfection of patients with hepatitis B infection. Finally, cytomegalovirus (CMV) infection is a cause of hepatitis particularly in immuno-compromised liver transplant recipients.

HEPATITIS B VIRUS INFECTION

About 350 million people worldwide have persistent hepatitis B virus (HBV) infection.

Cirrhosis occurs in 30–50% of patients with elevated aminotransferases and detectable HBeAg for more than 5 years. Hepatic failure may develop in patients with cirrhosis. Hepatocellular carcinoma may develop in patients with and without cirrhosis. HBV is the ninth leading cause of death worldwide. There is a wide variation in the prevalence of HBV ranging from 0.3% in the UK, 2% in the USA, to 20% in parts of Africa and Asia. HBV infection is declining in the West and infection rates have decreased in high prevalence areas where the universal immunization of infants has been introduced.

The clinical spectrum of HBV infection is wide. Infection in adult life generally causes acute hepatitis followed by viral eradication. Fulminant liver failure may occur in 2–3% of patients. Generally more than 90% of children infected as neonates develop chronic infection and appear to be relatively 'immunotolerant' during childhood, with high levels of replicating virus and little hepatic inflammation. However, for reasons that are poorly understood, as these children progress to adulthood they frequently develop exacerbations of hepatitis with elevated serum transaminases. The associated complications of HBV infection may ensue.

Transmission

The transmission of HBV has implications for treatment and prevention.

Perinatal transmission
Antepartum haemorrhage and ingestion or inoculation of maternal blood causes perinatal transmission of HBV. The neonatal route of transmission is particularly important in areas of high prevalence such as China. The risk of perinatal infection is highest for children born to HBeAg-positive mothers with high concentrations of virus in blood.

Horizontal transmission
Perinatal transmission only accounts for about one-half of the cases of childhood hepatitis. The remaining children acquire HBV from other children. In endemic regions, prevalence reaches a peak in children aged 7–14 years. Horizontal transmission of HBV was previously endemic in enclosed institutions and is more common in areas with poor socioeconomic conditions.

Intravenous transmission
Intravenous drug use, tattooing, laboratory accidents and accidental inoculation during surgical procedures are a cause of HBV transmission. Blood-bank screening of HBV came into effect in 1972 in Western society and infection via transfusion of blood products in the West is now uncommon.

Sexual transmission
HBV may be transmitted by both heterosexual and homosexual transmission and is particularly common in patients with high levels of replicating virus and during male homosexual intercourse.

Pathophysiology

HBV is a small, enveloped, partially double-stranded DNA virus. HBV is not thought to be directly cytopathic and hepatic inflammation represents an interaction between viral replication and a complex cellular immune response.

The replicative cycle of HBV is complex but an understanding of this is central to understanding the therapeutic approaches that have been adopted (Fig. 11.1). Although a DNA virus, replication occurs via reverse transcription of an intermediate RNA pregenome. After initial infection of the hepatocyte, viral genome DNA is converted to closed circular covalent molecule (cccDNA), which functions as a transcriptional template. Eradication of cccDNA has proved particularly problematical.

Therapeutic approaches

The following preventative approaches have been successful for prophylaxis of hepatitis B:

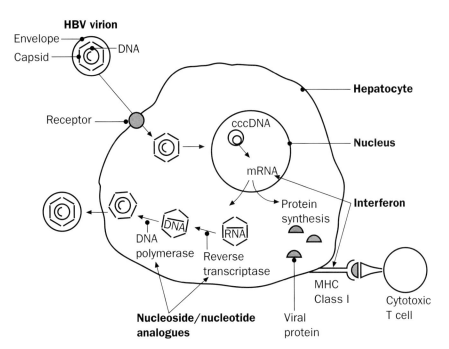

HBV virion

Envelope

Capsid

DNA

Receptor

cccDNA

Hepatocyte

Nucleus

mRNA

Protein
synthesis

Interferon

DNA
polymerase

Reverse
transcriptase

DNA

RNA

**Nucleoside/nucleotide
analogues**

Viral
protein

MHC
Class I

Cytotoxic
T cell

Figure 11.1 Site of
action of drugs during
HBV replication.

- Hepatitis B immunoglobulin
- Hepatitis B vaccine.

The following therapeutic approaches have been at least partially successful (Fig. 11.1):

- Inhibition of viral replication by α-IFN and nucleoside analogues such as lamivudine
- Augmentation of the cellular immune response (e.g. with α-IFN).

Treatment regimens

The treatment of HBV is evolving rapidly. Lamivudine, a new nucleoside analogue has been licensed for treatment of chronic hepatitis B. Several new nucleoside analogues are being developed and tested for efficacy in Phase III clinical trials in patients with chronic HBV infection. As with HIV infection, it is likely that the treatment of HBV in the future will involve combinations of nucleoside and nucleotide analogues. Individual drugs are, however, still being tested.

The success of each approach is dependent on the clinical setting, each of which will be described in turn. Treatment of children and other patient groups are described later in the chapter.

Acute hepatitis B infection and fulminant liver failure

Unlike hepatitis C virus infection, there is no evidence that antiviral therapy accelerates viral eradication in acute HBV infection or that it prevents chronic infection. Fulminant acute viral hepatitis is characterized by low levels of replicating virus at the time of presentation. α-IFN has not been found to be beneficial in patients with acute uncomplicated hepatitis B or in fulminant viral hepatitis. Preliminary data suggest that lamivudine is also ineffective in this setting.

Chronic hepatitis B virus infection

Chronic hepatitis B infection is defined arbitrarily by the detection of HBsAg for at least 6 months. An understanding of the serological markers characteristic of hepatitis B infection is central to determining the viral replicative state, underlying disease status, and the best treatment regimen.

Chronic HBV infection may be classified into predominantly 'replicative' and 'non-replicative' infection, although these are relative terms. α-IFN and lamivudine are currently available for the treatment of replicative chronic HBV. There is no efficacious treatment for predominantly non-replicative HBV infection, and treatment is not presently indicated for this group.

Replicative HBV infection

In the replicative phase of hepatitis B infection, readily discernible levels of viral replication are present. These patients are HBeAg-positive (unless infected with predominant pre-core variants), anti-HBe-negative and HBV DNA is detected in the serum by molecular hybridization assays. Serum aminotransferases are usually, but not always elevated in this group of patients.

Children and young adults may have normal serum aminotransferases with minimal inflammation at liver biopsy, despite high levels of replicating virus, attesting to the fact that it is the host immune response rather than the virus itself that is the cause of hepatic disease.

Approximately 10% of patients lose HBeAg and HBV DNA spontaneously and become anti-HBe positive each year, so that the benefits of any drug must be evaluated against the rate of spontaneous seroconversion within controlled trials.

A second major group of patients are infected with a predominance of circulating pre-core variant hepatitis B. The most common genomic alteration found with pre-core variant infection is the presence of a stop codon, in the pre-C region, preventing expression of HBeAg but not viral replication. Patients with a pre-core mutant are important to identify:

- They have detectable levels of circulating HBV DNA
- Undetectable HBeAg
- elevated transminases

- are at risk of liver injury
- may be amenable to treatment

The pre-core mutant is becoming increasingly common and in some countries is now the dominant type. Assessing replication by HBeAg status alone is therefore no longer acceptable.

Treatment should be aimed at patients before they develop cirrhosis. Liver biopsy should ideally be performed prior to treatment to assess the degree of inflammation and stage of fibrosis, since this will affect the likely outcome and side-effects of treatment.

Treatment options for predominantly replicative HBV infection include:

- α-IFN
- Nucleoside analogues
- Referral to a specialist unit for treatment within clinical trials

α-IFN

In 1992 α-IFN was licensed for use in chronic HBV infection. Several alpha-interferons including α-n1, α-2a and α-2b are now available (see p. 250 for pharmacology). Factors predictive of a response to α-IFN are as follows:

- Caucasian
- Female
- Heterosexual
- Acquired HBV over 6 years ago
- Disease duration less than 4 years
- History of jaundice
- Serum ALT over 100 IU/l
- High-grade hepatic inflammation
- HBV DNA in serum less than 200 pg/ml
- HBeAg-positive
- IgM anti-HBc-positive
- Absence of HIV/immunosuppression

None of these factors, either alone or in combination, allow accurate predictions at treatment outcome to be made in individual cases. Although these factors should be taken into consideration when planning treatment and randomization groups in clinical trials, no patients should be denied treatment on the basis of these factors alone. However, patients with mild chronic hepatitis and persistently normal serum aminotransferases seem less likely to respond, and are not generally unwell. Treatment should be deferred in these patients.

The aim of treatment in HBeAg-positive patients is to attain HBe-loss or anti-HBe sero-conversion, which is usually accompanied by normalization of serum aminotransferases. Approximately 30% of patients overall respond to α-IFN. Loss of HBsAg occurs in only 8% of patients and is usually observed in patients infected chronically for a relatively short period of time, rather than decades. The aim of treatment of anti-HBe-positive, HBV DNA-positive patients (infected with pre-core mutant variants) is loss of HBV DNA accompanied by normalization of serum aminotransferases. Relatively high response rates have been observed in this group of patients; unfortunately, however, most relapse after 1 year of treatment, and only 25% of patients have sustained loss of HBV DNA.

While α-IFN is appropriate for replicative HBV infection, it is poorly effective in patients with normal transaminases and in patients who are immunocompromised such as patients who are HIV-positive with low CD4 counts. It is generally not tolerated by patients with decompensated cirrhosis, because of the risk of leucopenia and thrombocytopenia, and an increased risk of sepsis. It is contraindicated in renal transplant patients because of the risk of graft rejection.

Nucleoside and nucleotide analogues

Following the success of nucleoside analogues in treating HIV infection, this group of drugs is currently under evaluation for use in chronic HBV infection. Nucleoside analogues are chain terminators, that is, they inhibit HBV reverse transcriptase and HBV DNA polymerase enzymes necessary for HBV replication. Lamivudine is the most extensively studied nucleoside analogue and has been licensed for treatment of chronic HBV. It is the negative enantiomer of 2′,3′-dideoxy-3′-thiacytidine. Lamivudine inhibits HBV DNA polymerase through chain termination of nascent proviral

DNA. Fortunately, it is only a weak inhibitor of host cellular enzymes, including DNA polymerase γ, which is required for mitochondrial DNA replication.

In a 1-year study of Chinese patients with elevated transaminases, 100 mg lamivudine daily was associated with significant histological improvement in 56% of patients and seroconversion to anti-HBe in 16% of patients versus 6% of the control group. HBV DNA levels fell to undetectable levels within 4 weeks of treatment in 90% of patients.[1] HBeAg loss has subsequently been shown to increase to 27% after 2 years' treatment and 33% after 3 years of treatment with loss of HBV DNA in 44% of patients.[2] Treatment responses are highest in patients with serum ALT concentrations greater than five times the upper limit of normal. Treatment with lamivudine has only rarely been associated with loss of HBsAg.

Unless seroconversion to anti-HBe occurs, the majority of patients became HBV DNA-positive again when treatment is stopped. Thus the optimal duration of treatment is not established and may be indefinite. In addition the durability of seroconversion remains to be established in a sizeable cohort of patients.

HBV variants associated with reduced drug sensitivity have been reported in patients treated with lamivudine. Lamivudine-resistant HBV is characterized by amino acid site mutations in the highly conserved YMDD motifs—part of the active site of the polymerase. These are analogous to the mutation seen in resistant human immunodeficiency virus. Such mutations had been observed in 14% of Chinese patients after 1 year of treatment but 38% of patients treated for 2 years, and this figure rises to more than 40% after 3 years of treatment.

The long-term clinical significance of these variants is not yet known. Although patients with these variants have a reduced therapeutic response, serum HBV DNA and serum aminotransferases tend to remain below pre-treatment levels. *In vitro* studies have suggested that several lamivudine variant HBV are less replication fit than the wild type virus.[3] It is uncertain whether improved histology with lamivudine will be maintained in the long term, after selection for resistant variants.

There are preliminary data on the effects of lamivudine in combination with α-IFN in previously untreated patients, and in patients who have previously failed to respond to α-IFN. Combination therapy compared with lamivudine monotherapy in naïve patients has been shown to enhance the HBeAg seroconversion rate, but these data did not achieve statistical significance.[4]

It should be emphasized that the seroconversion rate for patients with normal transaminases treated with lamivudine is less than 5%. At present, there are no good treatment options for this group of patients. Lamivudine has also been tested in patients with pre-core mutants— now the predominant type in many parts of the world. Interim results suggest that after 1 year of treatment, 65% of patients are HBV DNA-negative with normal transaminases compared with 9% of placebo recipients. However, relapse rates after discontinuing treatment have been high in this group of patients so that 6 months after the end of treatment only 30% of patients remain HBV DNA-negative and less than 17% of patients have normal transaminases.[5]

Famciclovir treatment results in low HBeAg seroconversion rates and is unlikely to have a role as monotherapy. HBV lacks a thymidine kinase, which may account for the lack of efficacy of this drug in HBV infection. Unfortunately famciclovir and lamivudine share cross resistance.

Adefovir dipivoxil is an adenosine nucleotide analogue, which is now in Phase III trials in HBV infection. Preliminary data suggest that the development of resistance may be less common than with lamivudine. Renal toxicity has been demonstrated in clinical trials in HIV infection when given in high doses.

Phase II studies of lobucavir have been suspended because of the carcinogenicity observed during extended preclinical testing.

There are several new nucleoside analogues beginning evaluation in Phase I trials including entecavir (BMS 200,475), emcitratibine (FTC), LdT LdC and LFMAU. These new agents cause a two to seven logarithmic drop or more in HBV DNA concentrations and can be administered orally.

Non-replicative HBV infection

'Non replicative' HBV infection is characterized by the detection of HBsAg, absence of HBeAg and negative HBV DNA (detectable by molecular hybridization assay) in the serum. Serum transaminases are usually normal and liver biopsy will show minimal hepatitis. This group of patients have been described as 'healthy carriers'; this is misleading since patients remain at risk of reactivation of viral replication and may later become HBeAg-positive or develop a fluctuating chronic hepatitis with intermittently detectable HBV DNA levels. They also remain a risk of hepatocellular carcinoma, particularly in the presence of cirrhosis. There is currently no treatment for this group of patients who have been excluded from clinical trials of interferon and lamivudine. The term 'non replicative' infection is a relative term and these patients merit regular follow-up since new, sensitive quantitative polymerase chain reaction (PCR) assays indicated a dynamic, fluctuating pattern of viral replication in some of these patients, accompanied by hepatic injury. Treatment may be indicated for patients with progressive disease.

Treatment of other groups

Children

Children with HBV infection are generally immunotolerant, and tend to have relatively high concentrations of hepatitis B DNA in serum, with normal transaminases and minimal inflammation on biopsy. These patients are unlikely to develop significant liver injury at this phase of the disease, and are also unlikely to respond to either α-IFN or lamivudine. It seems sensible not to treat such children at present but to wait until new, better alternatives are available.

Cirrhosis

Patients with compensated cirrhosis should be considered for treatment with lamivudine or α-IFN. Patients with decompensated cirrhosis should be considered for treatment with lamivudine. Seroconversion with α-IFN or lamivudine is unlikely but significant improvement in liver function and clinical benefit may be obtained. These patients must be monitored at least monthly during treatment. It must be remembered that treatment with lamivudine may have implications for future liver transplantation if resistance develops.

Transplantation

Patients with end-stage cirrhosis caused by HBV should be considered for liver transplantation. There is, however, a significant risk of graft re-infection associated with rapid progression to graft failure.

The introduction of hepatitis B immunoglobulin (HBIG) in 1993 as immunoprophylaxis reduced the recurrence rate to 33%, when given in the anhepatic stage during transplantation and continued indefinitely. Unfortunately, this beneficial effect was more limited in patients who were HBV DNA-positive pre-transplantation so that liver transplantation was only considered in patients who were HBV DNA-negative. In addition, the administration of HBIG is unpleasant, expensive and required life-long. Several other anti-viral therapies, including α-IFN, ganciclovir and foscarnet, were all found to be ineffective in preventing graft re-infection.

In 1996, lamivudine was shown to reduce HBV DNA to undetectable levels pre-transplantation and to prevent HBV recurrence in the graft, with loss of HBsAg, when continued indefinitely post-transplantation.[6]

The Achilles heel of lamivudine in transplantation is the development of resistance to the drug post-transplantation, with an associated resurgence of HBV DNA and graft failure. The timing of lamivudine treatment pre-transplantation is crucial: lamivudine must be given for long enough to render the patient HBV DNA-negative, while avoiding a protracted course before transplantation with the associated risk of resistance. Lamivudine therapy with HBIG should be considered to reduce recurrence rates. Clinical trials are presently underway to establish the optimum HBIG and lamivudine treatment regimen but there are good theoretical reasons to give these drugs together rather than sequentially (when drug resistance is more likely).

Adefovir dipivoxil may be given to patients who have developed lamivudine resistance post-transplantation on a compassionate basis (Gilead Sciences). It is likely that combinations of nucleoside analogues to prevent the development of resistance will be given to patients pre- and post-transplant in the future.

HIV and HBV infection

α-IFN treatment of HBV infection has been shown to be ineffective in patients co-infected with HIV.[7] Treatment of HBV infection with lamivudine in patients with HIV should be combined with other anti-retroviral therapies to avoid HIV resistance to lamivudine.

Glomerulonephritis and polyarteritis nodosa

Glomerulonephritis and polyarteritis nodosa are uncommon complications of chronic HBV infection. Treatment with α-IFN and subsequent loss of viral replication is associated with improvement of renal disease in the majority of patients. Similarly, lamivudine treatment may improve these extrahepatic complications.

Concomitant HDV infection

Patients co-infected with hepatitis D tend to progress more rapidly to cirrhosis. Trials with α-IFN have demonstrated a reduction in serum transaminases and HDAg and hepatitis D RNA; unfortunately, the majority of patients relapse when treatment is discontinued. Lamivudine has not been shown to be effective in hepatitis D-positive patients.

Immunosuppressed patients

Immunosuppression with chemotherapy (including prednisolone) is associated with a flare in viral replication and clinically with hepatitis or fulminant liver failure. Lamivudine prophylaxis is appropriate where immunosuppression is essential, or where cycled cytotoxic chemotherapy will be given. The course in these patients may still be complicated by exacerbations of hepatitis, despite a reduction in hepatitis B DNA in serum. HBcAg and other epitopes of hepatitis B may continue to be expressed for a considerable period after reduction of hepatitis B DNA in serum, since viral proteins are translated from the RNA pre-genome.

Pharmacology of drugs

α-IFN
Mode of action
The antiviral effect of α-IFN is probably mediated by effects on cellular immune responses: up-regulation of HLA Class I expression on hepatocytes (CD_8 cytotoxic T-cell pathway) and possible enhancement of HBV-specific T-cell activity. The mechanism of anti-proliferative and anti-fibrogenic effects is unclear. Direct anti-viral effects have also been described.

Dynamics/kinetics
After subcutaneous or intramuscular injection maximal serum levels are seen at 3–12 h, with undetectable levels 16 h after administration. Serum $T^{1/2}$ 2–3 h. Renal excretion is the predominant route of elimination.

Main indication
Chronic HBV infection, raised serum aminotransaminases, detectable HBV DNA and at least moderate hepatitis on liver biopsy.

Dosage
A dose of 9 million units is given three times per week, subcutaneously.

Duration of therapy
Therapy is given for 4 months.

Adverse reactions[8]
Side-effects are seen in 90% of patients (particularly 6–8 h post-dose influenza-like symptoms) but treatment due to side effects is discontinued in only about 10% of patients. Psychiatric problems are more common in, but not exclusive to, patients with a premorbid psychiatric history. Patients should be informed that most side-effects resolve after cessation of therapy but that thyroid derangement might persist.

Common adverse reactions that are mild and rarely require dose-modification include: influenza-like symptoms (e.g. fatigue, fever, malaise, arthralgia, headache), which are worst with the first injections; neuropsychiatric symptoms (e.g. mood change, cognitive impairment, poor sleep); alopecia; abdominal pain; and nausea. An aggravation of the chronic hepatitis and an increase in serum aminotransferases may occur during treatment. These are generally mild and resolve with continued treatment in responsive patients. However, the development of autoimmune hepatitis (see text following) usually necessitates discontinuation of treatment. Blood white cell, red cell and platelet counts are commonly decreased during treatment. These are usually mild if normal counts were present initially but may be dose-limiting in the presence of low counts.

Less common but serious and potentially life-threatening adverse reactions that require prompt dose-modification or cessation of therapy include: depression; suicidal ideation; psychosis; hepatic decompensation; bleeding; cardiac arrhythmia; dilated cardiomyopathy; hypotension; acute renal failure; retinopathy; hearing loss; pulmonary interstitial fibrosis; epilepsy, coma, skin disorders such as psoriasis and erythema multiforme; immune disorders such as autoimmune thyroid disease, autoimmune hepatitis, systemic lupus erythematosis, primary biliary cirrhosis; laboratory abnormalities including myelosuppression, neutropenia, thrombocytopenia, anaemia, proteinuria, and hepatotoxicity.

Drug interactions
Theophylline metabolism is impaired (i.e. increased circulating levels) with concomitant therapy; also there may be an increased risk of pneumonitis with herbal remedies.

Contraindications

Severe depression/psychiatric disease, decompensated cirrhosis, autoimmune hepatitis, hyperthyroidism, coronary artery disease, renal transplant, pregnancy (or absence of adequate contraception in patient or partner), epilepsy, diabetic retinopathy, active drug or alcohol dependency, severe thrombocytopenia (platelets <60), leucopenia, anaemia, high titres of auto-antibodies (anti-nuclear antibody, anti-smooth muscle antibody, anti-LKM1) are all contraindications. There is no safety information to guide use in breastfeeding patients. Renal function should be monitored closely in patients with mild/moderate renal impairment and α-IFN avoided in patients with severe renal impairment. Most contraindications are relative, and a balance of the risk of serious side-effects should be made with the potential benefit of the drug.

Monitoring

As a minimum, serum transaminases, haemoglobin levels and neutrophil count should be measured monthly. Patients with cirrhosis need particularly careful monitoring.

Lamivudine

There is no data in patients co-infected with HCV or delta virus, and limited data in pre-core mutants, in patients undergoing transplant and in patients receiving concurrent immunosuppressive regimens.

Mode of action

Lamivudine is a nucleoside analogue; it acts as a substrate for HBV viral polymerase.

Pharmacodynamics and kinetics

Lamivudine is metabolized to the triphosphate active derivative; it has a bioavailability of 85% and is excreted through the kidneys. $T^{1/2}$ is 5–7 h. Excretion is unaffected by hepatic impairment.

Indications

HBV viral replication with decompensated liver disease or histologically demonstrated active liver inflammation and/or fibrosis are indications for treatment.

Dosage

A dose of 100 mg daily is given with normal renal function. The dose is reduced if creatinine clearance is less than 50 ml/min. See data sheet for dose in renal impairment. There is no data on the use of lamivudine in children below 16 years of age.

Duration of treatment

Continue treatment until HBeAg seroconversion or HBsAg seroconversion occurs. Discontinue if there is loss of efficacy, that is if HBeAg-positive patients return to pre-treatment levels of serum transaminases or HBV DNA while on treatment. In HBeAg-negative patients with pre-core mutants, duration of treatment is unknown. Treatment should be continued until HBsAg seroconversion or loss of efficacy occurs. In patients who develop YMDD variant HBV, discontinue if seroconversion occurs or if not efficacious.

Patients may develop recurrent hepatitis when treatment is discontinued. In patients with decompensated liver disease treatment should not be discontinued since recurrent hepatitis and potentially fatal hepatic decompensation may ensue.

Adverse reactions

Lamivudine is generally very well tolerated but malaise, fatigue, respiratory tract infections, headache, abdominal discomfort, nausea, vomiting and diarrhoea have been reported.

Contraindications

This drug is not recommended in the first trimester of pregnancy, although animal studies have not demonstrated teratogenicity.

In patients co-infected with HIV there is a risk of HIV mutation if lamivudine monotherapy is used for the treatment of HBV.

Monitoring

As a minimum, ALT should be measured 3-monthly and HBV DNA and HBAg measured 6-monthly. Patients with decompensated liver disease should be monitored monthly.

Prevention of hepatitis B infection

Indications for active immunization and hepatitis B immunoglobulin (HBIG)

More than 10 years ago the World Health Organisation set a goal for universal active immunization against HBV in all countries by 1997. Unfortunately, we have failed to achieve this, even in relatively wealthy countries such as the UK. In 1996, the Department of Health recommended active vaccination for at-risk groups only, including:

- Close family contacts of a case or carrier, or families adopting children from countries with a high prevalence of HBV infection
- Babies born to mothers who are chronic carriers of HBV infection or to mothers who have had acute hepatitis B in pregnancy. In addition, babies born to mothers who have had acute hepatitis B in pregnancy or who are HBeAg-positive should receive HBIG (see later text). Currently, vaccine without HBIG is recommended to babies born to mothers who are HBsAg-positive but anti-HBeAb-positive
- Sexual contacts of patients with acute hepatitis B, who should also receive HBIG
- Parenteral drug abusers
- Patients with haemophilia (and others receiving regular blood transfusions or blood products) and carers responsible for the administration of blood products
- Patients with chronic renal failure
- Occupational risk groups: health care workers, staff and students of residential accommodation for those with severe learning difficulties, and members of the emergency and prison service plus inmates of custodial institutions
- Those travelling to areas of high prevalence

HBIG confers temporary passive immunity to HBV infection. Indications for HBIG include:

- Post exposure prophylaxis in persons who have not received prior vaccination, in those whose vaccination regimen is incomplete, or in those whose antibody titre is inadequate (<10 IU/l). The passive immunization of people at risk of exposure should be used in combination with hepatitis B vaccine
- Accidental exposure to blood or other material containing HBsAg; contamination of intact skin is not included unless it covers an extensive skin area
- Sexual contacts of patients with acute HBV infection
- Newborns of mother or are HBsAg and HBeAg-positive
- Newborns of mothers with acute HBV in the third trimester of pregnancy or early in the puerperium

Pharmacology of drugs

Hepatitis B vaccine

Recombinantly expressed HBsAg, the hepatitis B vaccine is adsorbed on aluminium hydroxide adjuvant. It is made biosynthetically using recombinant DNA technology.

Mode of action

This vaccine stimulates the production of HBV surface antibody. Antibody titres may be measured to ensure adequate response; it may take 6 months to mount adequate antibody response but protection lasts 3–5 years. Of people vaccinated, 80–90% respond; however, those aged over 40 years are less likely to respond. An antibody titre lower than 10 mIU/ml is a non-response and a repeat course of vaccine should be considered. An antibody titre over 100 mIU/ml is protective; those with levels from 10–100 mIU/ml should receive a booster. Higher doses of vaccine may be required in those who are immunocompromised.

Indication

See above 'Indications for active immunization and hepatitis B immunoglobulin'.

Dosage

If Energex B by SmithKline Beecham is used, three doses are required at all ages: the second 1 month and the third 6 months after the first injection. (H-B Vax II also available—doses not given—see data sheet if required).

The immunization is administered as follows:

- Adults: Intramuscular injection into the deltoid muscle, three doses of 1 ml (20 µg)
- Children (birth–12 years): Intramuscular injection into the anterolateral thigh, three doses of 0.5 ml (10 µg)
- Infants of HBsAg-positive mothers: Three doses of 0.5 ml (10 µg), first dose at birth with HBIG (at a separate site)

The subcutaneous route is preferred in patients with haemophilia and the dose is different—see the data sheet.

Adverse reactions

This vaccine is generally well tolerated.

Common reactions include redness at site of injection, and an intradermal injection may produce a persistent nodule.

Uncommon adverse reactions include fever, fatigue, rash, malaise, influenza-like syndrome, arthritis, arthralgia, myalgia, headache, dizziness, nausea, vomiting, diarrhoea, abdominal pain, lymphadenopathy, and elevated liver function tests.

Serious neurological reactions such as Guillain-Barré and demyelinating disease have been reported and, in France, the vaccine has been withdrawn; however, a causal relationship has not been demonstrated convincingly.

Drug interactions

None are known.

Contraindications

In general, vaccination should be postponed if patients are suffering from an acute illness. Minor infection without fever or systemic upset is not a contraindication.

HBIG

HBIG confers temporary passive immunity to HBV infection.

Mode of action

Prepared from pools of plasma with high titres of HBsAb. Neutralizing IgG antibodies binds to invading virus and are then phagocytosed or destroyed by complement.

Pharmocokinetics

Peak serum levels are reached in 2–3 days; $T_{1/2}$ is 21–22 days.

Indications

See guidelines on p. 244.

Dosage

Take a blood sample before giving HBIG to determine the carrier status of patient. Administration should not be withheld for more than 48 h while awaiting test result. Give intramuscular injection into the deltoid muscle (*not* buttock) as soon as possible after exposure but not more than 7 days after exposure.

Two doses 30 days apart should be given unless evidence of past HBV was found in the pre-immunoglobulin sample or that the HBsAg innoculum was anti-HBeAb-positive or if a course of HBV vaccine was begun at the same time as the first dose of immunoglobulin.

The immunization is as follows:

- Adult: Two doses of 500 IU each given 30 days apart
- Child (under 4 years): Two doses of 200 IU each given 30 days apart
  (5–9 years): Two doses of 300 IU each given 30 days apart
- Newborn: 40 IU/kg administered within 12 h of birth—two doses are given 30 days apart. HBV vaccine given at same time but in site with different lymphatic drainage

Adverse reactions

This vaccine is very well tolerated. There is usually pain over the injection site, but very rarely anaphylaxis.

Drug interactions

May interfere with live vaccines given before 5 weeks and up to 3 months.

Contraindications

If there is severe thrombocytopenia or a coagulation disorder that precludes intramuscular injections, injections may be given subcutaneously instead.

Experimental drugs and regimens

The following experimental drugs and regimens are under investigation for the prevention of hepatitis B infection.

- L-FMAU
- FTC
- BMS 200475—a novel guanosine analogue showing remarkable activity against woodchuck and duck HBV, reducing supercoiled HBV DNA; however, the safety in humans is presently unknown
- DNA vaccines
- CTL vaccines
- Therapeutic vaccines of surface antigen
- Immunomodulatory strategies:
  - Treatment 'holidays' with nucleoside analogues
  - Stimulation of viral replication and cellular immune responses following a short course of oral prednisolone prior to instituting therapy with nucleoside analogues

HEPATITIS C VIRUS INFECTION

Introduction

An estimated 150 million people worldwide are infected with hepatitis C virus (HCV). It is now recognized as a major cause of chronic hepatitis, cirrhosis, and hepatocellular carcinoma. It is predicated that within 20 years more deaths will occur annually in the USA from HCV than as a result of HIV infection. There are marked geographical variations in prevalence, with 0.5–2% of the population being anti-HCV antibody-positive in the USA and Europe but up to 15% in Egypt.

HCV may be transmitted parentally, with many cases following unscreened blood product transfusion; 90% of haemophiliac patients who received unsterilized factor-concentrates prior to 1985 are anti-HCV-positive. A history of intravenous drug abuse is an important risk factor, and other skin-piercing procedures have been shown to transmit the virus. Sexual transmission has also been described but it is an inefficient and infrequent route of infection. Mother-to-infant transmission occurs in 1–5% of cases but this rate is significantly higher after maternal co-infection with HIV where transmission rises up to 36% of cases. The precise mode of acquisition of HCV is uncertain in 20–30% of patients.

The natural history of HCV infection is complex and poorly understood and therapy for HCV infection is complicated by the wide individual variation in disease progression following infection. Up to 15% of patients may have an acute icteric hepatitis. The majority of infected patients (50–85%) develop chronic hepatitis, which may lead to cirrhosis and hepatocellular carcinoma (HCC). Up to 20% of chronically infected HCV patients may develop cirrhosis after 20 years, although only 4% of a large cohort of Irish women infected through hepatitis C-contaminated anti-D immunoglobulin have developed cirrhosis after 20 years of infection. Several host and viral factors are associated with more severe histological disease:

- Viral factors
  - Co-infection with HBV or HIV
  - High HCV viral load (over 2×10^6 copies/ml)
  - Quasispecies diversity
  - HCV genotype 1
- Host factors
  - Male gender
  - Alcohol excess
  - Older patient at time of infection
  - Long duration of infection
  - High liver iron content
  - Immunogenetic factors

Knowledge of these factors may aid decision-making with respect to therapy. A range of extra-hepatic manifestations of HCV infection may occur, which have a variable response to treatment. These are:

- Essential mixed (Type II) cryoglobulinaemia
- Porphyria cutanea tarda
- Membranoproliferative glomerulonephritis

- Autoimmune thyroiditis
- Sjögren's syndrome
- Idiopathic pulmonary fibrosis
- Focal lymphocytic sialadenitis
- Lichen planus

The assessment of patients has been advanced by the development of sensitive anti-HCV antibody tests, which allow confirmation of exposure to HCV, and PCR amplification to demonstrate the presence of HCV RNA in the serum, and therefore ongoing infection. Important advances in our understanding of the pathogenesis of HCV have also contributed to the significant improvements in treatment of chronic HCV infection that have been made over the last 10 years. There is now the prospect of inducing long-term suppression of viral replication and controlling disease progression in patients with chronic hepatitis C.

Pathophysiology

Hepatitis C virus is a member of the Flaviviridae family. The viral genomic RNA is a 9379 nucleotide, single-stranded, plus sense RNA, with a single long open reading frame. HCV contains several structural proteins, such as E1 and E2, which contain hypervariable regions, and are putative virion glycoproteins.

Sevেreal non-structural proteins that may be important for viral replication, and hence possible targets for therapy have been identified. They include a putative NS3 serine protease, RNA helicase, and a NS5a RNA-dependent RNA polymerase.

Sequence variability in the HCV genome has led to the classification of six main genotypes. Genotype 1 is common in Europe, is associated with a worse response to antiviral therapy, and may be responsible for more progressive disease than the other genotypes. Further subtype classifications may be performed (e.g. Type 1b, 3a) and, within a single individual patient, further minor HCV variants may exist as 'quasi-species'.

Hepatitis C is said to be a non-cytopathic virus and liver disease is thought to be immune mediated; however, this is probably over-simplistic since patients who are immunosuppressed (e.g. post liver transplantation or with HIV disease) have more severe, progressive liver disease than patients with a normal immune system.

The mechanisms of viral persistence and disease pathogenesis are not well understood and research is hampered by the lack of *in vitro* models for HCV infection. Antibodies to hepatitis C virus are a marker of infection or past exposure. Chimpanzees are not protected against recurrent infection with homologous or heterologous viral strains. In acute hepatitis C virus infection, a vigorous multi-specific cytotoxic and T-helper response can be demonstrated.[9] Despite this, chronic infection usually ensues. During chronic infection, T-cell responses may sometimes be demonstrated but are usually weak. Reasons for this are currently being investigated but may include antigenic variation, T-cell exhaustion, interference of T-cell function by HCV proteins or impaired T-cell response within the liver, which is known to be a tolerogenic organ.

Therapeutic approach

The aim of treatment in an individual infected with HCV is to prevent progression of liver disease to cirrhosis and end-stage liver disease. Other goals may include reducing the patient's infective risk to others, and the improvement of extra-hepatic manifestations associated with HCV. In clinical practice, it has become conventional to define response to treatment as normalization of ALT (biochemical response) or the development of negative HCV RNA by PCR (virological response). Treatment response is best considered as end of treatment response (ETR), sustained response (SR), or relapse. SR is usually defined as both a biochemical and virological response 6 months after stopping therapy. Sustained virological response, that is, HCV RNA undetectable by sensitive PCR (<100 copies/ml) for at least 6 months after cessation of treatment is the best correlate of response of hepatitis C disease to treatment. There is evidence that a long-term virological and biochemical response to treatment slows the progression of histological disease.

Pre-treatment assessment

In clinical practice, most patients with HCV infection present with chronic infection, that is, are HCV RNA-positive. In a patient who is anti-HCV antibody-positive, knowledge of HCV RNA status by PCR, HCV genotype, serum ALT, and the results of liver histology allow treatment (Fig. 11.2) to be planned.

A positive anti-HCV antibody test confirms previous exposure but cannot distinguish resolved from ongoing infection. PCR amplification of circulating HCV RNA allows a qualitative assessment of HCV RNA in the serum, and is required prior to treatment. Quantitation of HCV viral load is available in most specialist units, and may provide some further evidence concerning likely response to treatment; however, in a patient who is HCV RNA-positive using PCR, viral load measurement rarely influences the decision whether to treat, although very high viral load might suggest a longer treatment course in patients with genotype 1 infection.

HCV genotype should also be determined prior to treatment, since this factor significantly influences treatment responses and optimal duration of therapy.

Although patients who are HCV RNA-positive and have hepatitis on biopsy frequently have raised ALT, there is a poor correlation between level of serum transaminases and liver injury. A liver biopsy is therefore required to define the degree of hepatic necroinflammation (grade) and fibrosis (stage).

Who to treat

The NIH consensus document on hepatitis C management concluded that 'treatment is recommended for the group of patients with chronic hepatitis C who are at the greatest risk for progression to cirrhosis. These patients are characterized by persistently elevated ALT,

positive HCV RNA, and a liver biopsy with either portal or bridging fibrosis and at least moderate degrees of inflammation and necrosis'.[10] The merits of treating viraemic patients who have minimal histological disease is the subject of a large UK multicentre trial, and the EASL *International Consensus Conference on Hepatitis C*[11] recently concluded that HCV RNA-positive patients with normal ALT need not necessarily be considered for liver biopsy or treatment; however, some viraemic patients with normal ALT may have active and progressive liver disease. The treatment of other groups infected with HCV is considered in the text following.

Treatment regimens

Chronic hepatitis C infection

Although there are several new therapies in development, the only currently licensed treatments for chronic hepatitis C are α-IFN alone ('monotherapy') and recently, ribavirin in combination with α-IFN ('combination therapy'). The efficacy of these therapies have been considered for different patient groups, including:

- 'Naïve' or untreated patients
- Patients who have relapsed after a biochemical and virological ETR ('relapsers')
- Patients who have not responded to previous interferon treatment ('non-responders').

Interferon-naïve patients

In patients who receive a 12-month course of α-IFN monotherapy, 3 million units (MU) three times per week, up to 50% will have a biochemical ETR, but only 15–25% will have an SR. Meta-analysis has shown that virological SR is lower than biochemical SR.[12]

The publication in 1998 of several large trials of α-IFN therapy in combination with ribavirin as first-line therapy in chronic HCV confirmed significantly better response rates than have been seen with α-IFN:[13–15] McHutchinson *et al.* (Table 11.1) showed a virological SR in 38% of patients receiving combination therapy,

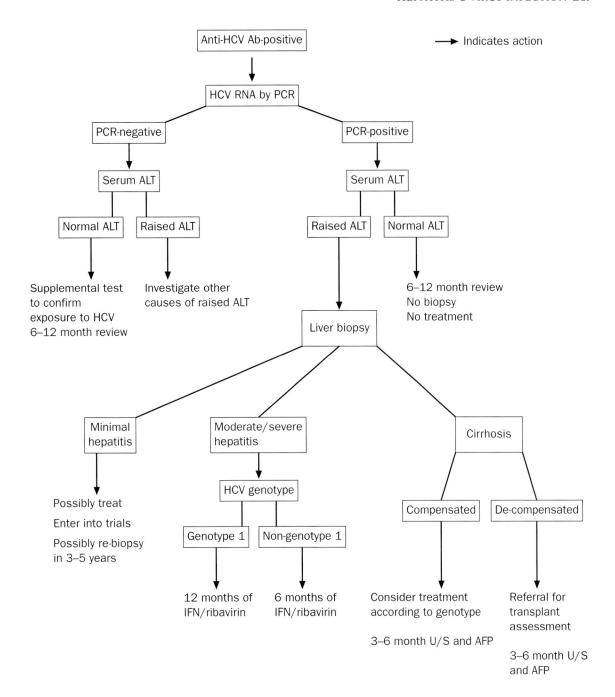

Figure 11.2 Management algorithm for anti-HCV antibody patients.
U/S, abdominal ultrasound scan; AFP, α-fetoprotein.

compared with 13% receiving α-IFN and placebo.[15] Response rates were worse for those with HCV genotype 1, in whom 12 months' combination therapy was clearly shown to have benefit over 6 months. No significant differences in SR were seen between 6 and 12 months treatment in those with non-genotype 1 infection, suggesting that 6 months' treatment with combination is as advantageous as 12 months' treatment for this group. This observation reinforced the cost-effectiveness of HCV genotype testing prior to therapy. There is now little place for α-IFN interferon monotherapy for hepatitis C in patients who do not have a contraindication to ribavirin.

'Relapsers'

In a study by Davies,[14] 345 patients who had relapsed after a previous course of α-IFN were randomized to 6 months of α-IFN and ribavirin or α-IFN alone. Combination therapy produced significantly improved biochemical and virological SR, and histological findings, compared with re-treatment with monotherapy. In 1999, the EASL *International Consensus Conference on Hepatitis C* concluded that 12 months of combi-

nation therapy, or possibly high-dose α-IFN monotherapy for 12 months should be considered for 'relapsers'.

Non-responders to interferon

Those patients who have shown no response to a previous course of α-IFN are very unlikely to achieve a SR with a further course, even using combination treatment. The use of long-term maintenance 'suppressive' treatment with combination therapy to reduce histological progression in non-responders remains controversial but is being investigated at present.

Pharmacology of drugs

α-IFN

Indication

Chronic hepatitis C, with HCV RNA-positive by PCR, raised serum aminotransaminases, and at least moderate hepatitis on liver biopsy. (See earlier text, p. 248, for other considerations.) Patients should be informed of the likely response rates to treatment, and of the factors predictive of a good response to treatment

Table 11.1 Sustained virological response rates to α-IFN/ribavirin combination therapy versus α-IFN therapy alone in treatment-naïve patients with chronic hepatitis C.[*]

	Treatment duration (weeks)	All patients	Genotype 1	Genotype non-1	HCV RNA >2 × 10⁶ copies/ml
α-IFN	24	13/231 (6%)	3/167 (2%)	10/64 (16%)	6/157 (4%)
	48	29/225 (13%)	11/162 (7%)	18/63 (29%)	11/162 (7%)
α-IFN/ribavirin	24	70/228 (31%)	26/164 (16%)	44/64 (69%)	44/166 (27%)
	48	87/228 (38%)	46/166 (28%)	41/61 (66%)	54/152 (36%)

[*] Data from McHutchinson JG, Gordon SC, Schiff ER, *et al.* 1998.[15]

before deciding on whether to undergo treatment. Factors predictive of a response to α-IFN are as follows:

- **Host factors**
  - Female gender
  - Young age (<40 years)
  - Low hepatic iron stores/serum ferritin
  - HIV negative
  - No cirrhosis on biopsy
- **Viral factors**
  - HCV genotype non-1
  - Low HCV RNA level in serum (<1 × 10⁶ genomes/ml)
  - Homogenous HCV quasispecies
  - Possible mutations in interferon-sensitive region in NS5a region of viral genome
  - Early normalization of alanine transferase (ALT) and clearance of HCV RNA after starting IFN therapy

Dosage
A dose of 3 million IU should be given three times/week, subcutaneously.

Duration of therapy
HCV genotype 1 should be given for 12 months; HCV genotype non-1 should be given for 6 months. Optimal therapy is in combination with ribavirin.

Mode of action, dynamics/kinetics, adverse reactions
See p. 242.

Drug interactions, contraindications
See p. 242.

Ribavirin
Mode of action
Ribavirin is a guanosine analogue, with action against RNA and DNA viruses, but its mode of action in hepatitis C is poorly understood. There is no sustained antiviral action when given alone but treatment is effective in combination with α-IFN. Ribavirin may deplete intracellular triphosphate pools by inhibiting inosine monophosphate dehydrogenase, or inhibit HCV RNA polymerase.

Dynamics/kinetics
Ribavirin is absorbed rapidly following oral ingestion (T_{max} = 1.5 h), with elimination $T_{1/2}$ of 79 h. With daily dosing of 1.2 g, the mean steady-state plasma levels are reached in 4 weeks. Bioavailability is 45–65%, and may be increased by food. The main determinants of drug clearance are body weight, gender, age, and serum creatinine.

Indications
Ribavirin should be taken in combination with α-IFN, for the already mentioned indications (p. 250).

Dose
A dose of 1–1.2 g/day should be taken orally (dose should be weight-adjusted) for as long as the α-IFN therapy.

Adverse reactions
Common reactions include haemolysis (Hb falls to <10 g/dl in 14% of patients, with a dose reduction required in 10–15% of cases), depression and fatigue.

Less common reactions include vertigo, insomnia, nausea, nasal congestion, metallic taste, dyspepsia, cough, dry mouth, hyperuricaemia.

Drug interactions
In vitro inhibition of zidovudine and stavudine phosphorylation occurs with concomitant therapy, perhaps leading to increased HIV plasma viraemia. Its clinical importance is not defined but monitoring of HIV RNA levels is recommended in patients on concomitant therapy.

Contraindications
These include:

- Pregnancy (teratogenicity shown in animal models, so drug should not be given during, or within 4 months prior to planned pregnancy. Adequate contraception in sexually active patients is essential, and male

patients on ribavirin should use condoms for 7 months after completing treatment, if there is a risk of pregnancy in partner, and also if partner is pregnant, to prevent transfer of ribavirin in semen)
- Haemoglobinopathies (but close monitoring and increased transfusion regimen may be sufficient for these patients)
- Coronary artery disease (anaemia may unmask undiagnosed cardiac disease)
- Renal failure (should be avoided in patients with creatinine clearance <50 ml/min)
- Severe psychiatric disease

Monitoring and supervision during combination treatment for hepatitis C

α-IFN treatment is self-administered by most patients, who should be taught correct drawing up of the drug, administration, and 'sharps' disposal. The first self-injection should be supervised. Rotation of injection sites is advised, and paracetamol 1 g orally prior to treatment usually alleviates influenza-like symptoms. Patients should be reviewed every 2 weeks for the first month, and then monthly. Clinical assessment should include serum transaminases, full blood count, serum glucose, and thyroid function tests. HCV RNA by PCR may be measured at 6 months but previous advice, on the basis of α-IFN monotherapy data, to check this at 3 months, and stop treatment if still positive, should be revised for combination therapy. On combination therapy, HCV RNA may become negative by the end of therapy, despite being positive after 3 months.

Anti-viral therapy in special groups

Acute hepatitis C

Small trials of α-IFN suggest that 3–6 MU 3 times a week, for at least 6 months, may reduce the severity of liver injury, and possibly progression to chronic disease. Trials of combination antiviral therapy have not been performed but extrapolation from results in chronic hepatitis C might suggest the logic in using combination therapy for acute hepatitis C.

Cirrhosis

Clinical trials of α-IFN monotherapy and combination therapy have excluded patients with decompensated cirrhosis as α-IFN is poorly tolerated in these patients. Patients with compensated cirrhosis may respond to combination therapy although the chance of a sustained response is less than 30%.[13] Cirrhotic patients must be monitored closely while on treatment, particularly for hepatic decompensation and thrombocytopenia.

Extrahepatic manifestations

Vasculitis, glomerulonephritis and cryoglobulinaemia related to HCV may respond well to α-IFN therapy but relapse is very common after cessation and maintenance therapy may be required.

Children

Serious complications of HCV usually take at least 20 years to develop, and since significant improvements in treatment are likely to be made during this period, it is difficult to justify instigating an α-IFN-based treatment with the inherent difficulties of administration and side-effect profile. A few studies of monotherapy in children with hepatitis C have been performed. Trials of combination therapy are in progress in this group.

HIV and HCV infection

Co-infection with hepatitis C and HIV is associated with a greater risk of cirrhosis and morbidity than hepatitis C infection alone. HCV infection and disease progression is particularly aggressive in these patients, perhaps owing to complex immune dysregulation. In view of the important advances made in treating HIV, and the high frequency of HCV co-infection, HCV threatens to have an increasing impact on morbidity and mortality in this group. There is no consensus, as yet, regarding the treatment of HCV in this group. Treatment may be indicated for patients with CD4 counts >200 but care is required to avoid potential drug interactions in patients whose HIV has been stabilized by antiretroviral combination therapy.

Liver transplantation

The number of patients being transplanted for HCV continues to increase. Five-year survival rates of 70% are similar to that for patients transplanted for non-malignant conditions. Re-infection of the transplanted liver is almost universal, and may lead to accelerated cirrhosis in the new graft. There is no consensus as to the optimal treatment of HCV in transplant recipients and currently most transplant centres are not treating post-transplantation HCV at this time.

New therapies for chronic hepatitis C

New anti-viral therapies under development should offer hope to the more than 50% of patients who fail to achieve a SR with present licensed treatments. New interferon formulations look promising, and the second generation of pegylated ('PEG') interferons appears to be more effective, and can be administered once weekly.

There is emerging evidence that pegylated interferon (PEG IFN) may be superior to α-IFN. PEG IFNs are derived by covalent attachment of 43 kD branched polyethylene glycol moieties to interferon. This chemical change substantially prolongs the plasma half-life and elimination half-life by decreasing enzyme degradation and renal elimination, giving a protracted effect. The net effect is increased drug exposure, permitting once-weekly dosing.

Importantly, preliminary data suggest that the altered pharmacokinetics of both PEG α-IFN 2a and PEG α-IFN 2b significantly improve their antiviral effect compared with recombinant interferon. Dose-ranging studies have been completed, which suggest a significantly superior efficacy of PEG α-IFN compared with α-IFN 2b and α-IFN 2a, and equivalent to the effect of recombinant α-IFN 2b combined with ribavirin. Also PEG α-IFN 2a 180 μg weekly in patients with cirrhosis has recently been shown to lead to sustained virological responses in 29% versus 6% of patients treated with α-IFN 2a. Of cirrhotic patients with non-1 HCV infec-tion 53% responded. It is not yet clear whether PEG IFN monotherapy will substantially improve the treatment of patients with Type 1 infection and high viral loads, where treatment responses are low; however, there is a reasonable expectation that the combination of PEG IFN and ribavirin will enhance responses, and these studies have begun. At least one PEG α-IFN has been filed for licence in the EU, and will probably be available for compassionate treatment shortly.

As has been shown in the treatment of HIV, combination therapy for HCV is the likely way forward. Other drugs being assessed in combination, including amantadine, non-steroidal anti-inflammatory agents (NSAIDs), and thymosin. Drugs to inhibit enzymes of HCV replication (serine protease, helicase or polymerase inhibitors), or HCV translation, are under development.

HEPATITIS A VIRUS INFECTION

Hepatitis A virus (HAV) infection occurs worldwide. Children aged 5–15 years are most commonly affected in developing countries. Infection in this group is often asymptomatic. In developing countries, 90% of children have HAV IgG antibodies by the age of 10 years. In developed countries, however, the mean age of infection has increased such that only 5–10% of young adults have serological evidence of previous exposure.

Transmission is faecal–oral so that infection is particularly common in areas of poor sanitation. The incubation is 3–5 weeks. Hepatitis A IgM is detectable in the serum for 45–60 days after the onset of symptoms and is the simplest way to establish the diagnosis. In adults, hepatitis may be severe and protracted. Approximately 5% of patients with clinically overt HAV infection develop cholestatic hepatitis. HAV may rarely cause fulminant liver failure (0.1%).

Pathophysiology

Hepatitis A virus (HAV) is a small RNA virus of the genus picornaviradae. The virus is not cytopathic and liver damage is caused by the host's immune response.

Therapeutic approach

There is no specific therapy for HAV infection. A short course of oral prednisolone has been shown to shorten the cholestatic phase of infection.[16] Hepatitis A vaccine and hepatitis A immunoglobulin are available.

Hepatitis A vaccine

Indications

Indications include:

- Travellers to areas of high HAV endemicity, particularly if sanitation and food hygiene are sub-optimum. Immunization is not considered necessary for those travelling to Northern or Western Europe or to North America, Australia or New Zealand. When practical, testing for antibodies to HAV prior to immunization may be worthwhile in those aged over 50 years, those born in areas of high HAV prevalence and those with a history of jaundice.
- Patients with chronic liver disease: these patients are at no greater risk of acquiring HAV than healthy individuals but the consequence of infection may be much more serious.
- Haemophiliac patients: transmission has been associated with factors VIII and IX concentrates where concentration procedures do not destroy the virus. Inject the vaccine subcutaneously in these patients.
- Occupational exposure: laboratory workers who work with the virus; institutions where standards of personal hygiene are poor; children's day care centres when local community outbreaks occur (after discussion with centre for disease control and prevention (CDC)).

- Homosexual behaviour: HAV occurs more commonly in homosexual men. Vaccine should be offered to anyone whose sexual practices put them at risk.
- Outbreaks: guidelines should be sought from the consultant in communicable disease control or from the PHLS Communicable Disease Surveillance Centre.

Mode of action

This vaccine is formaldehyde-inactivated, prepared from GBM or HM 175 strain of hepatitis A virus grown in human diploid cells. It is supplied as a suspension in pre-filled syringes and stored at 2–8°C.

Pharmacodynamics/kinetics

Antibodies persist for at least 1 year and may be prolonged by a booster dose of vaccine given 6–12 months after the initial course. Antibodies are protective 2–4 weeks post-vaccination. Human normal immunoglobulin may be administered at the same time if protection is required less than 10 days after the first dose of vaccine.

Dosage (HM 175 strain-HAVRIX)

- Adults: given a single dose of 1440 ELISA units (1 ml) of the HM 175 strain or 160 antigen units of the GBM strain. A booster dose after 6–12 months will give immunity for 10 years.
- Children and adolescents: Two doses of 720 ELISA units (0.5 ml) of the HM 175 strain are given 2 weeks to 1 month apart with a booster 6–12 months after the primary course.

Drug interactions

None are known.

Contraindications

Postpone vaccination in severe febrile illnesses. The effect of HAV vaccine on fetal development is not known. Since it is an inactivated virus, the risks to the fetus are negligible but, as with other vaccines in pregnancy, it should not be given unless there is a definite risk of infection.

Immunoglobulin

Mode of action

Human normal immunoglobulin (HNIG) offers short-term protection (up to 4 months) against infection with HAV. HNIG may modify disease rather than prevent infection but it also prevents secondary cases.

Main indication

Until recently HNIG, in addition to vaccination was indicated for patients requiring immediate protection against HAV, such as those travelling to endemic areas at short notice and immediate contacts of infected individuals. However, every batch of HNIG is manufactured from the pooled plasma of blood donors and there is a theoretical risk of human to human transmission of infective agents such as new variant Creutzfeld-Jacob Disease. In addition, as anti-HAV titres have fallen within the general population in developed countries, levels of specific antibody in pooled serum may be reduced.

The addition of HNIG was recommended because of concern about the time taken to develp neutralising antibodies with the vaccine. However, anti-HAV antibodies may be detected rapidly after vaccination and the recent demonstration of the efficacy of vaccination as post exposure prophylaxis against HAV attests to the immunogenicity of a single dose of vaccine.[17]

For these reasons we would recommend vaccination alone, rather than vaccination in addition to HNIG, for those individuals requiring immediate protection against HAV.

Dosage

The dose given to all ages is:

- a low dose (0.02–0.04 ml/kg) for travel lasting 2 months or less
- a high dose (0.06–0.12 ml/kg) for travel lasting 2–5 months and contacts.

Drug interactions

HNIG may interfere with the development of active immunity from live virus vaccines, which should be administered at least 3 weeks before HNIG. If immunoglobulin has been given first live vaccine should not be administered for 3 months.

OTHER VIRUSES CAUSING HEPATITIS

Hepatitis E

An enterically transmitted epidemic form of hepatitis was first recognized by epidemics of hepatitis unrelated to hepatitis A or B. Virus like particles (27–34 nm) in size were seen during the acute phase of hepatitis. A polyadenylated single-strand RNA of 8.5 kb was cloned by extracting nucleic acid from experimentally-infected macaque monkeys. Epidemics of hepatitis E have been observed in waterborne epidemics in several regions including the Indian subcontinent, South and Central Asia, Northern and Western Europe, Mexico and Eastern Europe. Hepatitis E is transmitted by the faecal–oral route. The highest attack rates have been observed in individuals between 15 and 40 years of age. In most outbreaks, the highest fatality rates have been in pregnant women (20%). Usually the disease is self-limiting. Chronic liver disease or persistent viraemia have not been observed. Serological assays have been developed to identify anti-HEV antibody in serum samples. PCR detection of HEV RNA is also possible. There is no specific treatment for hepatitis E.

Many viruses may infect the liver as part of a systemic infection causing a rise in transaminases, which settles as the virus is eradicated. Viral infections of the liver are a particular problem in immunosuppressed patients, such as liver and bone marrow recipients and patients with AIDS. Cocksackie virus, adenovirus, measles, varicella, varicella zoster and rubella may all cause hepatitis and treatment is supportive. CMV infection is a particular problem in liver transplant recipients.

CMV infection

Cytomegalovirus can cause a disease resembling EBV infection although patients do not have pharyngitis or cervical lymphadenopathy. Jaundice may last 2–3 weeks and sometimes months. Pyrexia, anorexia, tender hepatosplenomegaly are common features. CMV infection is a particular problem in liver transplant recipients. The infection is usually a primary infection from a CMV antibody-positive donor. Liver biopsy shows CMV intranuclear inclusions and clusters of polymorphs and lymphocytes. Infection usually presents within 90 days post-transplant and continues for months or years in patients who are heavily immunosuppressed. Ganciclovir may be used to treat CMV infection and, currently, we are conducting a trial to determine the efficacy of ganciclovir given in combination with foscarnet (see also Chapter 6).

Pharmacology of ganciclovir

Mode of action
Ganciclovir is a synthetic analogue of guanine that inhibits the replication of herpes viruses. It is phosphorylated by intracellular kinases. In CMV infected cells, there is an increase in intracellular kinases such that ganciclovir is preferentially phosphorylated inside these cells.

Dynamics/kinetics
Its major route of excretion is via glomerular filtration of the unchanged drug.

Indications
Patients with CMV infection diagnosed by CMV PCR in blood and inclusion bodies at liver biopsy. During treatment review and reduce immunosuppression if possible.

Dosage
A dose of 5 mg/kg twice daily should be given intravenously. Modify dose if renal insufficiency is present (see data sheet).

Adverse reactions
Common adverse reactions include neutropenia, thrombocytopenia, anaemia, diarrhoea, dyspepsia, nausea, anorexia, rash, headache, fever, and abnormal liver function tests.

Drug interactions
Interactions occur with:

- Probenecid: inhibits renal clearance
- Zidovudine: also causes neutropenia
- Imipenem-cilastatin: seizures with this combination have been reported.

Contraindications
Pregnancy and lactation are contraindications since ganciclovir is potentially carcinogenic and teratogenetic.

REFERENCES

1. Lai C-L, Chien R-N, Leung N, *et al.* A one-year trial of lamivudine for chronic Hepatitis B. *New Eng J Med* 1998; **339**: 61–68.
2. Leung NWY, Lai CL, Chang TT, *et al.* Three-year lamivudine therapy in chronic HBV. *J Hepatol* 1999; **30**: 59.
3. Ling R, Harrison TJ. Functional analysis of mutations confering lamivudine resistance on hepatitis B virus. *J Gen Virol* 1999; **80**: 601–606.
4. Schiff E, Karayalcin S, Grimm L. A placebo controlled study of lamivudine and alpha interferon 2b in patients with chronic hepatitis B who have previously failed interferon therapy. *Hepatology* 1998; **28**: 388A.
5. Tassopoulos NC, Volpes R, Pastore G, *et al.* Efficacy of Lamivudine in patients with hepatitis B e antigen-negative/hepatitis B virus DNA-positive (pre-core mutant) chronic hepatitis B. Lamivudine precore Mutant Study Group. *Hepatology* 1999; **29**: 889–896.
6. Grellier L, Multimer D, Ahmed M, *et al.* Lamivudine prophylaxis against re-infection in liver transplantation for hepatitis B cirrhosis. *Lancet* 1996; **348**: 1212–1215.
7. McDonald JA, Caruso L, Karayannis P, *et al.* Diminished responsiveness of male homosexual chronic hepatitis B carriers with HTLV-III antibodies, to recombinant alpha-interferon. *Hepatology* 1987; **7**: 719–723.
8. Dusheiko GM. Side-effects of alpha-interferon in hepatitis C. *Hepatology* 1997; **26**: 12S–21S.
9. Lechner F, Sullivan J, Spiegel H, *et al.* Success and failure of cytotoxic T lymphocytes in hepati-

tis C virus infection studied using HCA class I tetramers. *Philos Trans R Soc Lond* 2000; **355:** 1085–1092.

10. NIH Consensus development conference panel statement. *Hepatology* 1997; **26:** 2S–10S.

11. EASL International Consensus Conference on Hepatitis C. Consensus Statement. *J Hepatol* 1999; **30:** 956–961.

12. Carithers RJ, Emerson SS, Therapy of hepatitis C: meta-analysis of interferon alfa-2b trials. *Hepatology* 1997; **26:** 83S–88S.

13. Poynard T, Marcellin P, Lee S, *et al.* Randomised trial of interferon-2b plus ribavirin for 48 weeks or 24 weeks, versus interferon 2b plus placebo for 48 weeks for treatment of chronic infection with hepatitis C virus. *Lancet* 1998; **352:** 1426–1432.

14. Davis GL, Esteban-Mur R, Rustgi V, *et al.* Interferon alfa-2b alone or in combination with ribavirin for the treatment of relapse of chronic hepatitis C. *N Eng J Med* 1998; **339:** 1493–1499.

15. McHutchinson JG, Gordon SC, Schiff ER, *et al.* Interferon alfa-2b alone or in combination as initial treatment for chronic hepatitis C. *N Eng J Med* 1998; **339:** 1493–1499.

16. Gordon S, Reddy R, Schiff L, Schiff E. Prolonged intrahepatic cholestasis secondary to acute hepatitis A. *Ann Intern Med* 1984; **101:** 635–637.

17. Sagliocca L, Amoroso P, Stroffolini T, *et al.* Efficacy of hepatitis A vaccine in prevention of secondary hepatitis A infection: a randomised trial. *Lancet* 1999; **353:** 1136–1139.

12

Non-viral liver disease

John ML Christie, Roger WG Chapman

INTRODUCTION

The last decade has seen important advances in our knowledge of the diagnosis, natural history and treatment of non-viral-induced liver disease, including primary sclerosing cholangitis, primary biliary cirrhosis, autoimmune hepatitis, haemochromatosis, Wilson's disease, α_1-antitrypsin deficiency, alcoholic hepatitis, liver storage diseases, Budd-Chiari syndrome and drug-induced liver disease. Genes that cause hereditary liver disease have been discovered, including the gene for Wilson's disease and haemochromatosis. Therapies to prevent disease or progression are well-established for Wilson's disease, haemochromatosis and autoimmune hepatitis. As our understanding of the other liver diseases advances, so will further therapies be developed. We still have a long way to go, however, and many of the current therapies are aimed at symptom-control and treatment of complications rather than targeting the underlying disease process. Liver transplantation remains an essential therapy for end-stage disease.

PRIMARY SCLEROSING CHOLANGITIS

Introduction

Primary sclerosing cholangitis (PSC) is a progressive cholestatic disease characterized by stricturing and dilatation of the biliary system.[1] It usually progresses, by causing ductopenia, cholestasis, fibrosis and cirrhosis.[2] Approximately 20% of patients will develop cholangiocarcinoma.[3–5]

The diagnosis is made by cholangiography since liver histology is only diagnostic in one-third of cases. The generally accepted diagnostic criteria of primary sclerosing cholangitis are:

- Generalized beading and stenosis of the biliary system on cholangiography
- Absence of choleocholithiasis or a history of bile duct surgery
- Exclusion of bile duct cancer, usually by prolonged follow-up

Once considered to be rare, PSC occurs in approximately 6–8 cases per 100 000 of the population, and is strongly associated with inflammatory bowel disease, particularly ulcerative colitis, which is present in about 80% of patients with PSC. Of patients with ulcerative colitis, 3–10% will develop primary sclerosing cholangitis;[6] prevalence is greater in patients with substantial or total colitis than in those with distal colitis only.[7] The prevalence of primary sclerosing cholangitis is lower in patients with Crohn's colitis, being around 1%.[8] The lower prevalence may be related to less extensive colitis in patients with Crohn's disease.

The clinical course of PSC is highly unpredictable and unrelated to the clinical course of ulcerative colitis.[9][11] Primary sclerosing cholangitis is mainly a disease of young males, with a male to female ratio of 2:1. The majority of patients present between the ages of 25 and 40 years, although primary sclerosing cholangitis may be diagnosed at any age and has become recognized recently as an important cause of chronic liver disease in children. The clinical presentation is variable but commonly includes fatigue, intermittent jaundice, weight loss, right upper quadrant abdominal pain, and pruritus. The cause of pruritus in PSC, as in other cholestatic liver diseases, is not clear. Several hypotheses have been proposed including bile acid retention and endogenous opioids. Attacks of acute cholangitis are surprisingly rare, and usually follow instrumental biliary intervention. Physical examination is abnormal in approximately one-half of symptomatic patients. The most common findings are jaundice and hepatomegaly and splenomegaly. Many patients with primary sclerosing cholangitis are asymptomatic at diagnosis, which is made incidentally when a persistently raised serum alkaline phosphatase is discovered in patients with ulcerative colitis. The median survival for patients who are symptomatic is approximately 12–15 years. Most asymptomatic patients will progress.

Specific medical therapy has been disappointing and endoscopic therapy is reserved for patients with complications such as main duct stricturing and biliary stone formation. Orthotopic liver transplantation is effective therapy with 5-year survival rates of over 90% in recent series.[12,13] The presence of cholangiocarcinoma precludes liver transplantation because of a high recurrence rate and poor prognosis.[14] Recent reports have confirmed that PSC recurs in the transplanted liver in about 20% of cases at 1 year post-transplant.

Pathophysiology

In PSC, diffuse inflammation and fibrosis can involve the entire biliary tree. The progressive pathological process obliterates intrahepatic and extrahepatic bile ducts, ultimately leading to biliary cirrhosis, portal hypertension and hepatic failure.

The cause of primary sclerosing cholangitis remains unknown. Any proposed factors in aetiopathogenesis of primary sclerosing cholangitis clearly have to explain the close association in patients with inflammatory bowel disease. Current evidence suggests that primary sclerosing cholangitis is an immunologically mediated disease, probably triggered in genetically susceptible subjects by acquired toxic or infectious agents, which may gain access through the leaky diseased colon.

A close link with HLA A1, B8, DR3, DRW 52A, has been found.[15] This haplotype is found commonly in association with other organ-specific autoimmune diseases, such as autoimmune chronic active hepatitis. In patients who are DR3-negative, an increased prevalence of HLA DR2 and HLA DR6 has been found.[16]

The importance of immunological factors has been emphasized further by several reports, which have shown humoral and cellular abnormalities in primary sclerosing cholangitis. Perinuclear antineutrophil cytoplasmic antibodies (ANCA) have been detected in the sera of approximately 60–80% of patients with primary sclerosing cholangitis, with or without ulcerative colitis, and in approximately 30–40% of patients with ulcerative colitis alone.[17,18] The antibody is not specific for primary sclerosing cholangitis and is found in other chronic liver diseases, particularly in 50% of patients with autoimmune chronic active hepatitis. The antigen in the neutrophils has yet to be identified and it is unclear whether the presence of the antibody has any pathogenetic significance.[19]

In view of the link with inflammatory bowel disease, it has been hypothesized that portal vein bacterial cell wall products or absorption of toxins from the inflamed colon might be responsible for the biliary tract inflammation seen in PSC.[20]

Therapeutic approaches

There is no curative treatment for primary sclerosing cholangitis but a plethora of medical, endoscopic, and surgical approaches have been advocated. The treatment of primary sclerosing cholangitis can be divided into management of cholestasis, the management of complications, and lastly, specific treatments of the disease process.

Management of cholestasis
Symptomatic patients are frequently troubled by pruritus; this is best managed initially with cholestyramine and the dose should be increased until relief is obtained. In addition, fat-soluble vitamin replacement is necessary for jaundiced patients and metabolic bone disease, since osteoporosis is a frequent complication of advanced PSC. Prophylactic treatment with calcium and vitamin D_3 oral medication has been recommended.

Management of complications
Broad-spectrum antibiotics such as ciprofloxacin (see p. 128) should be given for acute attacks of cholangitis but they have no proven prophylactic value. If cholangiography shows a well-defined obstruction to the extrahepatic bile ducts, mechanical relief can be seen by either inducing a prosthesis or a balloon dilatation performed at endoscopic retrograde cholangiopancreatography (ERCP).[21]

Specific treatment
Medical
The medical treatment of primary sclerosing cholangitis has included trials of corticosteroids, immunosuppressive drugs and antibiotics, either alone or in combination. Ursodeoxycholic acid is a non-hepatotoxic hydrophillic bile acid that has been used widely for the treatment of cholestasis.[22] It reduces levels of cholestatic liver enzymes but controlled trials in conventional doses have shown no effect on symptoms, histology or survival. Larger doses may be needed to produce a more beneficial effect.[23] Several immunosuppressive agents have been tried, including prednisone, colchicine,[24] azathioprine,[25] methotrexate[26] and cyclosporin;[27] overall, the results have been disappointing.

Surgical treatment
Orthotopic transplantation is the only option available in young patients with primary sclerosing cholangitis and advanced liver disease. Five-year survival rates are between 80 and 90% in most centres. There are increasing reports of primary sclerosing cholangitis occurring in the transplanted liver but these have not yet led to any problems with liver decompensation. Proven cholangiocarcinoma is a contraindication to transplantation as the tumour rapidly recurs post-transplant with immunosuppression.

Treatment regimens

If the patient has pruritus cholestyramine therapy (4 g in the morning) should be commenced, increased to a usual maintenance dose of 12–16 g in two to three divided doses over 2–4 weeks. Cholestyramine should be mixed with water or juice and taken immediately after vigorous mixing. Patients should be advised to take other drugs at least 1 h before, or 4–6 h after, taking cholestyramine. Pruritus refractory to cholestyramine may respond, at least temporarily to rifampicin (150 mg twice daily) or the opioid antagonist, naltrexone (25 mg initially increasing to 50 mg daily).

Once patients have symptomatic disease, vitamin supplementation of fat-soluble vitamins, in particular vitamin A and D, may be required—especially if the patient is taking cholestyramine, which can also interfere with normal fat absorption.

The use of ursodeoxycholic acid remains controversial and ideally should be used in clinical trials.

Pharmacology

Cholestyramine

Mode of action

A major portion of the bile acids secreted into the intestine with the bile is reabsorbed and returned to the liver via the portal circulation in an entero-hepatic cycle. Cholestyramine resin binds with bile acids in the intestine to form an insoluble complex, which is excreted in the faeces. This process results in a continuous, although partial, removal of bile acids from enterohepatic circulation by preventing their reabsorption.

The increased loss of bile acids owing to cholestyramine leads to increased oxidation of cholesterol to bile acids and thus a decrease in serum cholesterol.

Kinetics

Cholestyramine is insoluble in water and is not absorbed from the gastrointestinal tract. Digestive enzymes do not affect it.

Indications

Relief of pruritus associated with partial biliary obstruction is an indication for treatment.

Adverse reactions

Cholestyramine may cause constipation, especially with higher doses and in the elderly. Less commonly, it may cause abdominal discomfort, flatulence, nausea, vomiting, heartburn, diarrhoea and anorexia. Fat-soluble vitamin (e.g. vitamin A, D and K) deficiencies may occur. Bleeding tendencies may be seen with vitamin K deficiency. Cholestyramine occasionally causes a rash and irritation to the skin, tongue and perianal area.

Drug interactions

Owing to the anion exchange resin properties of cholestyramine it has an affinity for acidic material; it may also adsorb neutral or basic material to some extent. Thus it may delay or reduce the absorption of concomitantly dosed medications, including warfarin, chlorothi-azide, tetracycline, phenobarbitone, thyroxine, digoxin and inorganic iron.

Contraindications

Hypersensitivity to any component of the drug, and complete biliary obstruction where no bile is secreted into the intestine are contraindications.

Naltrexone

Mode of action

This drug is an opioid antagonist.

Indications

Naltrexone prevents relapse in detoxified formerly opioid-dependent patients; it is also used to treat refractory pruritus.

Preparation and dose

Oral tablets are given, 25 mg initially, then 50 mg daily.

Adverse reactions

Nausea, vomiting, abdominal pain; anxiety, joint and muscle pain, chest pain, bowel disturbance, sexual dysfunction, rash, and abnormalities of liver biochemistry may occur.

Drug interactions

None are known.

Precautions and contraindications

Acute hepatitis, liver failure and patients currently dependent on opioids should not be treated with naltrexone.

Rifampicin

See Chapter 6, p. 131.

PRIMARY BILIARY CIRRHOSIS

Introduction

Primary biliary cirrhosis (PBC) is a chronic cholestatic liver disease that can result in fibrosis and biliary cirrhosis.[28] In common with other diseases that are thought to be immune-mediated, PBC occurs predominantly in females with a male to female ratio of 1:9. The disease usually presents in middle age. Estimates of prevalence range from 19–151/million of the population.[29]

The disease is strongly associated with the presence of anti-mitochondrial antibodies (AMA), which are detected in 95% of patients with PBC. Antimitochondrial antibodies are highly specific for PBC, although are also found in a small percentage of patients with drug-induced and autoimmune hepatitis.

Recent studies have suggested that there is a wide clinical spectrum of PBC, which ranges from patients presenting with an isolated anti-mitochondrial antibody, some of whom have an essentially normal prognosis, to patients who present with symptoms of pruritus and jaundice progressing rapidly to death from liver failure. Approximately 50% of patients are asymptomatic at presentation, and it has become apparent that, in addition to the environmental and genetic factors that lead to the onset of disease, there must be additional factors that determine whether the disease progresses. Most asymptomatic patients will develop symptoms within 2–4 years. Non-specific symptoms that occur in PBC are fatigue, which is present in approximately 80% of patients, and abdominal pain, which occurs in approximately 10–15% of PBC patients. The pain is typically in the right upper quadrant, and the aetiology of the pain remains unexplained. Approximately 50% of symptomatic patients will have isolated pruritus, which occurs typically at night, or after a hot bath and can effect predominantly the palms of the hands and soles of the feet, although it is often generalized. Cholestatic jaundice is seen decreasingly as the presenting feature of PBC.

Asymptomatic patients have longer life expectancies than symptomatic patients. Median survival for symptomatic patients ranges from 7–10 years, while it is 10–16 years in asymptomatic patients. Increasing jaundice is an important adverse prognostic sign in primary biliary cirrhosis, with levels of bilirubin of over 100 µmol/l should lead to referral for consideration of liver transplantation.[30]

Pathophysiology

PBC is characterized by the immunological destruction of interlobular and septal bile ducts leading to cholestasis, fibrosis, and biliary cirrhosis. PBC is considered to be one of the group of autoimmune liver diseases in which the biliary epithelial cells lining the interlobular and septal bile ducts form the target for key cell-related immune-mediated damage.[31] The pyruvate dehydrogenase complex has been identified as one of the major autoantigens.[32] The second process thought to be responsible for pathogenesis is the chemical damage to hepatocytes in areas of liver where bile drainage is impeded by the destruction of bile ducts. This results in retention of bile acids, bilirubin, copper and other substances normally excreted in bile, which may be the cause of further damage to liver cells.

Although the aetiological factors remain unknown, it is accepted widely that PBC arises in a susceptible individual, usually female, as a result of one or more environmental trigger factors. Evidence from family studies has shown that inherited factors play an important role in determining disease susceptibility.[33,34] Two studies have shown that the prevalence of PBC in first-degree relatives is 4–6%, significantly higher than the highest reported whole population prevalence.[35] Unlike the two other autoimmune diseases, autoimmune hepatitis and primary sclerosing cholangitis, PBC is not associated with an over representation of the HLA A1 B8 DR3 DR52a haplotype, nor are there secondary associations with HLA DR4 or DR2 as reported in these conditions. Several genotyping studies from different populations have demonstrated a positive association between HLA Class II antigen DR8 and PBC;[36] however, the association only accounts for a few patients with PBC. This may reflect the fact that the susceptibility allele lies some distance from the HLA DR genes.

Recent epidemiological studies have highlighted marked variations in the prevalence of PBC in certain geographical regions ranging from 1/1000 of urban women in Newcastle,

UK,[37,38] to a remarkable low prevalence of PBC in Victoria, Australia,[39] and Ontario, Canada[40] where, in both cases, the population is largely Caucasian of Western European origin. It is still unclear as to whether these variations are artifactual owing to variations in methods used for case finding. If these temporal and geographical variations in the prevalence of PBC prove to be correct, this has important implications in the investigation of aetiopathogenesis of the condition, suggesting there is a locally variable environmental factor.

Circumstantial evidence that an environmental agent may induce PBC was provided from a 3-year study of PBC in Sheffield, UK.[41] The prevalence of PBC was 10 times greater in one area of the city supplied by one water reservoir compared with five other areas of Sheffield supplied by different reservoirs. Chemical and bacteriological investigation failed to find any infectious or chemical factors unique to this reservoir but the Sheffield results have been repeated within the same city recently with similar results (Gleeson D, Personal communication 1998).

It has been suggested that antimitochondrial antibody and, ultimately PBC, are induced by exposure to enterobacterial antigens.[42,43] Immunoblotting studies have shown that PBC-specific antibodies recognize enterobacterial proteins, which correspond to mitochondrial target proteins.[44,45] On the current evidence, however, it is difficult to conclude that enterobacteriaceae are the trigger factors for PBC.[46]

Other possible causes of PBC that have been explored include *Mycobacteria* spp.[47] and retroviruses.[48,49] Although the *Mycobacteria* hypothesis is attractive, since *Mycobacteria* can induce granulomata and granulomata are commonly found in PBC, the results of studies have been conflicting. Similarly, the investigation of retroviruses have been inconclusive. It remains unproven as to whether Mycobacterium or retroviruses play any role in the pathogenesis of PBC.

Therapeutic approach

Therapy for PBC can be divided into management of the symptoms of chronic cholestasis and medical treatment of the underlying disease process. The symptoms of chronic cholestasis include pruritus, malabsorption of fat-soluble vitamins, steatorrhoea and osteoporosis, as discussed previously.

There have been many trials to establish a treatment for the underlying disease process in PBC. Many treatments have been found to be ineffective and even toxic. These include corticosteroids, which do not alter the course of the disease and accelerate osteoporosis.[50] Azathioprine has been shown to be safe but have little efficacy, with no improvement in liver function tests or histology in prospective trials.[51] Penicillamine has also been shown to be ineffective and was associated with a high (>25%) frequency of toxic side-effects.[52] Chorambucil was shown to improve bilirubin, albumin, immunoglobulin levels and improve histology in a pilot study but was associated with unacceptable side-effects, including bone marrow toxicity and leukaemia.[53] Cyclosporin was initially shown to improve symptoms, biochemical tests and histology but this was not confirmed in a subsequent 6-year, 349-patient, multicentre European study.[54]

Colchicine, methotrexate and ursodeoxycholic acid are the only drugs that demonstrated promise in clinical trials. Colchicine (oral 0.6 mg twice daily) has been evaluated in five prospective, double-blind randomized trials in PBC; three compared it with placebo, one with placebo and ursodeoxycholic acid and one with methotrexate. In one study there was significant improvement in biochemical liver function tests and survival,[55] and in three studies just improvement in biochemistry.[56] Biochemical improvement was less striking with colchicine than with methotrexate or ursodeoxycholic acid. Meta-analysis of the first three studies showed that colchicine reduced liver-related mortality.

Ursodeoxycholic acid (12–15 mg/kg/day in two to three divided doses) has been shown to improve serum bilirubin, alkaline phosphatase, aminotransferase and IgM levels in four controlled trials. In some studies, it decreased pruritus and prolonged time to clinical deterioration and liver transplantation.[57–60] Pooling of the data showed significant reduction in time to liver transplantation, although the time difference was modest (3.66 years compared with 3.45 years). These studies still have relatively short follow-up periods and reflect the results of patients with end-stage disease. Ursodeoxycholic acid may show greater benefits in patients with earlier disease, although this remains to be proven. Ursodeoxycholic acid is safe and well-tolerated.

Low-dose oral pulsed methotrexate has been shown to improve biochemical tests and histology in a pilot study.[61] Unfortunately there was a high incidence of interstitial pneumonitis (15%). Early results of combination studies of methotrexate and ursodeoxycholic acid have been promising and the results of further studies are awaited.

Treatment regimens

Pruritus is best managed with cholestyramine (see PSC, p. 262). Other drugs that have been shown to help are antihistamines when itching is mild, rifampicin and the opioid antagonist naltrexone (based on recent data suggesting that itching may be mediated by opioidergic neurotransmission).

Malabsorption of fat-soluble vitamins is proportional to the severity of the cholestasis. Vitamin A, D, E and K levels, if low, should be treated with oral supplementation, administered as far apart from cholestyramine: oral vitamin K 5–10 mg/day, vitamin A 10 000–25 000 IU/day, 25-OH vitamin D 20 µg three times weekly, supplemental calcium, vitamin E 400–1000 IU/day.

Although no medical therapy has been proven to alter the natural history of PBC, the benefit-risk ratio of ursodeoxycholic acid, methotrexate and colchicine appears to be more favorable than no treatment at all.

Ursodeoxycholic acid (13–15/mg/kg/day) in either divided doses or as a single daily dose) is safe and well-tolerated and is therefore widely used in all stages of PBC. Combination with colchicine 1 mg daily or methotrexate or both is still under evaluation.

Pharmacology

Ursodeoxycholic acid
Mode of action
Ursodeoxycholic acid is a naturally occurring bile acid that is present in small quantities in human bile. It is thought to reduce hepatocyte damage and cholestasis by acting as a cholorectic agent and by increasing the levels of hydrophilic non-hepatotoxic bile acids in bile. In addition, ursodeoxycholic acid has been shown to decrease histocompatibility antigen display by hepatocytes and may also have a direct cytoprotective effect.

Kinetics
Ursodeoxycholic acid is absorbed from the gastrointestinal tract and undergoes enterohepatic recycling.

Indications
Ursodeoxycholic acid is used in the treatment of PBC. It also is used in the treatment of cholestatic liver disease as a result of cystic fibrosis and primary sclerosing cholangitis. In addition, it may be used in the dissolution of cholesterol-rich gallstones in patients with functioning gallbladders.

Adverse reactions
Ursodeoxycholic acid may cause nausea, vomiting and diarrhoea. It may cause calcification of cholesterol gallstones.

Drug interactions
Concurrent use with cholestyramine may result in binding of ursodeoxycholic acid, thus decreasing its absorption. At least 4 hours should elapse between cholestyramine intake and ursodeoxycholic acid administration.

Contraindications

Sensitivity to ursodeoxycholic acid or to other bile acids are contraindications for its use. In pregnant women there is a theoretical risk that ursodeoxycholic acid may cross the placenta and cause toxicity to the fetus; however, it has been used in cholestatic disease of pregnancy with no apparent adverse effect. There is no evidence of safety with breastfeeding or renal impairment (but the drug is excreted in bile and faeces).

Colchicine

Mode of action

Colchicine is the active alkaloidal principle derived from various species of *Colchicum*. The precise mechanism of action has not been completely established. Colchicine inhibits microtubule assembly in various cells, including leukocytes, probably by binding to and interfering with polymerization of the microtubule subunit tubulin. Interference with microtubule formation may inhibit collagen production, thereby retarding the development of hepatic fibrosis. Colchicine may also increase degradation of collagen by stimulating production of collagenase. In addition, colchicine corrects some of the abnormalities of lymphocyte and monocyte function that have been identified in patients with active biliary cirrhosis.

Kinetics

Colchicine is absorbed rapidly after oral administration, although the rate and extent of absorption are variable. Colchicine is distributed rapidly to peripheral leukocytes and concentrations in these cells may exceed those in plasma. Colchicine also concentrates in the kidneys, liver, and spleen. It is metabolized in the liver and eliminated in bile, with enterohepatic recirculation and 10–20% through the kidney. Renal elimination may be increased in patients with hepatic disease. Owing to the high degree of tissue uptake, only 10% of a single dose is eliminated within 24 h; elimination of colchicine from the body may continue for 10 days or more after cessation of administration. Elimination is slower in patients with biliary disease.

Indications

Colchicine has primarily been used in the treatment of gout and familial Mediterranean fever because of its anti-inflammatory properties. Its role in PBC has already been discussed.

Adverse reactions

Colchicine has been reported to cause hypersensitivity reactions including skin rashes and angiodema; however, a skin rash that is not associated with hypersensitivity may occur, especially with long-term treatment in patients with renal or hepatic function impairment. With prolonged or long-term use, colchicine can cause bone marrow depression with agranulocytosis, aplastic anaemia and thrombocytopenia. In addition, myopathy and neuropathy can occur. Myopathy is more likely to occur in patients with impaired renal or hepatic function who are receiving long-term treatment with prophylactic doses of colchicine. This condition is characterized by proximal muscle weakness, spontaneous activity in the electromyelogram, and elevated creatinine kinase values.

Drug interactions

Concurrent alcohol use with orally administered colchicine increases the risk of gastrointestinal toxicity, especially when alcohol is taken in excess. Non-steroidal anti-inflammatory drugs (NSAIDs) may increase the risk of leukopenia, thrombocytopenia, or bone marrow depression and cause gastrointestinal bleeding. Absorption of vitamin B_{12} may be impaired by chronic administration or high doses of colchicine.

Contraindications

Colchicine should be avoided if there is concurrent severe hepatic and renal disease. Avoid or reduce dose by 50% in severe renal impairment. Colchicine is contraindicated in pregnancy and breastfeeding.

Methotrexate

See Chapter 5, p. 99.

AUTOIMMUNE HEPATITIS

Introduction

Autoimmune hepatitis can be defined as a self-perpetuating hepatic inflammation characterized by interface hepatitis on histological examination, hypergammaglobulinaemia and liver-associated autoantibodies in the serum.[62] The cause is unknown. The diagnosis requires exclusion of other causes of chronic liver disease that can give similar features, such as chronic viral infection, Wilson's disease, alpha$_1$ antitrypsin deficiency, haemochromatosis, non-alcoholic steatosis, and the immune cholangiopathies of primary biliary cirrhosis, primary sclerosing cholangitis and autoimmune cholangitis. Recently, criteria for diagnosis have been coded and a quantitative scoring system exists to predict definite or probable diagnosis (Table 12.1).[63]

The prevalence of autoimmune hepatitis ranges from 50–200/million in North European and North American populations and is seen more commonly in women with a male to female ratio of 1:4. It can present either acutely, which may result in fulminant hepatic failure, or insidiously. It can present at any age but is seen more commonly between the ages of 10 and 30 years, with a second peak in late middle age. Common presenting symptoms are of anorexia, fatigue, amenorrhoea, abdominal pain and fever. Hepatic inflammation leads to fibrosis, cirrhosis and liver failure. Between 30 and 80% of patients have cirrhosis at presentation of which 10–20% have evidence of decompensation. The most common physical signs are hepatomegaly (78%) and jaundice (69%). Splenomegaly may occur in patients with or without cirrhosis, as may spider naevi. Polyclonal hypergammaglobulinaemia is required for diagnosis, of which IgG predominates. Autoantibodies are present and include smooth muscle antibody (SMA), antinuclear antibody (ANA) and anti-liver, kidney, microsomal antibody (anti-LKM1). Other autoantibodies are possible. There is frequently (41%) concurrent immunological disease that involve other organs such as the thyroid.

Autoimmune hepatitis can be subclassified into Types 1 and 2.[64] Type 1 is characterized by the presence of SMA and ANA in the serum and is the most commonly seen form. Type 2 is characterized by anti-LKM and is mainly seen in children (age range 2–14 years). Type 2 is more likely to progress to cirrhosis and probably carries a worse prognosis.

Severity of the inflammation, judged both biochemically and histologically, can predict prognosis. In addition, HLA type predicts outcome. Serum aspartate aminotransferase (AST) and gammaglobulin levels are the most useful biochemical test; serum AST level of over 10 times normal predicts a 10-year mortality of 90%. HLA B8 and DR3 identify younger patients with more severe inflammation and less response to corticosteroid therapy and greater frequency of liver transplantation. HLA DR4 patients tend to be older, female and respond better to treatment than patients with DR3.[65]

Pathophysiology

A loss of tolerance against the patient's own liver is regarded as the pathogenic mechanism.[66] Two hypotheses have been proposed:

1. Autoantigen-driven cell-mediated cytotoxicity and
2. Antibody-dependant cell-mediated cytotoxicity.

The first hypothesis requires the aberrant display of HLA class II antigens on hepatocyte surface because of viral, drug, toxic, environmental or idiopathic factors (although none of these factors have been elucidated). There is enhanced presentation of normal liver cell constituents as autoantigens. Activation of antigen processing cells stimulates clonal expansion of autoantigen-sensitized cytotoxic T lymphocytes, which results in liver destruction and release of harmful cytokines. Only one autoantigen has, however, been incriminated

Table 12.1 Scoring system for the diagnosis of autoimmune hepatitis.

Parameter	Score
Gender	
· Female	+2
· Male	0
Serum biochemistry	
· Ratio of elevation of serum alkaline phosphatase versus aminotransferase	
>3.0	−2
<3.0	+2
· Total serum globulin, γ-globulin or IgG (times upper limit of normal)	
>2.0	+3
1.5–2.0	+2
1.0–1.5	+1
<1.0	0
· Autoantibodies (titres by immunofluorescence on rodent tissues)	
—*Adults*: ANA, SMA, or LKM-1	
>1:80	+3
1:80	+2
1:40	+1
<1:40	0
—*Children:* ANA or LKM-1	
>1:20	+3
1:10 or 1:20	+2
<1:20	0
· SMA	
>1:20	+3
1:20	+2
<1:20	0
· Antimitochondrial antibody	
Positive	−2
Negative	0
· Viral markers	
IgM, anti-HAV, HbsAg origM anti-HBC-positive	−3
Anti HCV-positive by ELISA or RIBA	−2
HCV-positive by PCR for HCV RNA	−3
Positive test indicating active infection by any other virus	−3
Seronegative for all the above	+3
Other aetiological factors	
· History of recent hepatotoxic drug usage or parenteral exposure to blood products	
Yes	−2
No	+1
· Alcohol (average consumption)	
Male <35 g/day; female <25 g/day	+2
Male 35–50 g/day; female 25–40 g/day	0
Male 50–80 g/day; female 40–60 g/day	−1
Male >80 g/day; female >60 g/day	−2
· Genetic factors: HLA DR3 or DR4	
Other autoimmune disease in patient or first-degree relatives	+1

Interpretation: Definite AIH: >15 before treatment and >17 after treatment: probable AIH: 10 to 15 before treatment and 12 to 17 after treatment.

(P_{450} IID6), which relates to one rare form of the disease (Type 2 autoimmune hepatitis).[67]

The second hypothesis proposes an intrinsic defect in suppressor T-lymphocyte function, which facilitates unmodulated B-cell production of IgG against normal hepatocyte membrane proteins. Antigen–antibody complexes form, which are then targeted by natural killer cells. However none of the autoantibodies that are detected in autoimmune hepatitis are pathogenic.

Therapeutic approaches

The treatment of choice is immunosuppression.[68] Treatment is indicated for the hepatic inflammation rather than the synthetic liver function, in other words prolonged prothrombin and low albumin is not an indication for treatment in the absence of severe inflammation, nor is cirrhosis a contraindication to treatment if severe inflammation is ongoing. Ascites and hepatic encephalopathy at presentation indicate a poor prognosis but are not a contraindication to therapy.

Standard treatment is either prednisolone or a combination of prednisolone and azathioprine. The combination treatment is the preferred choice since there is a lower risk of corticosteroid side effects. Once in remission, drug withdrawal can be attempted, usually not before 2 years of therapy, although relapse is common. Alternatively, maintenance treatment with low-dose prednisolone or azathioprine alone, or in combination, can be continued indefinitely.

Other immunosuppressive drugs have been used but further studies are required to judge their efficacy and safety in the treatment of autoimmune hepatitis. These include cyclosporin,[69] tacrolimus,[70] 6-mercaptopurine and budesonide.[71]

Treatment regimens

The two standard treatment regimens are shown in Table 12.2.

Combination therapy is the usual treatment of choice. Single therapy is considered in pregnancy and in patients with azathioprine intolerance or cytopenia.

The average treatment interval until remission is 22 months. Remission is defined as 'no symptoms and an AST <2-fold normal and inactivity on biopsy'. This is accomplished in 65% of patients. At this stage, patients can be withdrawn slowly from treatment; however, at least 50% will relapse within 6 months and 70–86% within 3 years. Reinstitution of therapy induces another remission but the consequences of relapse and retreatment is the development of drug-related complications owing to the high steroid dose, as well as disease

Table 12.2 Standard treatment regimens for autoimmune hepatitis.

Combination regimen		Single regimen
Prednisolone	**Azathioprine**	**Prednisolone**
30 mg once daily for 1 week	50 mg once daily until remission	60 mg once daily for 1 week
20 mg once daily for 1 week		40 mg once daily for 1 week
15 mg once daily for 2 weeks		30 mg once daily for 2 weeks
10 mg until remission		20 mg once daily until remission

progression. Patients who have relapsed more than twice require indefinite therapy. Long-term therapy is often considered for patients obtaining remission to avoid the known high relapse rate.

Of those treated, 13% of patients will have an incomplete response to therapy—they improve with therapy but not enough to satisfy complete remission as already defined. It is recommended that they remain on low-dose prednisolone indefinitely in the same way as patients who relapse after stopping therapy.

Despite compliance with conventional therapy 9% of patients deteriorate. High-dose prednisolone 60 mg or 30 mg in combination with azathioprine, induces clinical and biochemical improvement in 70% within 2 years; however, the histology resolves in only 20% and long-term therapy is usually necessary. Liver transplantation is recommended at the first sign of decompensation.

Thirteen per cent of patients will not tolerate standard therapy. Typical adverse effects include obesity, osteoporosis, psychosis with corticosteroids and cytopenia and nausea with azathioprine. Dose reductions with indefinite low-dose regimens are required or alternative investigational treatment.

If long-term therapy is advocated, treatment is aimed at reducing medication to the lowest possible dose without causing relapse. Two alternative regimens have been used widely. The first is prednisolone alone. Azathioprine, if used initially, is stopped and the prednisolone dose is reduced by 2.5 mg/month until the lowest possible dose is reached to prevent symptoms and to maintain serum AST below 5-fold normal. Alternatively azathioprine can be increased to 2/mg/kg and then prednisolone is discontinued in a tapering fashion. Azathioprine is continued indefinitely. This second approach has been shown to result in fewer relapses and lower hepatic mortality (1% versus 9%) than using prednisolone monotherapy.[72]

Pharmacology

Prednisolone
See Chapter 5 p. 91.

Azathioprine
See Chapter 5 p. 96.

WILSON'S DISEASE

Introduction

Wilson's disease, or hepatolenticular degeneration, is a rare autosomal disorder of copper accumulation.[73] The Wilson's gene is located on chromosome 13 and encodes a copper-transporting P-type ATPase protein.[74,75] Deficiency of the gene product is likely to be responsible for the lack of copper incorporation into caeruloplasmin and the defective biliary excretion of copper seen in Wilson's disease. This results in excess copper accumulation in the liver, brain and other organs including the kidney and cornea, resulting in Kayser-Fleischer rings (a golden-brown or greenish discoloration in the limbic area seen best during slit-lamp examination). The copper accumulation eventually leads to tissue damage.

The majority of symptomatic patients present with hepatic or neuropsychiatric features. The hepatic manifestations range from acute fulminant hepatic failure, chronic hepatitis and cirrhosis. Clinical symptoms are rarely observed before the age of 5 years and usually present in the second and third decades. Clinical hepatic features tend to occur at a younger age (mean 8–12 years) than neurological manifestations.

Ninety per cent of all patients with Wilson's disease and 65–85% of patients presenting with the hepatic manifestations, will have a low serum concentration of ceruloplasmin (normal range 20–35 mg/dl). The diagnosis of Wilson's disease can be made if the patient has a low ceruloplasmin concentration and Kayser-Fleischer rings. Otherwise hepatic copper concentration greater than 250 μg/g dry liver usually confirms the diagnosis.

In fulminant hepatic failure from Wilson's disease, patients tend to be young and the clinical picture may be indistinguishable from that of virally-induced massive hepatic necrosis. Characteristic clinical features include intravascular haemolysis, splenomegaly, Kayser-Fleischer rings and a fulminant course: patients rarely survive longer than days to weeks unless liver transplantation is performed. Serum aminotransferases are mildly to moderately elevated, with marked elevation of the serum bilirubin, a low serum alkaline phosphatase level and evidence of haemolytic anaemia. Serum caeruloplasmin may be in the normal range; however, 24 h urinary copper (normal range ≤30 μg/day) and free plasma copper levels are usually elevated (normal range 50–100 μg/l).

Pathophysiology

Copper toxicity plays a primary role in the pathogenesis of this disorder.[76] Affected organs invariably exhibit elevated copper levels, and reduction in the copper content results in improvement. Maintenance of normal copper homeostasis depends on the balance between gastrointestinal absorption and biliary excretion. Intestinal copper absorption is not different from normal individuals in Wilson's disease; however, biliary excretion is reduced. Studies in a rat model (Long-Evans Cinnamon rat) indicate a possible defect in the entry of copper into lysosomes but with normal delivery into bile. It is thought that the Wilson gene product may be essential for the routing of copper into the trans-Golgi apparatus and thus be essential for copper excretion by the lysosomal pathway.[77] The low ceruloplasmin level seen in Wilson's disease is unlikely to have a pathological role and it is now believed that the low level is simply the result of a lack of incorporation of copper into apocaeruloplasmin, which has a shorter half-life than the copper-bound caeruloplasmin. Excess copper appears to exert toxic effects by the generation of free radicals.

Therapeutic approach

Effective treatment of Wilson's disease depends upon establishing a negative copper balance thereby preventing deposition of more copper and mobilizing for excretion excess copper already deposited. This is achieved with copper-reducing drugs. Once negative copper balance is achieved, maintenance treatment must be continued life-long and effectiveness and compliance must be monitored regularly. Interruption of treatment can have serious consequences, including fatal liver failure.

Dietary restriction is now also considered to be important, with restriction of copper rich foods such as shellfish and liver.

Symptomatic recovery is often slow but if the treatment is started early enough is usually complete and life-expectancy will be normal. However, if the disease is detected late such that cirrhosis has already occurred, symptom relief is often only partial but treatment is essential to prevent further deterioration. Patients with end-stage liver disease often do not benefit from copper reducing therapy and liver transplantation is necessary. Liver transplantation is required for patients presenting with fulminant hepatitis.[78] The drugs used in the treatment of Wilson's disease are penicillamine, trientine and zinc.[79]

Treatment regimens

Penicillamine is a chelating agent, which aids the elimination from the body of certain heavy metal ions including copper by forming stable, soluble complexes that are readily excreted by the kidney. It is generally regarded as the agent of choice for the initial management of Wilson's disease as it brings about rapid reduction in copper levels. The usual dosage of penicillamine is 0.75–2 g daily in four divided doses. The optimal dose to reach a negative copper balance should be determined initially by regular analysis of 24-h urinary copper excretion. The initial goal of treatment is urinary copper excretion of 2000 μg/day. Values usually fall to below 500 µg/day after 4–6 months of treatment. A maintenance dose of 0.75–1 g daily may be adequate once remission is achieved and must be continued indefinitely. In children, a suggested dose is up to 20 mg/kg in divided doses. Small doses of pyridoxine (25 mg daily) should be given daily with penicillamine owing to the weak antipyridoxine effect of D-penicillamine.

In patients with neurological symptoms, penicillamine can worsen the symptoms and some experts advocate zinc as first-line therapy. This worsening of neurological signs is thought to be caused by transient increased copper concentrations in blood and brain after initiating therapy. Zinc, however, has a slow onset of action and is not suitable when rapid reduction of copper is required. Trientine is an alternative to penicillamine and is used in patients who are intolerant of penicillamine.

Once a negative copper balance has been achieved, treatment must be continued for life. Penicillamine, trientine or zinc can be used for maintenance therapy.

Pharmacology

Penicillamine

Mode of action

D-Penicillamine is a characteristic degradation product of penicillin, being the D-isomer of 3-mercaptovaline. It is the stable thiol group that gives penicillamine its biological activity, making it an effective chelating agent for heavy metals, such as copper. Two molecules of copper bind to one molecule of penicillamine. Penicillamine also reduces the affinity of copper for proteins and polypeptides, thus allowing removal of copper from tissues. It also induces synthesis of metallothionein in the liver, a protein that combines with copper to form a non-toxic product.

In addition to its chelating properties, penicillamine can also reactivate enzymes blocked by copper; copper blocks the sulphydryl groups of certain enzymes, which are reactivated by the free sulphydryl group of penicillamine.

Kinetics

Penicillamine is rapidly absorbed from the gut following oral administration. It is metabolized in the liver and up to 80% is excreted in the urine mainly as penicillamine disulphide or as a mixed disulphide; 80% is bound to plasma proteins. The initial half-life in blood is 20 min but this phase lasts for less than 1 h. It is also bound by tissues, especially by the skin, which delays final clearance by several weeks.

Indications

Penicillamine is used as a chelating agent in Wilson's disease and lead poisoning. It is also used in severe rheumatoid arthritis and in the treatment of cystinuria.

Adverse events

Side-effects are frequent but many are reversible when the drug is withdrawn. Up to 20% of patients will develop side-effects in the first month of treatment. Gastrointestinal disturbances, include anorexia, nausea and vomiting. Stomatitis, taste impairment and oral ulceration have been reported.

Allergic skin rash can occur early in treatment but is usually transient and responds to temporary withdrawal of the drug. Some patients may experience drug fever, associated with malaise, rash and lymphadenopathy usually in the second or third week after initiation. Most patients can be desensitized of these symptoms by gradual reintroduction of the drug. Lupus erythematosus and pemphigus have also been reported. A Stevens-Johnson-like syndrome has been reported.

Prolonged use of the drug at high dosage may effect skin collagen and elastin, resulting in skin friability and eruptions resembling perforans serpiginosis and acquired epidermolysis bullosa.

Haematological side-effects include thrombocytopenia and, to a lesser extent, leucopenia, which are usually reversible. Agranulocytosis, aplastic anaemia and haemolytic anaemia have occurred and fatalities have been reported.

Proteinuria occurs frequently and, in some patients, may progress to glomerulonephritis or nephrotic syndrome. Penicillamine-induced haematuria is rare and usually requires discontinuation of the drug.

Rare side-effects include Goodpasture's syndrome, myasthenia gravis, polymyositis, intrahepatic cholestasis and pancreatitis.

Patients should be told to report promptly fever, sore throat, chills, bruising or bleeding. Patients should also be monitored carefully for side-effects. One recommendation is to perform weekly full blood counts and urinalysis for the first 2 months of treatment and after any change in dosage, and then monthly thereafter. Treatment should be withdrawn if there is a decrease in white cell count or platelet count or if progressive proteinuria or haematuria occur.

Drug interactions

Plasma concentrations are reduced by antacids and iron. Penicillamine should not be given with other drugs capable of causing serious haematological or renal adverse effects; for example, gold salts or immunosuppressive drugs.

Contraindications

Penicillamine is contraindicated in patients with lupus erythematosus or a history of penicillamine-induced agranulocytosis, aplastic anaemia or severe thrombocytopenia. It should be used with care in patients with renal insufficiency.

Patients who are allergic to penicillin may react similarly, although this is rare.

Fetal abnormalities have been reported rarely in pregnant patients taking high doses of penicillamine; however, the dose of penicillamine used in the maintenance treatment of Wilson's disease appears to be well-tolerated by mother and infant during pregnancy, and continued treatment is recommended. Interruption of therapy may be associated with haemolytic anaemia and liver failure. No ill effects have been reported in breastfed infants of treated patients, although there may be reduced breast milk concentrations of zinc and copper.

Trientine

Mode of action

Trientine was introduced in 1969 as an alternative chelating agent to D-penicillamine. It competes for copper that is bound to albumin, resulting in copper chelation and detoxification.

Indications

Trientine is less potent than penicillamine and should only be used as a second-line agent in patients intolerant of penicillamine. Most of the side-effects of penicillamine, with the exception of elastosis perforans serpiginosa subside when patients are converted to trientine.

Kinetics

Trientine is administered orally and is well-absorbed, metabolized in the liver and excreted by the kidneys. The usual initial dose is 750–1250 mg daily in two to four divided doses increasing to a maximum of 2 g daily if required. In children, the initial dose is 500–750 mg daily, increasing to a maximum of 1.5 g daily if required.

Adverse events

Trientine may cause iron deficiency. Recurrence of systemic lupus erythromatosis (SLE) has been reported in a patient who had been treated previously with penicillamine. Other reported side-effects include gastrointestinal disturbance and rhabdomyolysis.

Drug interactions

If iron supplements are given, an interval of 2 h between administration of iron and trientine has been recommended.

Contraindications

Rheumatoid arthritis, biliary cirrhosis, and cystinuria are contraindications. No adverse effects on the fetus have been documented in pregnant patients with Wilson's disease who are taking trientine.

Zinc

Mode of action

The rationale of using zinc is its ability to induce intestinal and hepatic metallothionein synthesis. Zinc decreases copper absorption by increasing the formation of copper-metallothionein in intestinal epithelial cells: copper is not absorbed in this form but is excreted when the intestinal epithelial cells are shed. In the hepatocyte, the increase in metallothionein synthesis appears to be protective, since copper-metallothionein complex is non toxic.

Kinetics

Zinc is poorly absorbed from the gastrointestinal tract. Zinc is widely distributed throughout the body and is excreted in the faeces, with only traces occurring in the urine. The kidneys have little or no role in regulating zinc. The usual dose is 150 mg daily in two to three divided doses in between meals.

Adverse reactions

Zinc may cause gastrointestinal upset and headaches. Zinc poisoning has not been identified in man but may cause anaemia (and copper deficiency).

Indications

The experience with zinc in Wilson's disease is limited. It tends to be reserved for presymptomatic patients or for maintenance treatment once negative copper balance has been achieved in patients who have troublesome symptoms with penicillamine.

Drug interactions

Concurrent administration with penicillamine may reduce penicillamine levels.

HAEMOCHROMATOSIS

Introduction

Hereditary haemochromatosis is the most common genetic disease in people of North European descent, with a prevalence of 1/300.[80]

The disease is caused by excess iron deposition in multiple organs, with the liver affected predominantly. The disease is inherited in an autosomal recessive manner. The gene (named the HFE gene) was identified in 1996[81] and is found on the short arm of chromosome 6. Two mutations within the gene have been shown to be associated with the disease, with the commonest mutation being the substitution cys282tyr. Of patients with haemochromatosis, 85% are homozygote for this mutation.

The presentation of the disease has changed over the last 30 years. Previously patients would present with the classic 'bronze diabetes', arthritis, liver disease and cardiac failure. Now many patients are asymptomatic and have been detected because of investigation of abnormal serum liver biochemistry. Common symptoms include fatigue, joint symptoms, right upper quadrant pain and impotence in men. Other symptoms include symptoms of diabetes, cardiac failure and increased skin pigmentation.

The diagnosis should be suspected in patients with unexplained elevation of ferritin and iron saturation. Diagnosis is confirmed by determination of hepatic iron concentration on liver biopsy[82] and by genetic testing. Liver histology not only assesses the deposition of iron but also judges the severity of liver disease.

The liver disease seen in haemochromatosis tends to progress slowly. Fibrosis or cirrhosis tends not to occur before the age of 40 years in men and 50 years in women. Of patients in early reports, 25% died of complications of liver disease.[83] The risk of hepatocellular carcinoma in cirrhotic patients is increased by 200.[84]

Pathophysiology

Iron absorption is inappropriately high in patients with haemochromatosis. The transferrin receptor in the intestinal mucosa is upregulated and iron is transported into plasma at an increased rate. Increased transport of iron from the serosal side of the intestinal cell drives the increased absorption.

The excess iron is deposited in multiple organs including the heart, liver, pancreas, joints, skin, pituitary gland and other endocrine organs. The major site of iron deposition is the liver. Excess iron mediates liver damage and promote fibrogenesis via several possible mechanisms, such as formation of free radicals, direct damage of DNA and increasing collagen synthesis. Liver histology shows progressive fibrosis and iron deposition with little inflammation. Eventually cirrhosis and hepatocellular carcinoma may develop.

Treatment approach

Iron reduction by venesection is the cornerstone of treatment. Chelation therapy with desferrioxamine is less effective and may have adverse side-effects. Patients without cirrhosis at the start of treatment have a normal life expectancy. Patients with cirrhosis, although they have a reduced life-expectancy, still improve with venesection with improvement of liver function, even in patients with decompensation. Liver transplantation may be required for end-stage liver disease.

Treatment regimens

Removal of one unit of blood should be performed weekly until the serum ferritin is under 50 ng/ml. This usually results in a moderate fall in haemoglobin to a plateau of 11 g, which then remains stable until the patient becomes iron-deficient. The serum ferritin should be checked 3-monthly. Patients often require 1–2 years of weekly venesection to deplete their iron stores. Once iron stores have been mobilized, venesection four times a year should be adequate.

ALPHA₁ ANTITRYPSIN DEFICIENCY

Introduction

Alpha₁ antitrypsin (α_1AT) is an enzyme encoded by a gene on the long arm of chromosome 14 that protects tissues from proteases.[85] The phenotype is transmitted by autosomal co-dominance. There are about 75 different α_1AT alleles.[86] The phenotype protease inhibitor (Pi) MM is present in 95% of the population and is associated with normal serum levels of α_1AT. A single nucleotide substitution (glu→lys) leads to Zα_1AT protein. PiZZ is prevalent in 1/2000 of the population and is accompanied by severe deficiency of α_1AT. PiMZ leads to intermediate deficiency. Deficiency of α_1AT in the serum leads to emphysema, while, in contrast, the liver disease relates to the presence of the abnormal Z protein in the liver as opposed to the serum level of α_1AT. Liver disease is seen in both patients with PiZZ and PiMZ.

Children with α_1AT deficiency are often identified in the newborn period because of persistent jaundice. Of these children, 10% will develop moderate to severe liver disease during the first few years of life, although a large proportion will improve with time. The incidence of liver disease of individuals with α_1AT deficiency is 2% by age 20–40 years, 5% by age 40–50 years and 15% thereafter.

Patients may present with chronic hepatitis, cirrhosis, portal hypertension or hepatocellular carcinoma. Diagnosis is established by a serum α_1AT phenotype determination (Pi typing). α_1AT levels may be misleading since levels may be normal in patients with PiMZ and may even be normal in patients with PiZZ owing to increased levels due to inflammation. Histologically, eosinophilic periodic acid-Schiff-positive, diastase-resistant globules are seen in the endoplasmic reticulum of periportal hepatocytes.

Pathophysiology

The pathogenesis of α_1AT deficiency remains unclear but the most widely accepted theory is that the liver disease is a result of accumulation of the mutant $\alpha_1 AT$ molecule in the endoplasmic reticulum of liver cells, rather than caused by proteolytic attack, which is probably the cause of the lung disease.[87]

Treatment approaches

The most important treatment is to avoid cigarette smoking, which markedly accelerates the lung disease. Infusions of $\alpha_1 AT$ derived from pooled plasma or by recombinant DNA methods are being investigated for the treatment of the lung disease but are ineffective for the treatment of liver disease.

Liver transplantation is the treatment for advancing liver disease and should be performed before serious lung disease develops. Transplantation corrects the genetic defect and long-term survival after transplantation is excellent.

LIVER STORAGE DISEASES

Gaucher's disease

Introduction
Gaucher's disease is a lysosomal storage disease, inherited in an autosomal recessive manner.[88] The disease is most common in Askenazi Jews, with an incidence of 1/1000. Gaucher's disease presents usually with painless hepatosplenomegaly and elevated aminotransferase levels or with osteoporotic skeletal fractures. The outcome of Gaucher's disease is very variable with the severity of the liver disease matching the severity of extrahepatic disease. Liver failure is rare. The definitive diagnostic test is glucocerebrosidase activity in blood leucocytes or urine.

Pathophysiology
Gaucher's is caused by a disorder of the haematopoetic stem cell resulting in deficiency of the enzyme glucocerebrosidase. This leads to the accumulation of the enzyme substrate (glucosylceramide) in the reticuloendothelial cells throughout the body.

Treatment approaches
Treatment of Gaucher's disease is with enzyme replacement with alglucerase,[89] which has been shown to decrease the size of the liver and spleen over relatively short time intervals. The disease can be cured by bone marrow transplantation.

Liver transplantation may be performed for end-stage liver disease. This also improves the extrahepatic manifestations of Gaucher's disease, probably as a result of liver cell migration (microchimerism).[90]

Treatment regimens
The standard initial dose of alglucerase is 60 units/kg body weight infused intravenously over 1–2 every 2 weeks. The dose and frequency of infusions are then adjusted according to response.

Pharmacology
Alglucerase
Alglucerase is a modified form of human placental β-glucocerebrosidase. A recombinant version has now been developed (imiglucerase) and slow-release forms such as PEG-glucocerebrosidase are being developed.

Glycogen storage diseases

Glycogen storage diseases are characterized by an abnormal accumulation of glycogen in tissues including liver, heart, skeletal muscle, kidney and brain. There are several different types of glycogen storage disease described, most of which are inherited in an autosomal recessive fashion. Patients present in childhood with failure to thrive or with organ failure, including liver failure.

The main treatment is liver transplantation.

ALCOHOLIC LIVER DISEASE

Introduction

Alcohol is the most common cause of cirrhosis in the Western world. Over 50% of deaths from cirrhosis in the UK are a result of alcohol. The amount of alcohol ingested and the duration of intake correlate with the incidence of alcohol-related liver disease.[91] The risk of developing liver disease, however, varies from individual to individual for the same quantity of alcohol ingested: less than 20% of men consuming more than 12 units per day for 10 years will become cirrhotic. Separate factors, other than the quantity of alcohol, influence the development of alcoholic liver disease.[92] Women are at greater risk of liver disease from alcohol intake, which cannot be explained solely by differences in body composition or alcohol distribution. One possible theory is that gastric mucosal alcohol dehydrogenase is lower in women, resulting in higher quantities of absorbed alcohol. Genetic variability is thought to be important, although the genes responsible remain to be elucidated. Other predisposing factors include poor nutrition, co-infection with hepatropic viruses and co-exposure to drugs or toxins.

The clinical features of alcoholic liver disease vary from no symptoms to those of florid features of advanced liver cell failure and portal hypertension. Patients may complain of fatigue, anorexia, fever, confusion, vomiting, abdominal pain and weight loss. Physical signs include spider naevi, Dupuytren's contracture, gynaecomastia, testicular atrophy, parotid enlargement, hepatomegaly, splenomegaly, ascites and jaundice. None of these are specific or pathognomonic of alcoholic liver disease.

Elevated serum gamma glutamyltransferase (γGT), aspartate aminotransferase (AST), alanine aminotransferase (ALT), with an AST greater than ALT elevation are common with alcoholic liver disease. Macrocytosis, which occurs in other types of liver disease, is enhanced by the toxic effect of alcohol on the bone marrow. Leucocytosis in the absence of infection may occur as a result of the liver inflammation and thrombocytopenia can arise from the toxic effect of alcohol. Elevated bilirubin, prolonged prothrombin time and low albumin indicates more severe disease. Liver histology ranges from fatty liver (steatosis) to alcoholic hepatitis to cirrhosis. Often the features of all three are seen at once. Steatosis is considered fully reversible and alcoholic hepatitis at least partially reversible. Alcoholic hepatitis has been shown to be an important precursor to fibrosis and cirrhosis, although more recent studies have shown that alcohol can stimulate fibrosis without alcoholic hepatitis.

Pathophysiology

Nutritional, metabolic and immunological factors are thought to be important in the pathogenesis of alcoholic liver disease, although the relative importance of these factors remain unknown and thus to what degree these factors should be targeted with treatment is uncertain.[93,94] In the past, malnutrition was thought to play a key role in causing the disease; however it is now recognized that disease can occur despite good nutrition, and obesity may even be a predisposing factor. These findings suggest that the toxic effects of alcohol or the metabolic state induced by alcohol is responsible for the liver injury.

In the liver, alcohol is metabolized to acetaldehyde, which plays a pivotal role in liver injury. Acetaldehyde causes cellular necrosis, stimulates fibrosis and can alter protein structure and thereby protein function. This can result in intracellular disarray, with microfilaments being sheared allowing fat to be deposited. The fat is a result of alcohol oxidation, which results in the intracellular-redox potential and redox-sensitive nutrient metabolism being disturbed. An excessive accumulation of reducing equivalents favours metabolic pathways that lead to the accumulation of intracellular lipid. When alcohol is withdrawn, however, these processes are reversible.

In addition, the disruption of protein by

acetaldehyde causes the formation of neoantigens, which initiate immune reactions. Acetaldehyde has also been shown to stimulate Kupfer cells to produce proinflammatory cytokines, such as tumour necrosis factor-α (TNF$_\alpha$) and interleukin-8 (IL-8). The severity of alcoholic hepatitis has been shown to correlate with these cytokines. TNF$_\alpha$ causes direct damage to hepatocytes and IL-8 causes neutrophil infiltration that produces reactive oxygen species and hepatocyte damage. Oxygen radical scavengers that defend against this oxidative stress, such as vitamin E, selenium, glutathione and zinc, are reduced during long-term alcohol ingestion.

Therapeutic approach

Stopping alcohol consumption is the cornerstone of treatment. Resumption of a nutritious diet and supporting the patient while the liver recovers from the effects of alcohol are essential, in particular recognizing and treating infection. Hospitalization benefits those patients with significant extrahepatic complications of alcoholism, notably electrolyte abnormalities, cardiac dysfunction, pancreatitis, and major alcohol withdrawal symptoms. Patients with evidence of hepatocellular failure require hospitalization and mortality is high despite full support.

Diet is an important part of treatment. Alcohol reduces appetite, interferes with intestinal absorption and storage of nutrients, which results in protein, mineral and vitamin deficiencies. Thiamine should be given to prevent Wernicke's encephalopathy, along with multivitamins.[95] Nutritional support is best administered orally and if oral intake is poor a fine-bore nasogastric feeding tube should be considered. Although dietary protein may contribute to encephalopathy, protein content should rarely be restricted. Trials of supplemental amino acid therapy have been conflicting. Although nutritional therapy has been shown to improve malnutrition and liver function, the effect on mortality has seldom been shown to be statistically significant.

Specific therapies for both acutely decompensated and chronic alcoholic disease remain controversial. Despite abstinence of alcohol and nutritional support, some patients with alcoholic hepatitis have ongoing liver damage as a result of intense immune-related inflammation. Suppression of this immune response would thus be a logical therapeutic target.

Corticosteroids have been the subject of multiple studies and several meta-analyses.[93] Two recent prospective randomized, placebo-controlled trials[96,97] and one meta-analysis[98] have demonstrated that steroids benefit patients with severe alcoholic hepatitis, if patients with gastrointestinal haemorrhage and infection are excluded. The Maddrey discriminant function (DF = 4.6 × [patient's prothrombin time(s) − control prothrombin time(s)] + serum bilirubin (mg/dl)) that was determined to assess the outcome of alcoholic liver disease, has been used to predict which patients benefit from steroids. Patients with a DF greater than 32 have a 50% chance of dying during their current hospitalization and it is these patients who benefit from corticosteroids. The patients in these trials represent a selected group as co-morbid disease was excluded, such as diabetes and pancreatitis. Corticosteroids have been shown to reduce short-term mortality but the effect on long-term mortality remains unclear.

Propylthiouracil has been proposed as a treatment of alcoholic hepatitis, despite reports of hepatotoxicity, including some fatalities, in an attempt to slow the hypermetabolic state and relative hypoxia that occurs in the central vein areas of the liver. Following an early study that indicated that propylthiouracil hastened clinical improvement in patients with alcoholic liver disease, Orrego et al. conducted a double-blind placebo-controlled study to determine the effect of long-term treatment on survival.[99] In contrast to Halle et al.[100] who failed to find any beneficial effect, Orrego et al. found that, during their 2-year study, the 13% mortality rate in patients receiving propylthiouracil 300 mg daily was significantly lower than the 25%

mortality rate in patients receiving placebo. The main effect of propylthiouracil appeared to be on acute alcoholic hepatitis since the difference in mortality rate was greatest during the first 12 weeks. Although subgroup analysis indicated that the effect was greater in severely ill patients, the validity of this result is considered to be uncertain as the patients had not been randomized according to the severity of their disease on entry to the study. Lashner and Baker criticized the results of Orrego *et al.* on the basis that their statistical analysis was inappropriate to the objective of the study and they suggested there was no convincing evidence for a beneficial effect of propylthiouracil in alcoholic liver disease.[101] Sherlock has commented that propylthiouracil has not gained general acceptance for the treatment of alcoholic liver disease.[102]

Other treatments that have been studied have been anabolic steroids and drugs aimed at preventing fibrosis, such as penicillamine and colchicine[103] but they have not been shown to improve survival.

Treatment regimens

Abstinence and critical supportive care is the mainstay of treatment.

Thiamine hydrochloride 100 mg should be given as soon as possible to prevent development of Wernicke's encephalopathy. It should be given before dextrose administration, which may deplete inadequate stores of thiamine. Thiamine should be given parenterally initially, since oral thiamine may not be absorbed dependably or quickly enough to prevent Wernicke-Korsakoff syndrome. Thiamine is often given along with an infusion of other multivitamins.

Alcohol withdrawal is usually treated with either chlordiazepoxide or chlormethiazole. Chlordiazepoxide is given orally in a dose of 20–100 mg, repeated as needed up to a dose of 300 mg/day. The dose is then tapered after the first 48 h until the drug is discontinued after 5–7 days. Chlormethiazole is administered in a similar fashion starting with a dose of up to 9–12 tablets/day. Both should be reduced or stopped if excess drowsiness or signs of encephalopathy occur.

In severe alcoholic hepatitis, patients with a Maddrey discriminant score of greater than 32 benefit from corticosteroids. Patients with gastrointestinal bleeding, severe co-morbid disease, such as diabetes, and those with infection, should be excluded. A typical corticosteroid regimen is prednisolone 40 mg daily for 4 weeks and then tapered over several days to weeks.

Pharmacology

Thiamine (vitamin B_1)

Mode of action

Thiamine is a water-soluble vitamin that plays a vital role as a co-enzyme in carbohydrate metabolism. Deficiency can lead to severe neuromuscular syndromes such as beri-beri and Wernicke's encephalopathy and Korsakoff syndrome. Wernicke's encephalopathy and Korsakoff syndrome are a manifestation of thiamine deficiency seen most commonly in alcoholic patients. Wernicke's symptoms consist of ataxia, ophthalmoplegia and nystagmus. The manifestations of Korsakoff's are short-term memory loss, learning deficits and confabulation. The condition is associated with demyelination, glial proliferation, as well as haemorrhagic lesions, mainly in the periventricular regions of the brain.

Kinetics

Small amounts are well-absorbed from the gastrointestinal tract but the absorption of larger doses above 5 mg is limited. It is widely distributed around the body and, within the cell, it is present as the diphosphate. It is not stored in the body and excess above the body's requirements is excreted via the kidneys as unchanged thiamine or its metabolites.

Indications

Thiamine is used for the treatment and prevention of thiamine deficiency.

Adverse reactions

Adverse reactions seldom occur following oral administration. Parenteral administration has been associated with hypersensitivity reactions, which have varied from mild to severe anaphylaxis.

Drug interactions

None are known.

Contraindications

Previous hypersensitivity to thiamine is a contraindication.

Chlordiazepoxide

Mode of action

Chlordiazepoxide is a benzodiazepine with general properties similar to those of diazepam.

Kinetics

Chlordiazepoxide is well-absorbed, with 90% bound to plasma proteins. Reported values for the elimination half-life range from 5–30 h. It is excreted in the urine mainly as conjugated metabolites.

Indications

Chlordiazepoxide, as well as being used for alcohol withdrawal, is used for treatment of anxiety and for premedication.

Adverse reactions

Excess doses produce drowsiness, respiratory depression, hypotension and hypothermia.

Drug interactions

Administration with other sedative drugs may cause drowsiness.

Chlormethiazole

Mode of action

Chlormethiazole is a hypnotic and sedative with anticonvulsant effects.

Kinetics

Chlormethiazole is rapidly absorbed from the gastrointestinal tract with peak concentration 15–90 min after oral administration; 65% is bound to plasma proteins. It undergoes extensive first-pass metabolism in the liver and is excreted in the urine as metabolites.

When oral administration is not possible, intravenous chlormethiazole can be given as a continuous infusion, usually with a loading dose (0.8% solution chlormethiazole disulphate, 3–7.5 ml [24–60 mg]/min) until the desired effect has been attained followed by a slower maintenance infusion (0.5–1.0 ml [4–8 mg]/min) to achieve lowest possible rate to maintain shallow sleep and adequate spontaneous respiration. The patient needs careful monitoring to avoid over sedation. Cessation of the infusion usually results in rapid reversal of the sedation although prolonged recovery can occur.

Indications

Chlormethiazole is indicated for alcohol withdrawal, status epilepticus and pre-eclampsia.

Adverse reactions

Chlormethiazole may cause nasal, conjunctival irritation and gastrointestinal disturbance. Excess doses produce drowsiness, respiratory depression, hypotension and hypothermia. On intravenous infusion, localized thrombophlebitis, tachycardia and a transient fall in blood pressure may occur. With rapid infusion apnoea may occur.

Drug interactions

Administration of chlormethiazole with other sedative drugs can cause drowsiness. Cimetidine has been shown to reduce clearance of chlormethiazole leading to increased sedation.

Contraindications

Chlormethiazole is contraindicated in patients with acute pulmonary insufficiency and should be given with care in patients with chronic lung disease, cardiac, liver and renal disease.

Prednisolone

Chapter 5, p. 91 and p. 267.

BUDD-CHIARI SYNDROME

Introduction

Hepatic vein occlusion, known as the Budd-Chiari syndrome, is a rare disorder that presents with hepatomegaly, high protein ascites and abdominal pain. The natural history of untreated patients is progression of symptoms with death due to the complications of portal hypertension.[104] The syndrome can be classified according to the duration of symptoms and signs (e.g. acute, subacute or chronic), the site of obstruction (e.g. small hepatic veins, large hepatic veins or hepatic inferior vena cava) and the cause of the obstruction (e.g. membranous webs, direct infiltration of the veins by tumour or thrombosis).

Diagnosis is usually made by colour-flow Doppler ultrasound. Hepatic venography helps confirm the diagnosis and guides surgical treatment. Liver biopsy also has characteristic appearances and helps to judge the extent of the fibrosis.

Pathophysiology

Membranous occlusion of the hepatic veins is the most common cause of the Budd-Chiari syndrome worldwide, although is rarely seen in the UK. It is unclear whether these webs are congenital or are a result of a post-thrombic event. Most patients present with subacute or chronic disease and the majority of patients (70%) have an underlying thrombotic diathesis. Thrombotic disorders associated with the Budd-Chiari syndrome include:

- Haematological disorders (e.g. polycythaemia rubra vera, myeloproliferative disorders),
- Inherited thrombotic tendencies (protein C deficiency, protein S deficiency, antithrombin III deficiency, Factor V Leiden mutation)
- Pregnancy or the oral contraceptive pill
- Chronic infections
- Chronic inflammation
- Tumours

Treatment approaches

Medical therapy provides only short-term symptomatic benefit with 2-year mortality being as high as 90% with medical therapy alone. Diuretics can be helpful in relieving the symptoms of ascites but do not affect long-term outcome. Anticoagulation may help prevent further thromboses but has not been shown to help symptoms or affect mortality. There have been a few reported successes with anti-thrombolytic therapies, although the long-term outcome remains to be established.[105] Since the majority of patients do not present acutely, thrombolysis is unlikely to have a major role.

Portosystemic shunting or liver transplantation are the mainstay of treatment of patients with the Budd-Chiari syndrome.[106] If the patient is not cirrhotic and the overall hepatic function is good, surgical portosystemic shunting or transjugular intrahepatic portal shunt (TIPS) should be considered, while liver transplantation is the treatment of choice for patients with cirrhosis or hepatic decompensation.[107,108]

VENO-OCCLUSIVE DISEASE

Introduction

Hepatic veno-occlusive disease (VOD) may present acutely following bone marrow transplantation or chronically following toxicity of pyrrolizidine alkaloids from plants, often ingested in the form of herbal teas.[109] The drugs associated with VOD are listed in Table 12.3. Histologically, there is subendothelial sclerosis of the terminal hepatic venules with thrombosis secondary to the sclerosis. This then leads to perivenular and sinusoidal fibrosis. The acute form presents typically with jaundice and hepatomegaly, while the chronic form presents in a similar way to the Budd-Chiari syndrome.

Table 12.3   Drugs causing veno-occlusive disease.

Alcohol
Arsenic (inorganic) poisoning
Azathiopine
Cyclophosphamide
Dacarbazine
Daunorubicin
Dimethylbusulfan
Floxuridine
Pyrrolizidine alkaloids
Thioguanine
Urethane

Pathogenesis

Cytoreductive therapy is toxic primarily to both sinusoidal and vascular endothelial cells. Cytokine release, including TNF_α, has been shown in response to these cytoreductive drugs and is thought to play a role in the pathogenesis by increasing coagulation.

Treatment approach

Treatment following bone marrow transplantation is largely supportive. Pentoxifylline, which inhibits TNF_α release, has been used experimentally but requires further investigation. Chronic VOD often requires transplantation because of the extensive fibrosis present at the time of diagnosis, although it may be treated with portosystemic shunting if diagnosed early.

DRUG-INDUCED LIVER DISEASE

Introduction

Drug-induced liver disease can range from minor abnormalities of serum liver function tests in asymptomatic patients to hepatitis, jaundice and hepatic failure.[110] It has been estimated that up to 5% of jaundice seen in hospital patients is caused by drug reactions. Drug-induced liver disease may occur as an idiosyncratic reaction to a therapeutic dose of a drug or may be a result of the known toxicity of a drug. A detailed drug history is essential in any patient presenting with liver disease, including dosage, duration of therapy and concomitant drug use. Other causes of liver disease need to be excluded.

The list of drugs that have been implicated in causing liver injury is large and includes over-the-counter and herbal preparations. It is beyond the scope of this book to list all the implicated drugs. The cornerstone of treatment is to recognize the drug toxicity and stop the medication. Paracetamol (acetaminophen) is the most common cause of drug-induced liver injury and fulminant hepatic failure. Drug overdose is treated with N-acetylcysteine, which is discussed in later text.

Pathophysiology

Multiple factors can influence a patient's susceptibility to drug hepatoxicity, including age, gender, nutritional status, renal and liver function and comorbid disease. One important factor is the induction of liver enzymes involved in the metabolism of drugs.[111] The liver is exposed to high concentrations of ingested drugs, in particular those drugs with a high first-pass metabolism. Normally the liver metabolizes drugs to a more polar, hydrophilic form that allows excretion in aqueous forms. This usually takes place in two steps, known as Phase 1 and Phase 2 reactions. Phase 1 reactions are mediated by cytochrome P_{450} enzymes found primarily in the liver within the endoplasmic reticulum. Phase 1 reactions are mainly oxidative and result in aliphatic and aromatic hydroxylation, dealkylation or dehydrogenation. This often results in more active metabolites of the drug, which can be toxic. Phase 2 reactions are predominantly conjugative, converting the more active metabolites to non-toxic hydrophilic products that are more readily excreted. Drug injury may result from increased Phase 1 reaction, resulting in increased active metabolites or due to inadequate detoxification. There are many medications that may alter P_{450} activity and thus promote drug toxicity.

Paracetamol is normally metabolized by conjugation to glucuronide and sulphate with a relatively small amount being metabolized by the cytochrome P_{450} system to form oxidative metabolites, which are further conjugated prior to elimination. In overdose, the conjugation pathways become saturated and increased oxidation occurs via the cytochrome P_{450} system. One of the metabolites, N-acetyl-*p*-benzo-quinoneimine (NAPQI) leads to glutathione depletion, allowing it to bind covalently to cell macromolecules, disrupting mitochondrial function. Malnutrition and alcohol ingestion increase NAPQI toxicity by further reducing glutathione.

Treatment approaches

The main treatment of drug-induced liver disease is to stop any suspected medication. N-Acetylcysteine is used in the treatment of choice of paracetamol toxicity.[112] Methionine is an alternative treatment.

Treatment regimens

Paracetamol overdosage
With paracetamol overdose prompt treatment is essential. Gastric lavage should be undertaken especially if within 4 h of ingestion. Plasma paracetamol concentration should be determined (but not within the first 4 h to ensure peak concentrations). The patient's paracetamol level is compared against a standard nomogram reference line on a plot of plasma-paracetamol concentration against hours after ingestion. Treatment is required if

the patients level is above this line. Patients receiving enzyme-inducing drugs or with a history of alcohol excess should receive treatment if their plasma concentrations are up to 50% below the standard reference line.

Treatment should, however, be started as soon as paracetamol overdose is suspected, before paracetamol levels are obtained and stopped or continued according to subsequent levels. Treatment within 8 h of ingestion is very effective. Previously it was considered that treatment greater than 15 h after ingestion was not beneficial but more recent studies have shown N-acetylcysteine to still have some benefit even when administered late.[113] Intravenous acetylcysteine is the treatment of choice in the UK, while oral administration is preferred in the USA. In the UK, an initial dose of 150 mg/kg body weight of acetylcysteine as a 20% solution in 200 ml of 5% glucose is given intravenously over 15 min, followed by an intravenous infusion of 50 mg/kg in 500 ml of 5% glucose over the next 4 h and then 100 mg/kg in 1 l over the next 16 h.

Pharmacology

Acetylcysteine

Mode of action
Acetylcysteine works by several mechanisms, enhancing glutathione synthesis and the non-toxic sulphation pathway, and acting as a substitute to glutathione to inactivate NAPQI. It may also act as an antioxidant and modify secondary effects of inflammation and may improve liver oxygenation.

Kinetics
Acetylcysteine is absorbed rapidly from the gut and undergoes extensive first-pass metabolism; as a result, oral bioavailability is low. Intravenous administration is preferred in the UK, because of concerns over absorption in patients who are vomiting and who have received charcoal. Nausea and vomiting can be exacerbated by the foul taste of acetylcysteine.

Indications

In addition to paracetamol overdosage, acetylcysteine is used as a mucolytic agent in the treatment of respiratory and ocular disorders.

Adverse reactions

Adverse effects include bronchospasm, nausea, vomiting, stomatitis, rhinorrhoea, headache, tinnitus, urticaria, rashes and fever. Anaphylactic reactions have been reported but are rare. If a reaction is suspected, antihistamine should be administered, after which acetylcysteine may be able to be reintroduced at a slower infusion rate. Resumption of intravenous therapy is acceptable following all but life-threatening reactions.

Drug interactions

Acetylcysteine is physically incompatible with or can inactivate some antibiotics if mixed together.

Contraindications

Acetylcysteine should be used with caution in asthmatic patients and also patients with a history of peptic ulceration since acetylcysteine may disrupt the gastric mucosal barrier.

REFERENCES

1. Chapman RWG, Arborgh BAM, Rhodes JM, *et al*. Primary sclerosing cholangitis: a review of its clinical features, cholangiography, and hepatic histology. *Gut* 1980; **21**: 870–877.
2. Weisner RH, LaRusso NF. Clinicopathologic features of the syndrome of primary sclerosing cholangitis. *Gastroenterology* 1980; **79**: 200–206.
3. Converse CF, Reagan JW, DeCosse JJ. Ulcerative colitis and carcinoma of the bile ducts. *Am J Surg* 1975; **121**: 39–45.
4. Wee A, Ludwig J, Coffey RJ, *et al*. Hepatobiliary carcinoma associated with primary sclerosing cholangitis and chronic ulcerative colitis. *Human Pathol* 1985; **16**: 719–726.
5. Rosen CB, Nagorney DM, Wiesner RH, Coffey RJ, LaRusso NF. Cholangiocarcinoma complicating primary sclerosing cholangitis. *Ann Surg* 1991; **213**: 21–25.
6. Olsson R, Danielson A, Jarnerot G, Lindstrome, Loof L, Rolny P. Prevalence of primary sclerosing cholangitis in patients with ulcerative colitis. *Gastroenterology* 1991; **100**: 1319–1323.
7. Lundgrist K, Broome U. Differences in colonic disease activity in patients with primary sclerosing cholangitis. *Dis Colon Rectum* 1997; **40**: 1–6.
8. Eade MN, Cooke WT, Brooke BN, Thompson H. Liver disease in Crohn's colitis. A study of 21 consecutive patients having colectomy. *Ann Intern Med* 1970; **74**: 518–528.
9. Schrumpf E, Fausa O, Kolmannskog F, Elgjo K, Ritland S, Gjome E. Sclerosing cholangitis in ulcerative colitis. A follow-up study. *Scand J Gastroenterol* 1982; **17**: 33–39.
10. Sandberg-Gertzen H, Wallerstedt S, Lindberg G. Natural history and prognostic factors in 305 Swedish patients with primary sclerosing cholangitis. *Gut* 1996; **38**: 610–615.
11. Aadland E, Schrumpf E, Fausa O, Elgio K, Heilo A, Aakhus T. Primary sclerosing cholangitis: a long-term follow-up study. *Scand J Gastroenterol* 1987; **2**: 655–664.
12. Narumi S, Roberts JP, Emond JC, *et al*. Liver transplantation for sclerosing cholangitis. *Hepatology* 1995; **22**: 451–457.
13. Esquivel CO, Marsh JW, Fan Thiel DH. Liver transplantation for chronic cholestatic liver disease in adults and children. *Gastroenterol Clin N Am* 1988; **17**: 145–155.
14. Stieber AL, Marino IR, Iwatsuki S, Starzl TE. Cholangiocarcinoma in sclerosing cholangitis: the role of liver transplantation. *Int Surg* 1989; **74**: 1–3.
15. Chapman RW, Varghese Z, Gaul R, Patel G, Kokinon N, Sherlock S. Association of primary sclerosing cholangitis with HLA-B8. *Gut* 1983; **24**: 38–41.
16. Donaldson PT, Farrant JM, Wilkinson MK, Hayllar K, Portmann BC, Williams R. Dual association of HLA DR2 and DR3 with primary sclerosing cholangitis. *Hepatology* 1991; **13**: 129–133.
17. Duerr RH, Targan SR, Landers CJ, LaRusso NF, Lindsey KL, Wiesner RH. Neutrophil cytoplasmic antibodies: a link between primary sclerosing cholangitis and ulcerative colitis. *Gastroenterology* 1991; **100**: 1381–1385.
18. Lo SK, Fleming KA, Chapman RW. Prevalence of antineutrophil antibody in primary sclerosing cholangitis and ulcerative colitis using an

alkaline phosphatase technique. *Gut* 1992; **33:** 1370–1375.

19. Lo SK, Fleming KA, Chapman RW. A two-year follow-up study of antineutrophil antibody in primary sclerosing cholangitis. *J Hepatol* 1994; **21:** 974–978.

20. Palmer KR, Duerden BI, Holdsworth CD. Bacteriological and endotoxin studies in cases of ulcerative colitis submitted to surgery. *Gut* 1980; **21:** 851–854.

21. May GR, Bender CE, LaRusson NF, Wiesner RH. Non-operative dilatation of dominant strictures in primary sclerosing cholangitis. *Am J Radiol* 1985; **145:** 1061–1064.

22. Lindor KD. Ursodiol for primary sclerosing cholangitis. *N Engl J Med* 1997; **336:** 691–695.

23. Mitchell S, Lo SK, Douley J, Fleming K, Chapman RW. High-dose ursodeoxycholic acid in the treatment of primary sclerosing cholangitis *Gastroenterology* 2000; in press.

24. Lindor KD, Wiesner RH, Colwell LJ, Steiner BL, Beaver S, LaRusso NF. The combination of prednisolone and colchicine in patients with primary sclerosing cholangitis. *Am J Gastroenterol* 1991; **85:** 57–61.

25. Wagner A. Azathioprine in primary sclerosing cholangitis. *Lancet* 1971; **2:** 663–664.

26. Knox TA, Kaplan MM. Treatment of primary sclerosing cholangitis with oral methotrexate. *Am J Gastroenterol* 1991; **86:** 546–552.

27. Weisner RH, Steiner B, LaRusso NF, Lindor KD, Baldus WP. A controlled clinical trial evaluating cyclosporine in the treatment of primary sclerosing cholangitis [Abstract]. *Hepatology* 1991; **14:** 63A.

28. Kaplan MM. Primary biliary cirrhosis. *N Engl J Med* 1987; **316:** 521–528.

29. Myszor M, James OF. The epidemiology of primary biliary cirrhosis in north-east England: an increasingly common disease? *Quart J Med* 1990; **75:** 377–385.

30. Markus BH, Dickson ER, Grambsch PM, *et al.* Efficacy of liver transplantation in patients with primary biliary cirrhosis. *N Engl J Med* 1989; **320:** 1709–1713.

31. Weisner RH, LaRusso NF, Ludwig J, Dickson ER. Comparison of the clinicopathologic features of primary sclerosing cholangitis and primary biliary cirrhosis. *Gastroenterology* 1985; **88:** 108–114.

32. Van der Water J, Turchany J, Leung PS, *et al.* Molecular mimicry in primary biliary cirrhosis: evidence for biliary expression of a molecule cross with pyruvate dehydrogenase complex-E2. *J Clin Invest* 1993; **91:** 2653–64.

33. Bach N, Schaffner F. Familial primary biliary cirrhosis. *J Hepatol* 1994; **20:** 698–701.

34. Brind AM, Bray GP, Portmann BC, Williams R. Prevalence and pattern of familial disease in primary biliary cirrhosis. *Gut* 1995; **36:** 615–617.

35. Kaplan MM, Robson AR, Lee YM. Discordant occurrence of primary biliary cirrhosis in monozygote twins. *N Engl J Med* 1994; **331:** 932.

36. Gores GJ, Moore SB, Fisher LD, Powell FC, Dickson ER. Primary biliary cirrhosis association with class II major histocompatibility complex antigens. *Hepatology* 1987; **7:** 889–892.

37. Metcalf JV, Bhopal RS, Gray J, James OJ. Incidence and prevalence of primary biliary cirrhosis in the city of Newcastle upon Tyne, England. *Int J Epidemiol* 1997; **26:** 830–836.

38. Metcalf JV, Bhopal RS, Scott LMD, Gray J, Howel D, James OF. Temporal and geographical variations in the prevalence of primary biliary cirrhosis (PBC) in a stable population. *Hepatology* 1995; **22:** 384A.

39. Watson R, Angus PW, Dewar M, Goss B, Sewell RB, Smallwood RA. Low prevalence of primary biliary cirrhosis in Victoria, Australia. *Gut* 1995; **36:** 927–930.

40. Witt-Sullivan H, Heathcote EJ, Couch K. The demography of primary biliary cirrhosis in Ontario, Canada. *Hepatology* 1990; **12:** 98–105.

41. Trigger DR. PBC: an epidemiological study. *Br Med J* 1980; **281:** 772.

42. Burroughs AK, Rosenstein IJ, Epstein O, Hamilton-Miller JMT, Brumfitt W, Sherlock S. Bacteriuria and primary biliary cirrhosis. *Gut* 1984; **25:** 133–137.

43. Butler P, Falle F, Hamilton-Miller JMT, Brumfitt W, Baum H, Burroughs A. M2 mitochondrial antibodies and urinary rough mutant bacteria in patients with primary biliary cirrhosis and in patients with recurrent bacteriuria. *J Hepatol* 1992; **17:** 483–488.

44. Lindenborn-Fotinos J, Baum H, Berg PA. Mitochondrial antigens in primary biliary cirrhosis; further characterization of the M2 antigen by immunoblotting, revealing, species and non-species determinants. *Hepatology* 1985; **5:** 763–769.

45. Fussey SPM, Lindsay JG, Fuller C, *et al.* Autoantibodies in primary biliary cirrhosis: analysis of reactivity against eukaryotic and

prokaryotic 2-oxo-acid dehydrogenase complexes. *Hepatology* 1991; **13**: 467–474.

46. Hopf U, Stemerowicz R. Can enterobacterial antigens induce a primary biliary cirrhosis? In: *Immunology and Liver*. Zum Meyer, K-H Büschenfelde, J Hoofnagle, M Manns (Eds), Kluwer, London, 1993, 447–458.

47. O'Donohue J, McFarland B, Bromford A, Yates M, Williams R. Antibodies to atypical mycobacteriae in primary biliary cirrhosis. *J Hepatol* 1994; **21**: 887–889.

48. Van de Water J, Gershwin ME, Garry RF. Detection of retroviral antibodies in primary biliary cirrhosis and other idiopathic biliary disorders. *Lancet* 1998; **351**: 1620–1624.

49. Munoz SJ, Ballas SK, Norberg R, Maddrey WC. Antibodies to human immunodeficiency virus (HIV) in primary biliary cirrhosis. *Gastroenterology* 1988; **94**: A574 [Abstract].

50. Mitchison HC, Palmer JM, Bassendine MF, Watson AJ, Record CO, James OFW. A controlled trial of prednisolone treatment in primary biliary cirrhosis: three-year results. *J Hepatol* 1992; **15**: 336–344.

51. Crowe J, Christensen E, Smith M, *et al.* Azathioprine in primary biliary cirrhosis: a preliminary report of an international trial. *Gastroenterology* 1980; **78**: 1005–1010.

52. James OFW. D-Penicillamine for primary biliary cirrhosis. *Gut* 1985; **26**: 109–113.

53. Hoofnagle JH, Davis GL, Schafer DF, *et al.* Randomised trial of chlorambucil for primary biliary cirrhosis. *Gastroenterology* 1986; **91**: 1327–1334.

54. Lombard M, Portmann B, Neuberger J, *et al.* Cyclosporin A treatment in primary biliary cirrhosis: results of a long-term placebo controlled trial and effect on survival. *Gastroenterology* 1993; **104**: 519–526.

55. Kaplan MM, Alling DW, Zimmerman HJ, *et al.* A prospective trial of colchicine for primary biliary cirrhosis. *N Engl J Med* 1986; **315**: 1448–1454.

56. Neuberger J, Lombard M, Galbraith R. Primary biliary cirrhosis. *Gut* 1991; **32**: S73–S78.

57. Poupon RE, Balkau B, Eschwege E, *et al.* A multicentre, controlled trial of ursodiol for the treatment of primary biliary cirrhosis. *N Engl J Med* 1991; **324**: 1548–1554.

58. Poupon RE, Poupon R, Balkau B. Ursodiol for the long-term treatment of primary biliary cirrhosis. *N Engl J Med* 1994; **330**: 1342–1347.

59. Leuschner U, Fischer H, Kurtz W, *et al.* Ursodeoxycholic acid in primary biliary cirrhosis: results of a controlled double-blind trial. *Gastroenterology* 1989; **97**: 1268–1274.

60. Lindor KD, Dickson ER, Baldus WP, *et al.* Ursodeoxycholic acid in the treatment of primary biliary cirrhosis. *Gastroenterology* 1994; **106**: 1284–1290.

61. Kaplan MM, Knox TA. Treatment of primary biliary cirrhosis with low-dose weekly methotrexate. *Gastroenterology* 1991; **101**: 1332–1338.

62. Czaja AJ. Autoimmune hepatitis: evolving concepts and treatment strategies. *Dig Dis Sci* 1995; **40**: 435–456.

63. Johnson PJ, McFarlane IG. Meeting report of the International Autoimmune Hepatitis Group. *Hepatology* 1993; **18**: 998–1005.

64. Czaja AJ, Manns MP. The validity and importance of subtypes in autoimmune hepatitis: a point of view. *Am J Gastroenterol* 1995; **90**: 1206–1211.

65. Czaja AJ, Carpenter HA, Santrach PJ, Moore SB. Significance of HLA DR4 in type 1 autoimmune hepatitis. *Gastroenterology* 1993; **104**: 1755–1761.

66. Manns M, Kruger M. Immunogenetics in liver diseases. *Gastroenterology* 1994; **106**: 1676–1697.

67. Manns M, Griffin KJ, Sullivan KJ, Sullivan KF, Johnson EF. LKM-1 autoantibodies recognize a short linear sequence in P_{450} II D6, a cytochrome P_{450} mono-oxygenase. *J Clin Invest* 1991; **88**: 1370–1378.

68. Cjaza AJ. Current therapy of autoimmune hepatitis. In: *Liver Injury Update: Clinical Implications and Mechanistic Role of Cells of the Liver*. N Kapowitz (Ed.), Syllabus of the AASLD 1997 Postgraduate Course, 1997, 111–119.

69. Hayams JS, Ballow M, Leichtner AM. Cyclosporin treatment of autoimmune chronic active hepatitis. *Gastroenterology* 1987; **93**: 890.

70. Van Thiel DH, Wright H, Carroll P, *et al.* Tacrolimus: a potential new treatment for autoimmune hepatitis, chronic active hepatitis: results of an open label preliminary trial. *Am J Gastroenterol* 1995; **90**: 771–776.

71. Danielson A, Prytz H. Oral budesonide for treatment of autoimmune chronic active hepatitis. *Alim Pharm Ther* 1994; **8**: 585–590.

72. Johnson PJ, McFarlane IG, Williams R. Azathioprine for long-term maintenance of remission in autoimmune hepatitis. *N Engl J Med* 1995; **333**: 958–963.

73. Nazer H, Ede RJ, Mowat AP, Williams R. Wilson's disease: clinical presentation and use of prognostic index. *Gut* 1986; **27:** 1377–1381.

74. Petrukhin K, Fischer SG, Pirastu M, *et al.* Mapping, cloning and genetic characterization of the region containing the Wilson's disease gene. *Nature Genetics* 1993; **5:** 338–343.

75. Bull PC, Thomas GR, Rommens JM, Forbes JR, Cox DW. The Wilson's disease gene is a putative copper transporting gene P-type ATP-ase similar to Menkes gene. *Nature Genetics* 1993; **5:** 327–237.

76. Tankanow RM. Pathophysiology and treatment of Wilson's disease. *Clin Pharm* 1991; **10:** 839–849.

77. Sternlieb I, van den Hamer CJA, Morell AG, *et al.* Lysosomal defect of hepatic copper excretion in Wilson's disease. *Gastroenterology* 1973; **64:** 99–105.

78. Schilsky ML, Scheinberg IH, Sternlieb I. Liver transplantation of Wilson's disease: indications and outcome. *Hepatology* 1994; **19:** 583–587.

79. Brewer GJ. Practical recommendations and new therapies for Wilson's disease. *Drugs* 1995; **50:** 240–249.

80. Adams PC, Kertesz AE, Valberg LS. Clinical presentation of hemochromatosis: a changing scene. *Am J Med* 1991; **90:** 445–449.

81. Feder FN, Gnirke A, Thomas W, *et al.* A novel MHC class-1-like gene is mutated in patients with hereditary hemochromatosis. *Nature Genetics* 1996; **14:** 399–408.

82. Bassett ML, Halliday JW, Powell LW. Value of hepatic iron measurements in early hemochromatosis and determination of the critical iron level associated with fibrosis. *Hepatology* 1986; **6:** 24–29.

83. Niederau C, Fischer R, Sonnenberg A, Stremmel W, Trampisch HJ, Strohmeyer G. Survival and causes of death in cirrhotic and noncirrhotic patients with primary hemochromatosis. *N Engl J Med* 1985; **313:** 1256–1262.

84. Deugnier TM, Guyader D, Crantock L, *et al.* Primary liver cancer in genetic hemochromatosis: a clinical, pathological and pathogenetic study of 54 cases. *Gastroenterology* 1993; **104:** 228–234.

85. Rabin M, Watson M, Kidd V. Regional location of α-1-antichymotrypsin and α-1-antitrypsin genes on chromosome 14. *Somat Cell Mol Genetics* 1986; **12:** 209–214.

86. Brantly M, Nukiwa T, Crystal RG. Molecular basis of α-1-antitrypsin. *Am J Med* 1988; **84:** 13–31.

87. Carlson JA, Rogers BB, Sifers RN, *et al.* Accumulation of α-1-antitrypsin causes liver disease in transgenic mice. *J Clin Invest* 1988; **83:** 1183–1190.

88. Lavine JE, Jonas MM. Pediatric liver disease. *Semin Liver Dis* 1994; **14:** 213–217.

89. Whittington R, Goa KL. Alglucerase; a review of its therapeutic use in Gaucher's disease. *Drugs* 1992; **44:** 72–93.

90. Starzl TE, Demtris AJ, Trucco M, *et al.* Chimerism after liver transplantation for type IV glycogen storage disease and type 1 Gaucher's disease. *N Engl J Med* 1993; **328:** 745–749.

91. Orholm M, Sorensen TI, Bentsen K, *et al.* Mortality of alcohol abusing men prospectively assessed in relation to history of abuse and degree of liver injury. *Liver* 1985; **5:** 253–260.

92. Chedid A, Mendenhall CL, Gartside P, French SW, Chen T, Rabin L. Prognostic factors in alcoholic liver disease. *Am J Gastroenterol* 1991; **86:** 210–216.

93. Maddrey WC. Alcoholic hepatitis: clinicopathologic features and therapy. *Semin Liver Dis* 1998; **8:** 91–102.

94. Lindros KO. Alcoholic liver disease: pathobiological aspects. *J Hepatol* 1995; **23 (Suppl. 1):** 7–15.

95. Reuler JB, Girard DE, Cooney TG. Wernicke's encephalopathy. *N Engl J Med* 1985; **312:** 1035–1039.

96. Ramond MJ, Poynard T, Rueff B, *et al.* A randomized trial of prednisolone in patients with severe alcoholic hepatitis. *N Engl J Med* 1992; **326:** 507–512.

97. Carithers RL, Herlong F, Diehl AM, *et al.* Methylprednisolone therapy in patients with severe alcoholic hepatitis. *Ann Intern Med* 1989; **110:** 685–690.

98. Imperiale T, McCullough AJ. Do corticosteroids reduce mortality from alcoholic hepatitis? A meta analysis of the randomized controlled trials. *Ann Intern Med* 1990; **113:** 299–307.

99. Orrego H, Kalant H, Israel Y, *et al.* Effect of short-term therapy with PTU in patients with alcoholic liver disease. *Gastroenterology* 1979; **20:** 105–115.

100. Halle P, Pare P, Kaptein E, Kanel G, Redeker AG, Reynolds TB. Double-blind, controlled trial of propylthiouracil in patients with severe acute alcoholic hepatitis. *Gastroenterology* 1982; **87:** 925–931.

101. Lashner BA, Baker AL. Propylthiouracil for alcoholic liver disease. *N Engl J Med* 1988; **318:** 1471.

102. Sherlock S. Alcoholic liver disease. *Lancet* 1995; **345:** 227–229.

103. Akriviadis EA, Steindel H, Pinto PC, *et al.* Failure of colchicine to improve short-term survival in patients with alcoholic hepatitis. *Gastroenterology* 1990; **99:** 811–818.

104. Tilanus HW. Budd Chiari Syndrome. *Br J Surg* 1995; **82:** 1023–1030.

105. Raju GS, Felver M, Olin JW, Satti SD. Thrombolysis for acute Budd Chiari syndrome: case report and literature review. *Am J Gastroenterol* 1996; **91:** 1262–1263.

106. Klein A, Sitzmann J, Coleman J, Herlong F, Cameron J. Current management of the Budd-Chiari syndrome. *Ann Surg* 1990; **212:** 144–149.

107. Ringe B, Lang H, Oldhafer KJ, *et al.* Which is best surgery for Budd-Chiari syndrome: venous decompression or liver transplantation? A single centre experience with 50 patients. *Hepatology* 1995; **21:** 1337–1344.

108. Blum U, Rossle M, Haag K, *et al.* Budd-Chiari syndrome: technical, haemodynamic and clinical results of treatment with transjugular intrahepatic portosystemic shunt. *Radiology* 1995; **197:** 805–811.

109. McDonald G, Hinds M, Fisher L, *et al.* Veno-occlusive disease of the liver and multiorgan failure after bone marrow transplantation: a cohort study of 355 patients. *Ann Intern Med* 1993; **118:** 255–267.

110. Lee WM. Drug-induced hepatotoxicity. *N Engl J Med* 1995; **333:** 1118–1125.

111. Watkins PB. Role of cytochromes P_{450} in drug metabolism and hepatoxicity. *Semin Liver Dis* 1990; **10:** 235–250.

112. Keays R, Williams R. Paracetamol poisoning and liver failure. *Prescribers J* 1989; **29:** 155–162.

113. Keays R, Harrison PM, Wendon JA, *et al.* Intravenous acetylcysteine in paracetamol induced fulminant hepatic failure; a prospective trial. *Br Med J* 1991; **303:** 1026–1029.

13

Drug therapy for portal hypertension

Àngels Escorsell, Juan Rodés

INTRODUCTION

Portal hypertension represents the most common and severe complication of chronic progressive liver diseases (including cirrhosis of the liver, hepatic schistosomiasis and portal vein thrombosis). The complications that occur as a consequence of portal hypertension determine, in most patients, the clinical course of their liver disease.

The two major clinical syndromes developing as a consequence of portal hypertension are variceal bleeding and ascites. Variceal bleeding is the final stage of a series of complications initiated by the increase in portal pressure, followed by the formation and progressive dilatation of gastroesophageal varices (Fig. 13.1) until these finally rupture and bleed. A less common cause of bleeding in chronic liver diseases is portal hypertensive gastropathy (PHG). Ascites develops from the combination of sinusoidal portal hypertension and systemic vasodilatation, leading to sodium and water retention. This complication causes severe metabolic and haemodynamic disturbances resulting in the development of refractory ascites, hepato-renal syndrome (HRS) and spontaneous bacterial peritonitis (SBP).

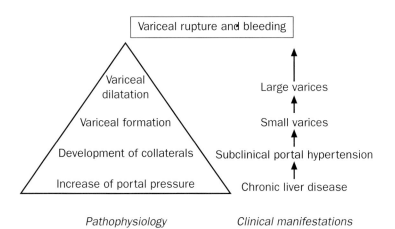

Pathophysiology   *Clinical manifestations*

Figure 13.1 Natural history of oesophageal varices according to the pathophysiological evolution of portal hypertension.

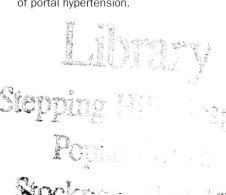

This chapter is an overview of drug therapy for portal hypertension, the pathophysiological basis and the therapeutic regimens used to treat this severe and, unfortunately, common complication of liver disease.

THE PATHOPHYSIOLOGICAL BASIS OF DRUG THERAPY FOR PORTAL HYPERTENSION

Elevated portal pressure is the event defining portal hypertension. Therefore, the rationale for drug therapy is to use pharmacological agents that might decrease pressure in the portal venous system and its collaterals.

As in any vascular system, the pressure gradient along the portal venous system is the result of the product of the portal blood flow and the vascular resistance that impedes that flow.[1] According to Ohm's law, this relationship is defined by the equation:

$$\Delta P = Q \times R$$

in which ΔP is the portal pressure gradient, Q is blood flow within the entire portal venous system (including the portosystemic collaterals), and R is the vascular resistance that opposes blood flow.

Factors influencing vascular resistance are interrelated by Poiselle's law in the equation:

$$R = 8\mu L/\pi r^4$$

in which μ is the coefficient of blood viscosity, L is the length of the vessel and r its radius. It follows that change in the radius of the vessels is the main factor influencing vascular resistance, and therefore, the development of portal hypertension.[1,2]

Portal pressure therefore may increase because of an increase in either portal blood flow, vascular resistance, or both. Consequently, we are able to reduce portal pressure with drugs that reduce portohepatic vascular resistance (vasodilators), portal blood flow (vasoconstrictors), or any combination of these parameters.

Portal hypertension is also characteristically associated with peripheral vasodilatation, which is thought to be due to three basic mechanisms:

1. Activation of neurohumoral systems (renin-angiotensin-aldosterone system, the sympathetic nervous system and vasopressin) leading to an increased concentration of circulating vasoconstrictors;
2. Increased endothelial production of local vasodilators;
3. Decreased responsiveness to endogenous vasoconstrictors.[3]

As a consequence of this disturbance, a hyperdynamic circulatory state, characterized by reduced arterial pressure, reduced peripheral resistance and increased cardiac output, develops. Systemic and splanchnic arterial vasodilatation leads to a circulatory hypovolaemia, that is to say, a decrease in central blood volume. This in turn leads to a further activation of neurohumoral systems, resulting in sodium and water retention by the kidneys and, subsequently, increased plasma volume. Finally, local changes in the portal venous bed result in the localization of the retained fluid within the peritoneal space as ascites.[4]

Treatment of ascites is primarily aimed at mobilizing the intrabdominal fluid by inducing a negative sodium balance; this can be achieved by:

- Bed rest and low-sodium diet
- Diuretic treatment
- Repeated paracentesis
- Peritoneovenous shunting or portosystemic shunting to reduce portal pressure

Ascites is associated with multiple complications requiring specific therapy; SBP must be treated (and prevented in high-risk patients) by the administration of antibiotics; HRS, which occurs in the setting of a profound derangement of systemic circulatory function leading to active renal vasoconstriction, can be treated by using systemic vasoconstrictors together with plasma volume expansion and, again, by treating portal hypertension and cirrhosis with portosystemic shunting and liver transplantation, respectively.

THERAPEUTIC APPROACHES

As previously stated, the clinical consequences of portal hypertension requiring specific therapy are:

- Variceal bleeding and the prevention of rebleeding
- haemorrhage from portal hypertensive gastropathy
- Ascites
- HRS
- spontaneous bacterial peritonitis

Pharmacological treatment of acute variceal bleeding

Haemorrhage from ruptured oesophageal varices is the main complication of portal hypertension and represents one of the leading causes of death in patients with cirrhosis. Despite the innovations in therapy introduced in recent years, the mortality of variceal bleeding episodes is still very high, averaging 35%.[5,6]

The major determinants of the poor prognosis of variceal haemorrhage are the magnitude of blood loss, the degree of liver failure and the occurrence of complications including infections, multi-organ failure and early rebleeding.[6] Early variceal rebleeding is specially important since it occurs in 30–50% of the patients during the first week of admission and is potentially preventable by therapy. For this reason, experts recommend that treatment for variceal bleeding should be aimed at arresting acute bleeding, and also at preventing very early rebleeding.[7]

Different techniques have been used to control variceal haemorrhage, including drugs, oesophageal tamponade, endoscopic sclerotherapy, banding ligation, transjugular intrahepatic portosystemic shunt (TIPS) and emergency surgery. None is perfect, and therefore the treatment frequently requires a combination of several of these procedures. Nevertheless, pharmacological therapy is the optimal treatment for variceal bleeding because it offers the unique advantage of not requiring sophisti-

cated equipment or specialized personnel and can thus be initiated immediately after admission or even at arrival to the emergency room, before diagnostic endoscopy, or while the patient is being transferred to hospital. Although currently available drugs do not entirely fulfil these requirements, it is useful to keep these advantages of pharmacological therapy in mind, since they point out the direction for future developments in the treatment of variceal haemorrhage.

Discussions at recent consensus conferences have indicated that drug therapy is an established and now widely accepted therapy for acute bleeding, which may be used as initial treatment before sclerotherapy or banding ligation.[8] However, recent guidelines issued by the British Society of Gastroenterology recommend that a patient with active variceal bleeding should be treated with endoscopic therapy as soon as the patient is haemodynamically stable (Fig. 13.1). Variceal band ligation is the method of first choice and sclerotherapy is used if banding is difficult because of continued bleeding or the technique is not available. Several drugs have been shown to be effective in this setting: vasopressin plus nitroglycerin, terlipressin and somatostatin; while other agents such as the somatostatin analogue, octreotide, require further investigation. It should be emphasized that correct initial management is crucial to reduce the mortality of an acute bleeding episode. This requires intensive resuscitation, adequate blood volume replacement, support of vital organ function, prevention of complications from hypovolaemic shock and to impending liver failure, and facilities for emergency diagnostic endoscopy.

Therapeutic regimens

Vasopressin

Vasopressin has been used in the treatment of variceal haemorrhage in the last three decades because of its ability to cause vasoconstriction. At pharmacological doses, it reduces blood flow to all splanchnic organs, and thereby decreases portal blood flow and portal pressure.[9] Vasopressin is also effective in reducing collateral blood flow and variceal pressure.[10] Adverse effects of vasopressin derive from systemic vasoconstriction increasing peripheral vascular resistance and reducing cardiac output, heart rate and coronary blood flow. These effects may result in serious complications such as myocardial ischaemia or infarction, arrythmias, mesenteric ischaemia, limb ischaemia and cerebrovascular accidents. In 25% of cases, vasopressin therapy must be withdrawn because of these complications.[11-22] Superior mesenteric artery infusions of smaller doses of vasopressin have failed to show a decrease in the systemic toxicity of the drug.[18] As a result, vasopressin is administered as a continuous intravenous infusion, starting at 0.4 U/min, which is increased if necessary to 0.6 and 0.8 U/min. Therapy is usually maintained until bleeding has been controlled for 12–24 h. If more than 0.4 U/min are required, the rate of infusion is decreased stepwise prior to discontinuation of therapy.

Vasopressin has been compared with non-active treatment or placebo in four randomized controlled trials (RCTs) including a total of only 157 patients and using different time points to assess its efficacy and incidence of side-effects.[11-14] Meta-analysis shows a significant beneficial effect of vasopressin in reducing failure to control bleeding, whereas the mortality rate was unaffected.[23] Complications appeared in 32–64% of vasopressin-treated patients, being the direct cause of death in three out of 78 patients.[23]

Vasopressin and endoscopic injection sclerotherapy (EIS) have been compared in five randomized control trials (RCTs).[24-28] Only one trial showed a significant, favourable effect of EIS in controlling bleeding.[27] However, in this study, the control of bleeding was assessed differently in the two groups of therapy, introducing a possible bias in the assessment of treatment outcome. The in-hospital rebleeding rate was almost significantly reduced by EIS.[23] Nevertheless, the different use of further EIS during admission in the two study groups makes it difficult to achieve a clear conclusion. The same applies to mortality for which the pooled odds ratio (POR) showed a beneficial effect of EIS when compared with vasopressin.[23]

Association of vasopressin and nitroglycerin
Nitroglycerin is a powerful venous dilator that was associated with vasopressin because it enhances the reduction in portal pressure (by decreasing portal venous resistance) while attenuating the systemic side-effects of vasopressin (by improving myocardial performance).[15]

Three RCTs have compared vasopressin plus nitroglycerin versus vasopressin alone. Nitroglycerin was given sublingually,[19] intravenously,[20] or transdermally[21] using continuous-release preparations. In two of these trials the side-effects were significantly reduced in the group treated with combined therapy.[19,20] All three studies showed that the association of vasopressin and nitroglycerin was more effective in controlling bleeding than vasopressin alone;[23] however, the decrease in mortality was not statistically significant. The only double-blind trial[21] showed that the association of transdermal nitroglycerin, but not of placebo, to vasopressin significantly reduced transfusion requirements, the need for balloon tamponade, and the number of patients requiring emergency surgery. These results suggest that the use of vasopressin should always be associated with nitroglycerin, although there are now better pharmacological options. Transdermal preparations are the easiest way of nitroglycerin administration.

Terlipressin
Terlipressin is a synthetic vasopressin analogue (triglycyl lysine vasopressin), which, in addition to an intrinsic vasoconstrictor activity, is slowly converted *in vivo* into vasopressin by enzymatic cleavage of the triglycyl residues. This allows a slow but continuous release of vasopressin resulting in a lower incidence of side-effects when compared with vasopressin, while maintaining a significant decrease in

portal pressure. In addition, terlipressin, unlike vasopressin, does not enhance fibrinolysis and has a longer biological activity, which makes continuous intravenous infusion unnecessary.[22] The preferred schedule of administration is intravenous injection of 2 mg/4 h until achieving a bleeding-free period of 24–48 h.

The clinical efficacy of terlipressin was assessed in three placebo-controlled trials (Table 13.1).[29-31] The pooled estimates showed a significant reduction in failure to control bleeding and also in mortality in terlipressin-treated patients. Terlipressin controlled the acute bleeding episode in 79% of the cases.[23] It is important to emphasize that this is the only pharmacological treatment that has been shown to reduce mortality from variceal bleeding.

Terlipressin was compared with vasopressin in five unblinded trials (Table 13.1),[32-36] in two

of which vasopressin was associated with nitroglycerin.[34,36] All studies reported a significantly lower complication rate with terlipressin, even when vasopressin was combined with nitroglycerin.[23] The control of bleeding was superior with terlipressin than with vasopressin, although this difference did not reach statistical significance.

Terlipressin may be considered to be equivalent to emergency EIS in both the control of variceal haemorrhage and the prevention of early variceal rebleeding with a lower incidence of side-effects.[37] Finally, terlipressin was found to be equally effective as both balloon tamponade[38,39] and somatostatin.[40,41]

Somatostatin

Somatostatin was introduced for the treatment of variceal haemorrhage because of its ability to

Table 13.1 **Results of randomized controlled trials of terlipressin for the treatment of variceal bleeding.**

Author (reference)	No. of patients (C/TP)	Control of bleeding (C/TP) (%)	Rebleeding rate (C/TP) (%)	Mortality rate (C/TP) (%)
Terlipressin versus placebo or non-active treatment				
Walker et al.[29]	25/25	52/80	20/20	32/12
Freeman et al.[30]	16/15	38/60	31/7	25/20
Soderlund et al.[31]	29/31	55/84	NR	38/10
Terlipressin versus vasopressin				
Freeman et al.[32]	11/10	9/70	27/30	27/20
Desaint et al.[33]	6/10	83/80	0/50	33/30
Lee et al.[34]	24/21	33/19	33/48	33/48
Chiu et al.[35]	28/26	54/50	11/15	36/46
D'Amico et al.[36]	55/56	76/91	33/37	16/25
Terlipressin versus emergency sclerotherapy				
CSFG[37]	114/105	68/62	13/15	14/18
Terlipressin versus balloon tamponade				
Colin et al.[38]	27/27	88/88	15/11	22/15
Fort et al.[39]	24/23	79/78	46/43	8/13

C, control group; TP, terlipressin-treated group; NR, not reported.

decrease portal pressure without the adverse effects of vasopressin on systemic circulation.[42] Somatostatin causes selective splanchnic vasoconstriction and thereby decreases portal and collateral blood flow and portal pressure.[42] This is probably due to the inhibition by somatostatin of the release of splanchnic vasodilator peptides such as glucagon.[43] A bolus injection of somatostatin causes a profound and rapid fall in both portal pressure and portocollateral (azygos) blood flow.[44] These changes are much greater than those induced by continuous infusion.[44] Thus it is recommended that three bolus injections are given during the first hours of therapy and also when there is rebleeding during treatment. The usual dose for a bolus injection is 250 μg, and 250 μg/h are given as continuous infusion. When successful, therapy is maintained for 5 days to prevent early variceal rebleeding.[45] The lack of significant side-effects from somatostatin represents its major advantage over other agents.

The results of RCTs evaluating the efficacy of somatostatin versus placebo or in comparison with other treatments are summarized in Table 13.2. Two placebo-controlled trials have assessed the effectiveness of somatostatin with divergent results; Valenzuela et al.[46] failed to show any beneficial effect, whereas Burroughs et al.[47] reported a significant reduction in bleeding with somatostatin. However, the Valenzuela study showed an extremely high rate of response (83%) in the placebo group, the highest ever reported; which may probably reflect some inadvertent bias. The two trials also differed in the duration of treatment (30 h versus 5 days, respectively) as well as in the definition of treatment success (bleeding-free periods of 4 h and 5 days, respectively), making it difficult to compare the two studies. Conversely, studies comparing somatostatin with 'non-active' treatments showed that somatostatin was equally effective as ranitidine[48] and significantly better than cimetidine.[49] Altogether, on pooling the results of studies comparing somatostatin with placebo or 'non-active' treatment, somatostatin was found to significantly reduce failure to control variceal bleeding.[23]

Somatostatin was compared with vasopressin in seven trials.[50–56] The results showed an important reduction of failure to control bleeding with somatostatin, which approached statistical significance. In all trials, complications were virtually absent with somatostatin (6%), whereas the median complication rate was 49% with vasopressin.[23] Two RCTs have compared somatostatin with terlipressin; both showed that the two drugs were highly effective in arresting variceal bleeding, there being no differences in the rate of control of bleeding, mortality or incidence of side-effects.[40,41]

Somatostatin was also shown to be equivalent to balloon tamponade in two trials.[57,58] Furthermore, trials versus sclerotherapy[59–61] showed somatostatin to be equally effective as this invasive technique for active bleeding (Table 13.2). Finally, a recent study has shown that a continuous somatostatin infusion for 5 days after controlling the initial haemorrhage was equally effective as sclerotherapy in preventing early rebleeding, while causing fewer complications.[45]

Therefore RCTs comparing somatostatin with other active treatments strongly suggest that somatostatin is highly effective in the treatment of variceal bleeding.

Octreotide

Octreotide is a synthetic long-acting somatostatin analogue that has been shown to be significantly more efficient than the native hormone in treating acromegaly and endocrine tumours.[62] This greater efficacy arises from the fact that octreotide is significantly more potent than natural somatostatin in inhibiting growth hormone and glucagon release.[62] This advantage, in addition to its long half-life and easy administration (octreotide can be administered subcutaneously), have led to the clinical use of octreotide in conditions other than those previously mentioned and in which somatostatin has clearly shown to be highly efficient, such as portal hypertension and its related complications. Although octreotide has been shown to reduce portal pressure in animals,[63] however, this effect is uncertain in cirrhotic patients.[63,64]

Table 13.2   Results of randomized controlled trials of somatostatin for the treatment of variceal bleeding.

Author (reference)	No. of patients (C/SMT)	Control of bleeding (C/SMT) (%)	Rebleeding rate (C/SMT) (%)	Mortality rate (C/SMT) (%)
Somatostatin versus placebo or non-active treatment				
Valenzuela et al.[46]	36/48	75/56	8/8	28/31
Burroughs et al.[47]	59/61	41/64	NR	12/15
Loperfido et al.[48]	25/22	32/32	52/59	32/32
Testoni et al.[49]	14/15	93/93	NR	0/7
Somatostatin versus vasopressin				
Kravetz et al.[50]	31/30	56/53	16/33	45/47
Jenkins et al.[51]	12/10	33/70	0/30	33/20
Bagarani et al.[52]	25/24	32/67	NR	40/25
Cardona et al.[53]	18/20	56/40	22/50	17/30
Hsia et al.[54]	24/22	37/55	29/41	62/63
Saari et al.[55]	22/32	50/66	5/19	36/34
Rodriguez Moreno et al.[56]	16/15	63/40	25/40	19/20
Somatostatin versus terlipressin				
Walker et al.[40]	53/53	83/72	36/24	21/21
Feu et al.[41]	80/81	80/84	30/28	16/16
Somatostatin versus emergency sclerotherapy				
Di Febo et al.[59]	24/33	92/79	NR	21/26
Shields et al.[60]	41/39	83/77	15/21	20/31
Planas et al.[61]	35/35	83/80	17/25	23/29
Somatostatin versus balloon tamponade				
Jaramillo et al.[57]	20/19	50/58	10/16	25/26
Avgerinos et al.[58]	30/31	67/68	47/16	33/23

C, control group; SMT, somatostatin-treated group; NR, not reported.

McKee et al.[65] reported a reduction in portal pressure after octreotide but this has not been confirmed by other authors using similar and even higher doses of octreotide.[66] A recent haemodynamic study showed that octreotide injection caused a marked but very transient reduction in portal pressure, azygos blood flow and glucagon levels, that could not be maintained or prolonged by adding a continuous infusion of octreotide.[66] In addition, the administration of repeated boluses caused significant tachyphylaxis.[66] The effect of octreotide on variceal pressure is also unpredictable, as increases of intra-variceal pressure have been reported.[67]

Similarly, the efficacy of octreotide in variceal haemorrhage has not been assessed adequately so far. Octreotide has been compared with placebo in four RCTs; in three studies, octreotide was administered immediately after performing EIS or banding ligation[68–70] whereas, in the remaining, larger study, EIS was used as a rescue therapy in cases of failure of octreotide or placebo.[71] Failure to control bleeding was reduced by using octreotide only in those studies combining octreotide with endoscopic techniques, suggesting that octreotide may improve the results of endoscopic therapy but has little effect if used alone.

Octreotide has been compared to balloon tamponade,[65] vasopressin,[72] terlipressin[73,74] or sclerotherapy,[75,76] in the treatment of oesophageal variceal bleeding. Although the results of these studies suggested a similar efficacy of octreotide as control therapies, the small sample sizes, different schedules of octreotide treatment, the significant heterogeneity of the results and the unclear end-points of these trials, not in accordance with a recent consensus conference,[8] indicate that there are insufficient data to support the use of octreotide in the treatment of acute variceal bleeding out of the context of RCT.

Conclusions

Pharmacological agents that decrease pressure and blood flow at the oesophageal varices may be used to treat variceal haemorrhage. According to recent consensus conferences, therapy should be aimed not only at arresting the bleeding but also at preventing early rebleeding within the first week of admission, which is a major determinant of prognosis.[8,77]

Pharmacological therapy has the theoretical advantage of allowing specific therapy, without requiring sophisticated equipment, immediately after admission or even prior to arrival at hospital, which may make it optimal as first-line therapy.

Vasopressin infusions should no longer be used unless associated with nitroglycerin (transdermal or intravenous). Terlipressin, which can be administered as a repeated bolus injection every 4 h, is definitely better than vasopressin alone or associated with nitroglycerin. Somatostatin injections followed by a con-tinuous intravenous infusion, are equally effective and are probably safer than terlipressin. These vasoactive drugs achieve an effective control of bleeding (i.e. a bleeding-free period of more than 24 h) in 75–90% of patients. Terlipressin is the only drug that has been shown to improve survival from variceal haemorrhage.

Somatostatin and terlipressin have also been shown to be equally effective as EIS in preventing early rebleeding when administered from 5–7 days following the initial control of bleeding.

Gastric varices

Gastric varices, which are continuous with oesophageal varices (gastro-oesophageal varices) are managed in the same way as oesophageal varices. In isolated gastric varices, drug therapy can be started before or at the same time as endoscopic therapy in order to improve the rate of haemostasis. The initial treatment is endoscopic injection of sclerosants, cyanoacrylate ('super-glue') or thrombin (1000 U/ml). In most studies, the rebleeding rate has been high after endoscopic treatment and TIPS or shunt surgery may be needed for long-term control of variceal bleeding. However, due to the low incidence of bleeding from isolated gastric varices, no definite studies exist.

Additional treatment in patients with bleeding varices

Bacterial infection is common after upper gastrointestinal bleeding in cirrhotic patients and a major cause of morbidity and mortality. All patients presenting with an episode of variceal bleeding should have antibiotic prophylaxis (e.g. norfloxacin 400 mg/12 h for 7 days). Treatment should be initiated to prevent and treat hepatic encephalopathy (see Chapter 14, *Hepatic failure*) which may be precipitated by gastrointestinal haemorrhage in a patient with chronic liver disease.

Pharmacological prevention of variceal rebleeding

Patients surviving an episode of variceal bleeding have a very high risk of rebleeding (63% within 1–2 years) and death (33%) if no further treatment is given.[23] For this reason, experts agree that all patients surviving an episode of acute variceal bleeding should receive active treatment to prevent rebleeding.[8,77]

Many drugs have been shown to reduce portal pressure in man. For practical purposes, only orally administered drugs are suitable for continuous administration. Among them, non-selective β-adrenoreceptor antagonists are the most and, until recently, the only drugs used to prevent rebleeding.

β-Adrenoreceptor antagonists (β-blockers)

Non-selective β-blockers such as propranolol and nadolol reduce portal pressure by lowering the portal and collateral blood flow as a result of both the decrease in cardiac output due to the blockade of cardiac β-1 adrenoceptors, and the splanchnic vasoconstriction due to the blockade of vasodilating β-2 adrenoceptors in the splanchnic vasculature.[78] This explains why cardioselective β-blockers have a lesser portal pressure reducing effect.

Propranolol and nadolol are given orally with doses adjusted for each patient according to clinical tolerance, heart rate and arterial blood pressure. In general, the dose is increased every 2–3 days until the heart rate decreases by 25%, but not below 55 beats/min, while maintaining a systolic blood pressure above 80 mmHg. Once the maintenance dose is reached, it is possible to give the total dose in a single administration of a long-acting preparation.

Contraindications to β-blockers in patients with cirrhosis include chronic obstructive lung disease, asthma psychosis, atrioventricular heart block, aortic valve disease and insulin-dependent diabetes with a past history of hypoglycaemia. Side-effects are reported in about

15% of the patients but severe events are rare. The most frequent complaints are fatigue, shortness of breath and sleep disorders. Although complications from propranolol therapy in cirrhosis have never been lethal, side-effects are important because their appearance may endanger the patient's compliance. Nadolol is easier to administer because of a more prolonged half-life (allowing once a day administration) and renal metabolism, implying easier dosage than that of propranolol. It has also been suggested that nadolol may cause fewer central effects than propranolol because of its inability to cross the blood–brain barrier; however, this has not yet been demonstrated.

Twelve RCTs, including a total of 809 patients, evaluating β-blockers versus placebo or non-active treatment have been reported.[79–90] Propranolol was assessed in 11 studies and nadolol in one; none was double-blind. Overall, β-blockers significantly reduce the risk of recurrent bleeding (from 63% in controls to 42%) and improve survival.[23] No patient had a fatal complication from treatment with β-blockers.

β-Blockers have been compared with long-term EIS in 10 RCTs including a total of 862 patients.[91–100] Although the therapeutic protocols, and consequently the results, were highly heterogeneous, the pooled data show no significant differences between the two treatments in either the rebleeding rate or mortality.[23] Side-effects were significantly less frequent and severe with β-blockers.

β-Blockers have also been used in combination with sclerotherapy to reduce the risk of rebleeding. Ten RCTs have compared EIS with the combination of EIS and β-blockers[23] and three have compared β-blockers alone with the association of EIS and β-blockers.[101–103] Overall, the rebleeding rate was significantly lower with the combination therapy without differences in mortality.[23] These results suggest that patients rebleeding on β-blockers or EIS might benefit from the combination of the two treatments.

A major inconvenience of non-selective β-blocker therapy is that over 60% of the patients do not obtain an adequate fall in portal pressure (a fall which adequately protects from rebleeding) despite adequate β-blockade.[104] Haemodynamic studies have demonstrated that to significantly reduce the risk of rebleeding, hepatic venous pressure gradient (HVPG) must decrease by more than 20% from baseline or below 12 mmHg.[104] Thus, there is a wide individual and clinically unpredictable variation in the reduction of portal pressure achieved with β-blockers. This makes it advisable to measure HVPG before and 1–3 months after achieving the final dose of propranolol or nadolol.

In order to improve the results of β-blockers, alternative therapies causing effective reductions in HVPG in a greater proportion of patients must be developed. This is the rationale for looking for new, powerful agents, that alone or in combination with β-blockers, may enhance the portal pressure reduction and decrease the number of non-responder patients.

Long-acting nitrovasodilators

Vasodilators reduce portal pressure by decreasing the vascular resistance to portal-collateral blood flow, and also, by promoting reflex splanchnic vasoconstriction as a response to reduced mean arterial pressure.[105] An advantage of vasodilators over β-blockers is that the former may allow portal pressure to be reduced without further impairing liver perfusion.

Nitrovasodilators used in the treatment of portal hypertension include isosorbide dinitrate and isosorbide 5-mononitrate. Both have been shown to markedly reduce HVPG in acute administration but significantly less after chronic administration, probably because of the development of partial tolerance.[106] Isosorbide-5-mononitrate, unlike isosorbide dinitrate, has minimal first-pass metabolism, which facilitates its dosage in patients with liver failure and portosystemic shunting. Indeed, this is the only vasodilator that has been evaluated for the prevention of variceal haemorrhage in a RCT.

The major concern with the use of vasodilators in patients with advanced cirrhosis is that, because of the reduction in arterial pressure, they may promote the activation of endogenous vasoactive systems, leading to water and sodium retention and, probably, to the worsening of renal function in patients with ascites.[107] Recent studies, however, have shown that long-term treatment with isosorbide-5-mononitrate is safe in compensated cirrhotic patients, without affecting renal function or sodium handling.

No study has evaluated the efficacy of isolated treatment with nitrovasodilators in the prevention of variceal rebleeding in cirrhotic patients.

Combination therapy: β-blockers combined with isosorbide-5-mononitrate

Haemodynamic studies have shown that the combination of isosorbide-5-mononitrate with β-blockers achieves greater reductions in portal pressure than propranolol alone.[108] This is the rationale for comparing the isolated treatment with β-blockers with the combined therapy. Two RCTs reported in abstract included 199 patients and compared β-blockers plus isosorbide-5-mononitrate with β-blockers alone and failed to show any benefit from the combination therapy.[109,110] Nevertheless, the inconsistency of the results does not allow definite conclusions to be made.

The combination treatment has been compared with EIS in one RCT[111] and with banding ligation in two others.[112,113] The rebleeding rate was reduced with the combination therapy (25% versus 50% with endoscopic treatment). This reduction was statistically significant compared with EIS and nearly significant with banding ligation. In addition, combined treatment has fewer complications related to therapy than EIS.[23]

Finally, propranolol plus isosorbide-5-mononitrate was found to be equally effective as shunt-surgery in good surgical risk patients[114] but less effective than TIPS in patients with advanced cirrhosis, although in the latter the extremely high risk of hepatic encephalopathy following TIPS precludes the use of this technique as a first therapeutic option.[115] All of these studies strongly suggest that the combination of β-blockers with isosorbide-5-mononitrate represents the most effective pharmacological treatment for the prevention of variceal rebleeding evaluated so far.

Conclusions

In summary, non-selective β-blockers significantly reduce the risk of variceal rebleeding and mortality. In addition, they are equivalent to EIS with fewer frequent side-effects. Combined treatment with β-blockers and EIS is superior to therapy alone, whereas the association of β-blockers with isosorbide-5-mononitrate is superior to endoscopic therapy.

These results suggest that patients surviving an episode of variceal bleeding should be treated with non-selective β-blockers. In case of contraindications or intolerance to β-blockers, patients should be treated with endoscopic therapy. Assessment of HVPG response during pharmacological therapy would be well advised.

Finally, further clinical studies with other drugs achieving greater reductions in portal pressure than β-blockers, associated or not with nitrovasodilators, are warranted.

Pharmacological prevention of first variceal bleeding

All cirrhotic patients with gastroesophageal varices are at risk of acute variceal bleeding. This risk is related to the tension exerted on the variceal wall (depending on portal pressure, variceal size and variceal wall thickness) and with the degree of liver failure. In this sense, a consensus has been reached on the need to treat all patients with large varices.[8,77]

Owing to its efficacy and lack of severe side-effects, pharmacological therapy is the established therapy for the prevention of first bleeding. Although other pharmacological options have been tested, non-selective β-blockers are the recommended drugs.

Non-selective β-blockers
Meta-analysis of the 11 published RCTs comparing β-blockers with non-active treatment and including a total of 1189 patients, shows that β-blockers significantly reduce the risk of variceal bleeding and reduce mortality.[23] The beneficial effect of β-blockers was found in all cirrhotic patients regardless of the presence of ascites and variceal size.[116] Unfortunately, contraindications or intolerance to treatment appeared in 15–20% of the patients, limiting the applicability of the therapy.

Long-acting nitrovasodilators (isosorbide-5-mononitrate)
One randomized study compared isosorbide-5-mononitrate with propranolol in the prevention of first bleeding.[117] Both were found to be equally effective. However, after long-term follow-up (7 years), there was an increased mortality in patients over 50 years of age receiving vasodilators.[117] Although this point needs further clarification, the results suggest that isosorbide-5-mononitrate should be reserved for patients with contraindications or intolerance to β-blockers.

Combination therapy: β-blockers combined with isosorbide-5-mononitrate
Three studies including a total of 552 have been reported comparing the efficacy of β-blockers with that of β-blockers plus isosorbide-5-mononitrate.[118–120] Overall, both treatments resulted in a remarkably low bleeding rate (15% in patients receiving β-blockers versus 10% in those receiving combined therapy) with no differences in mortality. Side-effects were more frequent in the combination therapy group.[23]

Conclusions
According to these results, we can recommend treatment in all patients with medium to large varices with β-blockers. Where there is a contraindication or intolerance to β-blockers, patients may be treated with isosorbide-5-mononitrate while strictly monitoring liver and renal function. Up to now, there is no evidence supporting the use of combined therapy in this situation.

Pharmacological treatment of portal hypertensive gastropathy

Portal hypertensive gastropathy (PHG) consists of a wide-spectrum of diffuse macroscopic lesions in the gastric mucosa of patients with portal hypertension. These lesions are classified as mild (mosaic-like pattern) or severe (diffuse cherry red spots) according to the endoscopic appearance. Clinically, PHG causes acute or chronic blood loss in 60–90% of patients with severe lesions.[121]

PHG is thought to be caused by a gastric venous congestion caused by an increase in both portal pressure and gastric blood flow. Therefore, drugs causing splanchnic vasoconstriction (and consequently decreasing portal pressure) may be of potential use in the treatment of this complication. In this sense, preliminary studies have demonstrated that intravenous administration of vasopressin, terlipressin or somatostatin are effective in the reduction of gastric blood flow in PHG patients;[121] however, no clinical data are available. Propranolol is the only pharmacological therapy that has been proven useful to prevent rebleeding from PHG;[122] however, despite propranolol, 50% of cirrhotic patients will develop rebleeding from PHG within 2 years of follow-up.[122] In these cases, endoscopic photo- or electrocoagulation (if lesions are confined to a restricted area of the stomach) or more aggressive approaches (such as TIPS or liver transplant) may be useful.

Pharmacological treatment of ascites

The aim of medical treatment of ascites is to remove the intrabdominal fluid by causing a negative sodium balance. In a few patients, this can be achieved by bed rest and reduced dietary sodium intake (40 mmol/day), whereas the remaining patients (more than 80%) need diuretic therapy in order to treat ascites.

In addition to their effects in removing ascites, a low sodium diet and diuretic therapy (spironolactone) have the advantage of reducing portal pressure, probably by preventing the development of plasma volume expansion, which characterizes portal hypertension.[123]

Diuretics

Spironolactone (a distal tubular-acting agent) and furosemide (a loop diuretic) are the most commonly used diuretics in the treatment of ascites. Spironolactone is a competitive aldosterone antagonist that can be administered alone or in combination with furosemide at a dose from 50–400 mg/day once daily. Furosemide acts by inhibiting the Na^+–K^+–$2Cl^-$ co-transporter in the loop of Henle; its dose ranges from 20–160 mg/day (in two doses).

From a pragmatic point of view, diuretic treatment usually begins with spironolactone. The addition of furosemide and the progressive increase in the dose of diuretics depend on the patient's response, which should be monitored by measuring body weight, urine volume and sodium excretion regularly.

Unfortunately, 10% of the patients with ascites develop refractory ascites either because of a lack of response to diuretic therapy or diuretic-induced complications precluding its use.[124] In this subgroup of patients, alternative therapies such as therapeutic paracentesis, peritoneovenous shunting or portosystemic shunts should be considered.

Common complications of diuretic therapy in cirrhotic patients include electrolyte disturbances (mainly hyponatraemia and hyperkalaemia), hepatic encephalopathy, renal impairment, gynaecomastia (with spironolactone) and muscle cramps.

Pharmacological treatment of hepatorenal syndrome

Hepatorenal syndrome (HRS) is a serious complication that results from extreme, functional vasoconstriction of the kidneys. Two types of HRS may be found:

1. Type I: characterized by a rapid progression of renal and hepatic failure leading to death within a few days or weeks

2. Type II: characterized by a moderate, steady impairment of renal function, which allows the patient to be included in a liver transplantation programme.[125]

Owing to its poor, rapid prognosis, considerable effort has been made to treat Type I HRS.

From a theoretical point of view, it can be treated by correcting the mechanisms leading to active renal vasoconstriction (i.e. increased activity of endogenous vasoconstrictor systems as a response to systemic vasodilatation and imbalance in the intrarenal synthesis of vasoconstrictors/vasodilators). Among the numerous treatments assessed, intravenous administration of vasoconstrictors (mainly vasopressin derivatives) associated with plasma volume expansion (preferably intravenous albumin) and TIPS are the most promising. Improvement in renal function associated with a trend to normalize the overactivated endogenous vasoconstrictor systems has been described with both therapies.[125] Therefore, the results of ongoing clinical trials will be of great interest.

Pharmacological treatment of spontaneous bacterial peritonitis

Spontaneous bacterial peritonitis (SBP) is a frequent bacterial infection complicating cirrhosis with ascites, which is defined as 'the infection of a previously sterile ascitic fluid'. Once diagnosis is confirmed (a polymorphonuclear cell count in ascitic fluid higher than 250 cells/mm^3),[126] empirical treatment should be started.

In clinical practice, cefotaxime, a third-generation cephalosporin, is considered the first-choice antibiotic therapy owing to its broad-spectrum covering the most common isolated organisms in SBP (Gram-negative bacilli) without causing adverse effects. Actually, cefotaxime is more effective than ampicillin plus tobramycin, with a negligible incidence of nephrotoxicity or superinfections.[127] The usual scheme of administration of cefotaxime is 2 g every 6 h for 5 days, although lower doses (2 g/12 h) have shown similar efficacy in the treatment of SBP (with a resolution rate of over 90% of the cases).[127]

Other parenteral antibiotics such as ceftriaxone, cefonicid or amoxycillin associated with clavulanic acid, have shown a similar efficacy to cefotaxime in treating SBP, although the small number of patients evaluated precludes definite conclusions.

A recent large study in patients with SBP without serious complications (i.e. no septic shock, ileus or serum creatinine level over 3 mg/dl), has demonstrated that, in this special subgroup of patients, oral administration of ofloxacin (a wide-spectrum quinolone) at a dose of 400 mg every 12 h is equally effective as intravenous cefotaxime in treating SBP.[128] Further studies are needed to confirm the potential role of oral antibiotics in the treatment of SBP.

Pharmacological prophylaxis of spontaneous bacterial peritonitis

Spontaneous bacterial peritonitis (SBP) is thought to be the result of the passage of intestinal bacteria into the general circulation and then into ascitic fluid, in otherwise immunocompromised patients. This is the rationale for using selective intestinal decontamination (SID) in patients with a high risk of developing SBP, namely:

- Cirrhotic patients with gastrointestinal haemorrhage
- Patients with low ascitic fluid total protein concentration
- Those recovering from an episode of SBP[127]

SID is the elimination of aerobic Gram-negative bacilli from the intestinal flora while preserving the remaining aerobic and anaerobic bacteria. This is achieved by the administration of oral non- or poorly absorbable antibiotic, the most commonly used being norfloxacin. In fact, norfloxacin (400 mg/day orally) dramatically reduces the incidence of SBP in all the subgroups of patients at risk of developing this complication.[127]

Initial hypotheses claiming for a potential development of bacterial resistance during long-term administration of quinolones have not been confirmed. Furthermore, patients developing SBP while on SID with quinolones should receive the same empirical approach as those not on SID. This is so because cefotaxime is also highly effective against most of the Gram-positive and Gram-negative organisms causing SBP in patients receiving quinolones.[129]

Pharmacology of drugs

Vasopressin
Mode of action
Vasopressin constricts mesenteric arterioles and decreases portal venous inflow, thereby reducing portal pressure.

Indications
Bleeding oesophageal and gastro-oesophageal are indications for treatment, always in association with nitroglycerin.

Preparations/dose
A 0.4 U bolus followed by 0.4–1.0 U/min is given as an intravenous infusion in combination with intravenous nitroglycerin (10–50 μg/min).

Dynamics/kinetics
Most of drug metabolized by the liver and kidney. Half-life 15–20 min.

Adverse reactions
Side-effects occur in up to 45% of patients. Extrasplanchnic vasoconstrictions may lead to myocardial, cerebral and intestinal ischaemia. Side-effects include pallor, nausea, belching, colicky abdominal pain, desire to defaecate, angina and myocardial ischaemia. Rarely, water intoxication and allergic reactions. Concurrent administration of nitroglycerin accentuates the portal hypotensive actions of vasopressin while reducing its systemic vasoconstrictor effects.

Precautions and contraindications
Caution should be exercised in patients with heart failure, asthma, epilepsy, migraine and renal impairment.

Contraindications include vascular disease—especially of the coronary arteries. No adequate studies have yielded results to guide its use in pregnant patients.

Terlipressin
Terlipressin is a synthetic analogue of vasopressin (triglycyl lysine vasopressin) with fewer side-effects and a longer biological half-life. Infrequent side-effects include abdominal cramps, headache and increase in arterial blood pressure. The dose is 2 mg over 1 min given intravenously followed by 1–2 mg every 4 h until bleeding is controlled for 24–48 h.

β-Blockers
Indications
These are:

- Primary and secondary prophylaxis of variceal bleeding
- Prevention of bleeding from portal hypertensive gastropathy

Mode of action
Non-selective β-blockers block adrenergic dilatory tone in mesenteric vessels resulting in unopposed α-adrenergic-mediated vasoconstriction and therefore a decrease in portal inflow and variceal pressure.

Preparations/dose
Oral propranolol 40 mg is given twice daily, increasing to a dose of 160 mg twice daily if necessary. Oral nadolol is given, 40 mg daily, increasing to 160 mg daily if necessary.

Dynamics/kinetics
- Propranolol: its onset of action is 1 h; its duration of action is 6 h and there is extensive first-pass metabolism in the liver to inactive and active metabolites; 99% is excreted in the urine
- Nadolol: its duration of effect is 24 h; it is excreted unchanged in the urine

Adverse reactions

These include bradycardia, myocardial depression and heart failure, hypotension, conduction defects, bronchospasm, peripheral vasoconstriction, gastrointestinal disturbances, fatigue, sleep disturbance, skin rash, and impotence; β-blockers may mask the symptoms of hypoglycaemia in diabetic patients.

Precautions and contraindications

In renal failure, 50% of the normal dose of nadolol should be given with moderate renal failure, 25% of the dose with severe renal failure. In pregnancy β-blockers may cause intrauterine growth retardation, neonatal hypoglycaemia and bradycardia. A small amount is excreted in breast milk; β-blockade is, however, considered compatible with breastfeeding but monitor infant for signs of β-blockade.

Contraindications include uncontrolled heart failure, asthma, chronic obstructive airways disease, marked bradycardia, sick-sinus syndrome.

Drug interactions

A decreased effect of β-blockers is seen with cholestyramine, NSAIDs and rifampicin. Increased effect/toxicity of β-blockers is seen with calcium-channel blockers, flecanide, haloperidol, cimetidine (propranolol), diuretics, phenothiazines and ciprofloxacin. β-Blockers may increase effect/toxicity of flecanide, amiodarone, calcium-channel blockers, cardiac glycosides, haloperidol, phenothiazines, warfarin, benzodiazepines and ACE inhibitors.

Isosorbide mononitrate
Mode of action

This drug decreases the vascular resistance to portal collateral blood flow.

Indications

It is used to prevent first variceal bleeding.

Precautions

One should always avoid abrupt withdrawal because of a rebound in portal and variceal pressure leading to variceal bleeding in myasthenia gravis and diabetes mellitus.

Preparations/dose

Oral isosorbide mononitrate 20 mg is given twice daily, which is increased up to 40 mg twice daily.

Dynamics/kinetics

Its onset of action is within 10–30 min; its half-life being 5–10 h; it is excreted via the kidneys.

Adverse reactions

Headache, flushing, dizziness, postural hypotension, palpitations, abdominal pain, diarrhoea, methaemoglobinaemia (rarely with high doses), renal failure (except when associated to β-blockers) are adverse reactions.

Drug interactions

With concomitant use with sildenafil, the hypotensive effect is enhanced, so avoid concomitant use.

Contraindications

Hypersensitivity to nitrates, hypertrophic obstructive cardiomyopathy, aortic stenosis, mitral stenosis, and closed-angle glaucoma are contraindications for treatment.

Somatostatin
Mode of action

Somatostatin inhibits the release of vasodilator hormones such as glucagon, indirectly causing splanchnic vasoconstriction and decreased portal inflow.

Indications

Bleeding gastro-oesophageal varices are indications for treatment.

Preparations/dose

A 250 μg bolus is followed by 250 μg/h, given by intravenous infusion, for 5 days.

Octreotide
Mode of action

Octreotide is a long-acting analogue of natural somatostatin.

Indications

Bleeding gastro-oesophageal varices as concomitant treatment in patients receiving endoscopic therapy are indications for treatment.

Preparations/dose

For bleeding gastro-oesophageal varices give 50 μg bolus followed by 50 μg/h by intravenous infusion for 5 days.

Dynamics/kinetics

Its duration of action is 6–12 h after subcutaneous injection. There is rapid absorption after subcutaneous administration, with 100% bioavailability. There is extensive hepatic metabolism, and approximately 30% excreted by the kidney.

Adverse reactions

Anorexia, nausea, vomiting, abdominal pain and bloating, diarrhoea, fat malabsorption, gallstones after long-term treatment, hyper- or hypoglycaemia, skin flushing, dizziness and drowsiness are adverse reactions. Pain and irritation may occur at the subcutaneous injection site and sites should be rotated. Injections should be given between meals to minimize gastrointestinal side-effects.

Drug interactions

Absorption of cyclosporin is reduced (decreased plasma concentrations) with concomitant octreotide. In diabetes mellitus, octreotide possibly reduces insulin and antidiabetic drug requirements.

Precautions and contraindications

During pregnancy avoid if possible since there is a possible effect on fetal growth. During breastfeeding, avoid unless it is essential; however, no information is available regarding presence in breast milk.

Spironolactone

Mode of action

Spironolactone competes with aldosterone for receptor sites in the distal renal tubule, increasing sodium chloride and water excretion, while conserving potassium and hydrogen ions.

Indications

Management of ascites and oedema associated with cirrhosis of the liver are indications for treatment.

Preparations/dose

Tablets and oral suspension, 100 mg, are given in the morning; the dose may be increased to a maximum of 400 mg daily.

Dynamics/kinetics

Spironolactone is 90–98% protein bound, metabolized in the liver to multiple metabolites, and has urinary and biliary excretion.

Adverse reactions

Gastrointestinal disturbances, painful gynaecomastia, impotence, increased hair growth and deepening of voice in females, menstrual irregularities, headache, rashes, confusion, hyperkalaemia and hyponatraemia are adverse effects.

Drug interactions

These comprise:

- Increased risk of hyperkalaemia with: potassium, potassium-sparing diuretics, indomethacin and possibly other NSAIDs, cyclosporin and angiotensin converting enzyme inhibitors may increase serum potassium levels
- NSAIDs antagonize diuretic effect
- Lithium excretion is reduced by spironolactone (increased plasma lithium and risk of toxicity)

Precautions/contraindications

These include:

- Hyperkalaemic patients or those receiving other potassium-sparing diuretics or potassium supplements
- Renal failure: owing to an increased risk of hyperkalaemia, avoid in moderate to severe renal failure
- Pregnancy: avoid this drug since there was toxicity in animal studies

Frusemide

Mode of action

Inhibits the $Na^+/K^+/2Cl^-$ co-transporter in the ascending loop of Henlé and distal renal tubule, thus inhibiting reabsorption of sodium and chloride.

Indications

Management of ascites and oedema associated with cirrhosis of the liver are indicators for treatment.

Preparations/dose

Tablets or solution are given by mouth: a dose of 40 mg in the morning, may be increased to a maximum of 160 mg daily.

Dynamics/kinetics after oral dosing

Its onset of action is within 1 h; its peak effect within 1–2 h; its duration of action: 6–8 h; its half-life is about 1 h (up to 9 h in severe renal impairment). Elimination is 50–80% excreted in the urine within 24 h, the remainder is metabolized in the liver.

Adverse reactions

Electrolyte imbalance (hyponatraemia, hypokalaemia, hypomagnesaemia, hypochloraemic alkalosis, increased calcium excretion, hyperuricaemia and gout), hyperglycaemia, orthostatic hypotension, dizziness, diarrhoea, loss of appetite and adverse reactions. Rarely: prerenal renal failure, photosensitivity, pancreatitis, tinnitus, deafness, bone marrow depression, hepatotoxicity and interstitial nephritis occur.

Drug interactions

These comprise:

- Antiarrhythmic drugs: risk of cardiac toxicity increased if hypokalaemia occurs
- Antihistamines: increased risk of ventricular arrhythmias if hypokalaemia occurs
- Halofantrine: increased risk of ventricular arrhythmias if hypokalaemia occurs
- Pimozide: increased risk of ventricular arrhythmias if hypokalaemia occurs

- Cardiac glycosides: increased toxicity if hypokalaemia occurs
- Furosemide increases ototoxicity of aminoglycosides, colistin and vancomycin
- Antidiabetics: hypoglycaemic effect is antagonized by frusemide
- NSAIDs antagonize the diuretic effect
- Lithium excretion is reduced by frusemide (increased plasma lithium and risk of toxicity)

Precautions/contraindications

In renal failure higher doses may be needed. Avoid in pregnancy. The amounts excreted in breast milk are too small to be harmful.

REFERENCES

1. Groszmann RJ, Atterbury CE. Portal hypertension: classification and pathogenesis. Semin Liver Dis 1982; **2:** 177–186.
2. Folkow B, Neil E (Eds). *Circulation*. Oxford University Press, London, 1971, 14–19.
3. Groszmann RJ. The pathophysiological basis of therapy in portal hypertension and ascites: an overview. In: *Therapy in Liver Diseases*. V Arroyo, J Bosch, M Bruguera, J Rodés (Eds), Masson, Barcelona, 1997, 13–20.
4. Schrier RW, Martin PY. Sodium and water retention in chronic liver diseases: causes and consequences. In: *Therapy in Liver Diseases*. V Arroyo, J Bosch, M Bruguera, J Rodés (Eds), Masson, Barcelona, 1997, 63–70.
5. Pagliaro L, D'Amico G, Pasta L, *et al.* Portal hypertension in cirrhosis: natural history. In: *Portal Hypertension: Pathophysiology and Treatment*. J Bosch, RJ Groszmann (Eds), Blackwell, Oxford, 1992, 72–92.
6. Graham DY, Smith JL. The course of patients after variceal hemorrhage. *Gastroenterology* 1981; **80:** 800–809.
7. Bosch J, D'Amico G, Luca A, García-Pagán JC, Feu F, Escorsell A. Drug therapy for variceal hemorrhage. In: *Portal Hypertension: Pathophysiology and Treatment*. J Bosch, RJ Groszmann (Eds), Blackwell, Oxford, 1992, 108–123.
8. Grace ND, Groszmann RJ, García-Tsao G, *et al.* Portal hypertension and variceal bleeding: an

AASLD single topic symposium. *Hepatology* 1998; **28:** 868–880.

9. Bosch J. Effect of pharmacological agents on portal hypertension: a haemodynamical appraisal. *Clin Gastroenterol* 1985; **14:** 169–183.

10. Bosch J, Bordas JM, Mastai R, *et al*. Effects of vasopressin on the intravariceal pressure in patients with cirrhosis: comparison with the effects on portal pressure. *Hepatology* 1988; **8:** 861–865.

11. Merigan TC, Plotkin GR, Davidson CS. Effect of intravenously administered posterior pituitary extract on hemorrhage from bleeding esophageal varices. *N Eng J Med* 1962; **266:** 134–135.

12. Conn HO, Ramsby GR, Storer EH, *et al*. Intra-arterial vasopressin in the treatment of upper gastrointestinal hemorrhage: a prospective controlled clinical trial. *Gastroenterology* 1975; **68:** 211–221.

13. Mallory A, Schaefer JW, Cohen JR, Holt AS, Norton LW. Selective intra-arterial vasopressin infusion for upper gastrointestinal tract hemorrhage. A controlled trial. *Arch Surg* 1980; **115:** 30–32.

14. Fogel RM, Knauer MC, Andres LL, *et al*. Continuous intravenous vasopressin in active upper gastrointestinal bleeding. A placebo-controlled trial. *Ann Intern Med* 1982; **96:** 565–569.

15. Groszmann RJ, Kravetz D, Bosch J, *et al*. Nitroglycerin improves the haemodynamic response to vasopressin in portal hypertension. *Hepatology* 1982; **2:** 757–762.

16. Johnson WC, Widrich WC, Ansell JE, Robbins AH, Nabseth DC. Control of bleeding varices by vasopressin: a prospective randomized study. *Ann Surg* 1977; **186:** 369–376.

17. Clanet J, Tournet R, Fourtanier G, Joncquiert F, Pascal JP. Traitement pour la pitressin des hémorragies pour rupture de varices oesophagiennes chez le cirrhotique. Etude contrôlée. *Acta Gastroenterol Belg* 1978; **41:** 539–543.

18. Chojkier M, Groszmann RJ, Atterbury CE, *et al*. A controlled comparison of continuous intra-arterial and intravenous infusion of vasopressin in hemorrhage from esophageal varices. *Gastroenterology* 1979; **77:** 540–546.

19. Tsai YT, Lay CS, Lai KH, *et al*. Controlled trial of vasopressin plus nitroglycerin vs vasopressin alone in the treatment of bleeding esophageal varices. *Hepatology* 1986; **6:** 406–409.

20. Gimson AES, Westaby D, Hegarty J, Alastair W, Williams R. A randomized trial of vasopressin plus nitroglycerin in the control of acute variceal hemorrhage. *Hepatology* 1986; **6:** 410–413.

21. Bosch J, Groszmann RJ, García-Pagán JC, *et al*. Association of transdermal nitroglycerin to vasopressin infusion in the treatment of variceal hemorrhage: a placebo-controlled clinical trial. *Hepatology* 1989; **10:** 962–968.

22. Blei AT. Vasopressin analogs in portal hypertension: different molecules but similar questions. *Hepatology* 1986; **6:** 146–147.

23. D'Amico G, Pagliaro L, Bosch J. Pharmacological treatment of portal hypertension. An evidence-based approach. *Semin Liver Dis* 1999; **19:** 475–506.

24. Soderlund C, Ihre T. Endoscopic sclerotherapy vs conservative management of bleeding esophageal varices. *Acta Chir Scand* 1985; **151:** 449–456.

25. Larson AW, Cohen H, Zwieiban B, *et al*. Acute esophageal variceal sclerotherapy. *J Am Med Assoc* 1986; **255:** 497–500.

26. El-Zayadi A, El-Din S, Kabil M. Endoscopic sclerotherapy versus medical treatment for bleeding esophageal varices in patients with schistosomal liver disease. *Gastrointest Endosc* 1988; **34:** 314–317.

27. Westaby D, Hayes P, Gimson AES, Polson R, Williams R. Controlled clinical trial of injection sclerotherapy for active variceal bleeding. *Hepatology* 1989; **9:** 274–277.

28. Alexandrino P, Alves MM, Fidalgo P, *et al*. Is sclerotherapy the first choice treatment for active oesophageal variceal bleeding in cirrhotic patients? Final report of a randomized clinical trial. *J Hepatol* 1990; **11 (Suppl.):** S1.

29. Walker S, Stiehl A, Raedsch R, Kommerell B. Terlipressin in bleeding esophageal varices. A placebo controlled double-blind study. *Hepatology* 1986; **6:** 112–115.

30. Freeman JG, Cobden MD, Record CO. Placebo-controlled trial of terlipressin (glypressin) in the management of acute variceal bleeding. *J Clin Gastroenterol* 1989; **11:** 58–60.

31. Soderlund C, Magnusson I, Torngren S, Lundell L. Terlipressin (triglycyl-lysine vasopressin) controls acute bleeding oesophageal varices. A double-blind, randomized, placebo-controlled trial. *Scand J Gastroenterol* 1990; **25:** 622–630.

32. Freeman JG, Cobden I, Lishman AH, Record CO. Controlled trial of terlipressin (glypressin)

versus vasopressin in the early treatment of esophageal varices. *Lancet* 1982; **2:** 66–68.

33. Desaint B, Florent C, Levy VG. A randomized trial of triglycyl-lysine vasopressin versus lysine vasopressin in active cirrhotic variceal hemorrhage. In: *Vasopressin Analogs and Portal Hypertension.* D Lebrec, AT Blei (Eds), John Libbey Eurotext, Paris, 1987, 155–157.

34. Lee YF, Tsay YT, Lai KH, *et al*. A randomized controlled study of triglycyl-vasopressin and vasopressin plus nitroglycerin in the control of acute esophageal variceal hemorrhage. *Chinese J Gastroenterol* 1988; **5:** 131–138.

35. Chiu WK, Sheen IS, Liaw YF. A controlled study of glypressin versus vasopressin in the control of bleeding from esophageal varices. *J Gastroenterol Hepatol* 1990; **5:** 549–553.

36. D'Amico G, Traina M, Vizzini G, *et al*. Terlipressin or vasopressin plus transdermal nitroglycerin in a treatment strategy for digestive bleeding in cirrhosis. A randomized clinical trial. *J Hepatol* 1994; **20:** 206–212.

37. Cooperative Spanish-French Group for the Treatment of Bleeding Esophageal Varices. Randomized controlled trial comparing terlipressin vs endoscopic injection sclerotherapy in the treatment of acute variceal bleeding and prevention of early rebleeding. *Hepatology* 1997; **26 (Suppl.):** 249A.

38. Colin R, Giuli N, Czernichow P, Ducrotte P, Lerebours E. Prospective comparison of glypressin, tamponade and their association in the treatment of bleeding esophageal varices. In: *Vasopressin Analogs and Portal Hypertension.* D Lebrec, AT Blei (Eds), John Libbey Eurotext, Paris, 1987, 149–153.

39. Fort E, Sautereau D, Silvaine C, Ingrand P, Pillegand B, Beauchant M. A randomized trial of terlipressin plus nitroglycerin vs balloon tamponade in the control of acute variceal hemorrhage. *Hepatology* 1990; **11:** 678–681.

40. Walker S, Kreichgauer HP, Bode JC. Terlipressin vs somatostatin in bleeding esophageal varices: a controlled double blind study. *Hepatology* 1992; **15:** 1023–1030.

41. Feu F, Ruiz del Arbol L, Bañares R, Planas R, Bosch J and Members of Variceal Bleeding Study Group. Double-blind randomized controlled trial comparing terlipressin and somatostatin in the treatment of acute variceal hemorrhage in patients with cirrhosis. *Gastroenterology* 1996; **111:** 1291–1299.

42. Bosch J, Kravetz D, Rodes J. Effects of somatostatin on hepatic and systemic haemodynamics in patients with cirrhosis of the liver: comparison with vasopressin. *Gastroenterology* 1981; **80:** 518–525.

43. Kravetz D, Bosch J, Arderiu MT, *et al*. Effects of somatostatin on splanchnic haemodynamics and plasma glucagon in portal hypertensive rats. *Am J Physiol* 1988; **254:** G322–G328.

44. Cirera I, Feu F, Luca A, *et al*. Effects of bolus injections and continuous infusions of somatostatin and placebo in patients with cirrhosis: a double-blind haemodynamic investigation. *Hepatology* 1995; **22:** 106–111.

45. Escorsell A, Bordas JM, Ruiz del Arbol L, *et al*. Randomized controlled trial of sclerotherapy versus somatostatin infusion in the prevention of early rebleeding following acute variceal hemorrhage in patients with cirrhosis. *J Hepatol* 1998; **29:** 779–788.

46. Valenzuela JE, Schubert T, Fogel MR, *et al*. A multicentre, randomised, double-blind trial of somatostatin in the management of acute hemorrhage from esophageal varices. *Hepatology* 1989; **10:** 958–961.

47. Burroughs AK, McCormick PA, Hughes MD, Sprengers D, D'Heygere F, McIntyre N. Randomized, double-blind, placebo-controlled trial of somatostatin for variceal bleeding. Emergency control and prevention of early variceal rebleeding. *Gastroenterology* 1990; **99:** 1388–1395.

48. Loperfido S, Godena F, Tosolini G, *et al*. La somatostatina nel trattamento dell'emorragia da varici esofago-gastriche. *Recent Prog Med* 1987; **78:** 82–86.

49. Testoni PA, Masci E, Passaretti S, *et al*. Comparison of somatostatin and cimetidine in the treatment of acute esophageal variceal bleeding. *Curr Ther Res* 1986; **39:** 759–766.

50. Kravetz D, Bosch J, Terés J, Bruix J, Rimola A, Rodés J. Comparison of intravenous somatostatin and vasopressin infusion in treatment of acute variceal hemorrhage. *Hepatology* 1984; **4:** 442–446.

51. Jenkins SA, Baxter JN, Corbett WA, Devitt P, Ware J, Shields R. A prospective randomized controlled clinical trial comparing somatostatin and vasopressin in controlling acute variceal haemorrhage. *Br Med J* 1985; **290:** 275–278.

52. Bagarani M, Albertini V, Anza M, *et al*. Effect of somatostatin in controlling bleeding from

esophageal varices. *Ital J Surg Sci* 1987; **17:** 21–26.

53. Cardona C, Vida F, Balanzó J, Cussó X, Farré A, Guarner C. Eficacia terapéutica de la somatostatina versus vasopresina más nitroglicerina en la hemorragia activa por varices esofagogástricas. *Gastroenterol Hepatol* 1989; **12:** 30–34.

54. Hsia HC, Lee FY, Tsai YT, *et al.* Comparison of somatostatin and vasopressin in the control of acute esophageal variceal hemorrhage. A randomized, controlled study. *Chinese J Gastroenterol* 1990; **7:** 71–78.

55. Saari A, Klvilaakso E, Inberg M, *et al.* Comparison of somatostatin and vasopressin in bleeding esophageal varices. *Am J Gastroenterol* 1990; **85:** 804–807.

56. Rodríguez-Moreno F, Santolaria F, Glez-Reimers E, *et al.* A randomized trial of somatostatin vs vasopressin plus nitroglycerin in the treatment of acute variceal bleeding. *J Hepatol* 1991; **13(Suppl.):** 162.

57. Jaramillo JL, de la Mata M, Miño G, Costán G, Gómez-Camacho F. Somatostatin versus Sengstaken balloon tamponade for primary haemostasia of bleeding esophageal varices. *J Hepatol* 1991; **12:** 100–105.

58. Avgerinos A, Klonis C, Rekoumis G, Gouma P, Papedimitriou N. Controlled trial of somatostatin and balloon tamponade in bleeding esophageal varices. *J Hepatol* 1991; **13:** 78–83.

59. Di Febo G, Siringo S, Vacirca M, *et al.* Somatostatin and urgent sclerotherapy in active esophageal variceal bleeding. *Gastroenterology* 1990; **98 (Suppl.):** A583.

60. Shields R, Jenkins SA, Baxter JN, *et al.* A prospective randomised controlled trial comparing the efficacy of somatostatin with injection sclerotherapy in the control of oesophageal varices. *J Hepatol* 1992; **16:** 128–137.

61. Planas R, Quer JQ, Boix J, *et al.* A prospective randomized trial comparing somatostatin and sclerotherapy in the treatment of acute variceal bleeding. *Hepatology* 1994; **20:** 370–375.

62. Bosch J, Lebrec D, Jenkins SA. Development of analogues: successes and failures. *Scand J Gastroenterol* 1998; **33 (Suppl.):** 3–13.

63. Jenkins SA, Baxter JN, Corbett WA, Shields R. Effects of a somatostatin analogue SMS 201–995 on hepatic haemodynamics in the pig and on intravariceal pressure in man. *Br J Surg* 1985; **72:** 1009–1012.

64. Eriksson LS, Brundin T, Söderlund C, Wahren J. Haemodynamic effects of a long-acting somatostatin analogue in patients with liver cirrhosis. *Scand J Gastroenterol* 1987; **22:** 919–925.

65. McKee R. A study of octreotide in oesophageal varices. *Digestion* 1990; **45:** 60–65.

66. Escorsell A, Bandi JC, François E, *et al.* Desensitization to the effects of intravenous octreotide in cirrhotic patients with portal hypertension. *Hepatology* 1996; **24(Suppl.):** 207A.

67. Primignani M, Nolte A, Vazzoler MC, *et al.* The effect of octreotide on intraesophageal variceal pressure in liver cirrhosis is unpredictable. *Hepatology* 1990; **12:** 989A.

68. Besson I, Ingrand P, Person B, *et al.* Sclerotherapy with or without octreotide for acute variceal bleeding. *N Eng J Med* 1995; **333:** 555–560.

69. Sung JJ, Chung SCS, Yung MY, *et al.* Prospective randomized study of effect of octreotide on rebleeding from esophageal varices after endoscopic ligation. *Lancet* 1995; **346:** 1666–1669.

70. Signorelli S, Paris B, Negrin F, Bonelli M, Auriemma M. Esophageal varices bleeding: comparison between treatment with sclerotherapy alone vs sclerotherapy plus octreotide. *Hepatology* 1997; **26 (Suppl.):** 137A.

71. Burroughs AK. Double-blind RCT of 5-day octreotide versus placebo, associated with sclerotherapy for trial failures. *Hepatology* 1996; **24 (Suppl.):** 352A.

72. Hwang JS, Lin CH, Chang CF, *et al.* A randomized controlled trial comparing octreotide and vasopressin in the control of acute esophageal variceal bleeding. *J Hepatol* 1992; **16:** 320–325.

73. Campisi C, Padula P, Peressini A, Boccardo F, Biraghi M, Casaccia M. Emorragie digestive alte confronto fra terlipressina e octreotide. *Minerva Chir* 1993; **48:** 1–5.

74. Silvain C, Carpentier S, Sautereau D, *et al.* Terlipressin plus transdermal nitroglycerin vs. octreotide in the control of acute bleeding from esophageal varices: a multicenter randomized trial. *Hepatology* 1993; **18:** 61–65.

75. Sung JJ, Chung SCS, Lai CW, Chan FKL, Leung JWC, Yung MY. Octreotide infusion of emergency sclerotherapy for variceal hemmorrhage. *Lancet* 1993; **342:** 637–641.

76. Jenkins SA, Copeland G, Kingsworth A, Shields R. A prospective randomized controlled clinical trial comparing Sandostatin and injection

sclerotherapy in the control of acute variceal haemorrhage: an interine report. *Gut* 1992; **33:** F221.

77. Groszmann RJ, Bendtsen F, Bosch J, *et al*. Baveno II Consensus Statements: Drug therapy for portal hypertension. In: *Portal Hypertension II: Proceedings of the Second Baveno International Consensus Workshop on Definitions, Methodology and Therapeutic Strategies.* De Franchis (Ed.), Blackwell Science, Oxford, 1996, 98–99.

78. Bosch J, Mastai R, Kravetz D, *et al*. Effects of propranolol on azygous venous blood flow and hepatic and systemic haemodynamics in cirrhosis. *Hepatology* 1984; **4:** 1200–1205.

79. Burroughs AK, Jenkins WJ, Sherlock S, *et al*. Controlled trial of propranolol for the prevention of recurrent variceal hemorrhage in patients with cirrhosis. *N Eng J Med* 1983; **309:** 1539–1542.

80. Lebrec D, Poynard T, Bernuau J, *et al*. A randomized controlled study of propranolol for prevention of recurrent gastrointestinal bleeding in patients with cirrhosis: a final report. *Hepatology* 1984; **4:** 355–358.

81. Villeneuve JP, Pomier-Layrargues G, Infante-Rivard C, *et al*. Propranolol for the prevention of recurrent variceal hemorrhage: a controlled trial. *Hepatology* 1986; **6:** 1239–1243.

82. Queuniet AM, Czernichow P, Lerebours E, Ducrotte P, Tranvouez JL, Colin R. Etude controlée du propranolol dans la prévention des récidives hémorragiques chez les patients cirrhotiques. *Gastroenterol Clin Biol* 1987; **11:** 41–47.

83. Gatta A, Merkel C, Sacerdoti D, *et al*. Nadolol for prevention of variceal rebleeding in cirrhosis: a controlled clinical trial. *Digestion* 1987; **37:** 22–28.

84. Colombo M, De Franchis R, Tommasini M, Sangiovanni A, Dioguardi N. Beta-blockade prevents recurrent gastrointestinal bleeding in well-compensated patients with alcoholic cirrhosis: a multicenter randomized controlled trial. *Hepatology* 1989; **9:** 433–438.

85. Sheen IS, Chen TY, Liaw YF. Randomized controlled study of propranolol for the prevention of recurrent esophageal varices bleeding in patients with cirrhosis. *Liver* 1989; **9:** 1–5.

86. Garden OJ, Mills PR, Birnie GG, Murray GD, Carter DC. Propranolol in the prevention of recurrent variceal hemorrhage in cirrhotic patients. *Gastroenterology* 1990; **98:** 185–190.

87. Rossi V, Calès P, Pascal B, *et al*. Prevention of recurrent variceal bleeding in alcoholic cirrhotic patients: prospective controlled trial of propranolol and sclerotherapy. *J Hepatol* 1991; **12:** 283–289.

88. Cerbelaud P, Lavignolle A, Perrin D, *et al*. Propranolol et prevention des recidives de rupture de varice oesophagienne du cirrhotique. *Gastroenterol Clin Biol* 1986; **18:** A10.

89. Colman J, Jones P, Finch C, Dudley F. Propranolol in the prevention of variceal hemorrhage in alcoholic cirrhotic patients. *Hepatology* 1990; **12:** 851A.

90. Kobe E, Schentke KU. Unsichere rezidivprophylaxe von osophagusvarizenblutungen durch propranolol bei leberzirrhotikern: eine prospective kontrollierte studie. *Z Clin Med* 1987; **42:** 507–510.

91. Fleig WE, Stange EF, Hunecke R, *et al*. Prevention of recurrent bleeding in cirrhotics with recent variceal hemorrhage: prospective, randomized comparison of propranolol and sclerotherapy. *Hepatology* 1987; **7:** 355–361.

92. Fleig WE, Stange EF, Schonborn W, *et al*. Propranolol versus endoscopic sclerotherapy for the prevention of recurrent hemorrhage in cirrhosis: final analysis of a randomized clinical trial. *J Hepatol* 1988; **7 (Suppl.):** 32.

93. Dollet JM, Champigneulle B, Patris A, Bigard MA, Gaucher P. Sclerotherapy endoscopique contre propranolol après hèmorrage par rupture de varices oesophagiennes chez le cirrhotique. *Gastroenterol Clin Biol* 1988; **12:** 234–239.

94. Alexandrino PT, Martin Alves M, Pinto Correia J. Propranolol or endoscopic sclerotherapy in the prevention of recurrence of variceal bleeding. A prospective, randomized clinical trial. *J Hepatol* 1988; **7:** 175–185.

95. Westaby D, Polson RJ, Gimson AES, Hayes PC, Hayllar K, Williams R. A controlled trial of oral propranolol compared with injection sclerotherapy for the long-term management of variceal bleeding. *Hepatology* 1990; **11:** 353–359.

96. Liu JD, Jeng YS, Chen PH, Siauw CP, Ko FT, Lin KY. Endoscopic injection sclerotherapy and propranolol in the prevention of recurrent variceal bleeding. *Gastroenterology World Congress Abstract Book* 1990; FP: 1181.

97. Andréani T, Poupon RE, Balkan B, Trinchet JC, Grange JD, Reigney N. Preventive therapy of first gastrointestinal bleeding in patients with cirrhosis: results of a randomized controlled trial comparing propranolol, endoscopic sclerotherapy and placebo. *Hepatology* 1990; **12:** 1413–1419.

98. Martin T, Taupignon A, Lavignolle A, Perrin D, LeBodic L. Prévention des récidives hémorragiques chez des malades atteints de cirrhose. Résultats d'une étude controlé comparant propranolol et sclérose endoscopique. *Gastroenterol Clin Biol* 1991; **15**: 833–837.

99. Dasarathy S, Dwivedi M, Bhargava DK, Sundaram KR, Ramachandran K. A prospective randomized trial comparing repeated endoscopic sclerotherapy and propranolol in decompensated (Child class B and C) cirrhotic patients. *Hepatology* 1992; **16**: 89–94.

100. Terés J, Bosch J, García-Pagán JC, Feu F, Cirera I, Rodés J. Propranolol vs sclerotherapy in the prevention of variceal rebleeding. A randomized controlled trial. *Gastroenterology* 1993; **105**: 1508–1514.

101. O'Connor KW, Lehman G, Yune H, Brunelle R, Christiansen P, Hast J, *et al.* Comparison of three nonsurgical treatments for esophageal varices. *Gastroenterology* 1989; **96**: 899–906.

102. Ink O, Martin T, Poynard T, *et al.* Does elective sclerotherapy improve the efficacy of long-term propranolol for prevention of recurrent bleeding in patients with severe cirrhosis? A prospective multicenter randomized trial. *Hepatology* 1992; **16**: 912–919.

103. Signorelli S, Negrini F, Paris B, Bonelli M, Girola M. Prevention of rebleeding from varices: trial of nadolol compared to nadolol plus sclerotherapy. *J Hepatol* 1996; **25(Suppl.)**: 92.

104. Feu F, García-Pagán JC, Bosch J, *et al.* Relation between portal pressure response to pharmacotherapy and risk of recurrent variceal hemorrhage in patients with cirrhosis. *Lancet* 1995; **346**: 1056–1059.

105. Navasa M, Bosch J, Chesta J, Rodés J. Isosorbide 5-mononitrate reduces hepatic vascular resistance and portal pressure in patients with cirrhosis. *Gastroenterology* 1989; **96**: 1110–1118.

106. García-Pagán JC, Feu F, Navasa M, *et al.* Long-term haemodynamic effects of isosorbide 5-mononitrate in patients with cirrhosis and portal hypertension. *J Hepatol* 1990; **11**: 189–195.

107. Salmeron JM, Ruiz del Arbol L, Ginès A, *et al.* Renal effects of acute isosorbide-5-mononitrate administration in cirrhosis. *Hepatology* 1993; **17**: 800–806.

108. García-Pagán JC, Feu F, Bosch J, Rodés J. Propranolol compared with propranolol plus isosorbide-5-mononitrate for portal hypertension in cirrhosis. A randomized controlled study. *Ann Int Med* 1991; **114**: 869–873.

109. Masilah C, Gournay J, Martin T, Schneo M, Graf E, Perrin D. 5-Mononitrate d'isosorbide associé au propranolol contre propranolol seul après hémorragie par rupture de varices oesophagiennes: un étude randomisée. *Gastroenterol Clin Biol* 1997; **21**: A87.

110. Patti R, D'Amico G, Pasta L, *et al.* Isosorbide mononitrate with nadolol compared to nadolol alone for prevention of recurrent bleeding in cirrhosis. A double-blind placebo controlled randomised trial. *J Hepatol* 1999; **30(Suppl.)**: 81.

111. Villanueva C, Balanzó J, Novella MT, *et al.* Nadolol plus isosorbide-5-mononitrate compared to sclerotherapy for the prevention of variceal rebleeding. *N Eng J Med* 1996; **334**: 1624–1634.

112. Gallego A, Villanueva C, Ortiz J, *et al.* A randomised trial comparing endoscopic ligation with nadolol plus isosorbide-5-mononitrate for the prevention of variceal rebleeding. Preliminary results. *J Hepatol* 1998; **28 (Suppl.)**: 74.

113. Goulis J, Patch D, Greenslade L, Gerunda G, Merkel C, Burroughs AK. RCT of variceal ligation vs propranolol-isosorbide for variceal rebleeding with target pressure reductions: methodological problems. *J Hepatol* 1998; **28 (Suppl.)**: 74.

114. Feu F, McCormick PA, Planas R, Burroughs AK, Bosch J and the Variceal Rebleeding Study Group. Randomised controlled trial comparing propranolol + isosorbide-5-mononitrate vs shunt surgery/sclerotherapy in the prevention of variceal rebleeding. *J Hepatol* 1996; **24 (Suppl.)**: 69.

115. Escorsell A, Bañares R, Gilabert R, *et al.* Transjugular intrahepatic portosystemic shunt (TIPS) vs propranolol + isosorbide-5-mononitrate for the prevention of variceal rebleeding in patients with cirrhosis. *Hepatology* 1998; **28 (Suppl.)**: 770A.

116. Poynard T, Cales P, Pasta L, *et al.* Beta-adrenergic-antagonists in the prevention of first gastrointestinal bleeding in patients with cirrhosis and oesophageal varices. An analysis of data and prognostic factors in 589 patients from four randomized clinical trials. *N Eng J Med* 1991; **324**: 1532–1538.

117. Angelico M, Carli L, Piat C, Gentile S, Capocaccia L. Effects of isosorbide-5-mono-

nitrate compared with propranolol on first bleeding and long-term survival in cirrhosis. *Gastroenterology* 1997; **113:** 1632–1639.

118. Merkel C, Marin R, Enzo E, *et al.* Randomised trial of nadolol alone or with isosorbide mononitrate for primary prophylaxis of variceal bleeding in cirrhosis. *Lancet* 1996; **348:** 1677–1681.

119. Pietrosi G, D'Amico G, Pasta L, *et al.* Isosorbide mononitrate with nadolol compared to nadolol alone for prevention of first bleeding in cirrhosis. A double-blind placebo-controlled randomised trial. *J Hepatol* 1999; **30 (Suppl.):** 66.

120. Spanish Variceal Bleeding Study Group. Propranolol + placebo vs propranolol + isosorbide-5-mononitrate in the prevention of the first variceal bleeding. A multicenter double-blind randomised clinical trial. *J Hepatol* 1999; **30 (Suppl.):** 55.

121. Piqué JM. Portal hypertensive gastropathy. In: *Baillière's Clinical Gastroenterology. Portal Hypertension.* J Bosch (Ed.), Baillière Tindall, London, 1997, 257–270.

122. Pérez Ayuso RM, Piqué JM, Bosch J, Panés J, González A, Pérez R. Propranolol in the prevention of rebleeding from portal hypertensive gastropathy. *Lancet* 1991; **337:** 1431–1434.

123. García-Pagán JC, Salmerón JM, Feu F, *et al.* Effects of low sodium diet and spironolactone on portal pressure in patients with compensated cirrhosis. *Hepatology* 1994; **19:** 1095–1099.

124. Ginès P, Fernández-Esparrach G, Arroyo V. Ascites and renal functional abnormalities in cirrhosis. Pathogenesis and treatment. In: *Baillière's Clinical Gastroenterology. Portal Hypertension.* J Bosch (Ed.), Baillière Tindall, London, 1997, 365–385.

125. Arroyo V, Bataller R, Guevara M. Treatment of hepatorenal syndrome in cirrhosis. In: *Ascites and Renal Dysfunction in Liver Disease.* V Arroyo, P Ginès, J Rodés, RW Schrier (Eds), Blackwell Science, Malden, 1999, 492–510.

126. Navasa M. Treatment of spontaneous bacterial peritonitis and other severe bacterial infections in the setting of cirrhosis. In: *Treatments in Hepatology.* V Arroyo, J Bosch, J Rodés (Eds). Masson, Barcelona, 1995, 109–115.

127. Navasa M. Treatment and prophylaxis of spontaneous bacterial peritonitis. In: *Ascites and Renal Dysfunction in Liver Disease.* V Arroyo, P Ginès, J Rodés, RW Schrier (Eds), Blackwell Science, Malden, 1999, 538–549.

128. Navasa M, Follo A, Llovet JM, *et al.* Randomised, comparative study of oral ofloxacin versus intravenous cefotaxime in spontaneous bacterial peritonitis. *Gastroenterology* 1996; **111:** 1011–1017.

129. Llovet JM, Rodríguez-Iglesias P, Moitinho E, *et al.* Spontaneous bacterial peritonitis in patients with cirrhosis undergoing selective intestinal decontamination. A retrospective study of 229 spontaneous bacterial peritonitis episodes. *J Hepatol* 1997; **26:** 88–95.

14

Hepatic failure

William Bernal, Julia Wendon

INTRODUCTION

Patients with liver failure frequently require drug therapy both for the primary hepatic disease and for other complicating conditions. The liver has a central role in drug metabolism and disposition and, consequently, impairment of hepatic function may have profound effects on drug handling. Since inappropriate drug administration may worsen hepatic failure or even precipitate serious complications, the administration of many drugs often needs to be modified radically in patients with hepatic failure.

In this chapter, general principles of prescribing for patients with liver failure will be discussed, areas of importance in their supportive care will be outlined and practical therapeutic approaches to the treatment of hepatic encephalopathy, a frequent and important complication of hepatic failure, will be examined in detail.

BACKGROUND

Hepatic failure may occur in two distinct settings, dependant upon the presence or absence of pre-existing liver disease. In patients without co-existing chronic liver disease, the abrupt loss of hepatic function can occur as a consequence of hepatotoxins, infection, vascular or auto-immune disease and may lead rapidly to the syndrome of acute liver failure (ALF). This comprises the consequences of hepatic functional impairment, with the loss of metabolic and synthetic capacity resulting in jaundice and coagulopathy, and severe encephalopathy, which is often accompanied by cerebral oedema. Hepatic failure in this setting has a short intense course, frequently in association with a rapidly progressive multiple-organ systems failure.

Systemic or hepatotoxic insults to patients with chronic impairment of liver function may provoke decompensation of chronic liver disease (CLD), with a more gradual deterioration of hepatic function and the development of encephalopathy. Encephalopathy in patients with CLD is infrequently accompanied by cerebral oedema and, although progression to multiple organ failure may also occur, it seldom develops so rapidly as that seen in ALF.

The management of both these clinical scenarios is essentially supportive. It aims to remove or ameliorate the insult leading to impairment of hepatic function, while preventing or limiting the severity of the associated complications. Conditions needed for hepatic regeneration to occur must be optimized to promote a return to premorbid levels of hepatic function. In some patients with ALF, sufficient hepatic recovery may not be possible and, in such cases, without emergency liver transplantation survival is poor. The two distinct conditions therefore share common features in their management, and an important aspect of this is the approach to the prescription of drug therapy.

GENERAL PRESCRIBING GUIDELINES IN PATIENTS WITH LIVER FAILURE

Most commonly used drugs are dependant upon hepatic biotransformation for their activation or elimination, a function that is disturbed in hepatic failure. Hepatic extraction of drugs absorbed from the intestine may also be altered by changes in liver blood flow and portosystemic shunting, and their biliary excretion by the presence of cholestasis. Drug effects may be complicated further by the simultaneous changes in extrahepatic organ function and associated drug sensitivity. All of these factors may be abnormal to varying degrees in different liver diseases. Consequently, the effects of liver failure upon pharmacokinetics and pharmacodynamics are extremely complex and drug effects may be increased, decreased or changed in other ways. Despite this complexity, several straightforward principles may be applied in the approach to drug treatment of patients with hepatic failure:

- Administer drugs only if absolutely necessary
- Avoid or withdraw all potentially hepatotoxic drugs
- Avoid all drugs that may worsen the complications of liver failure
- Monitor drug levels where possible

Administer drugs only if absolutely necessary

In hepatic failure it should generally be assumed that drugs will have reduced clearance, and that most will have enhanced activity. There is consequently considerable potential for enhanced hepatic and extrahepatic toxic effects, which may worsen already compromised hepatic function and precipitate or worsen complications of hepatic failure. Consequently, drugs should only be administered if considered absolutely necessary, and enhanced and prolonged drug effects anticipated.

Avoid or withdraw all potentially hepatotoxic drugs

These include those with dose-related effects including paracetamol, and anti-tuberculous medication or any drug that may result in idiosyncratic hepatotoxicity. If paracetamol must be prescribed in patients with CLD it should be at a reduced dose. Non-steroidal anti-inflammatory drugs (NSAIDs) can both result in hepatotoxicity and have a dramatic effect on renal function and are contraindicated. Where treatment for active mycobacterial infection is necessary, hepatic function must be monitored closely and alternative anti-tuberculous drugs with minimal hepatotoxicity used where possible.

Avoid all drugs that may worsen the complications of liver failure

Patients with liver disease may have enhanced responses to sedatives, and encephalopathy may be precipitated by benzodiazepines, opioids and barbiturates. Where possible, drugs causing hypokalaemia, hyponatraemia or constipation should also be avoided for similar reasons.

Fluid retention and renal dysfunction may be worsened by the use of NSAIDs or corticosteroids. Aminoglycoside antibiotics and angiotensin converting enzyme (ACE)-inhibitors have increased nephrotoxicity in patients with liver disease and can cause renal failure.

Monitor drug levels where possible

Where relatively contraindicated drugs must be given, such as aminoglycoside or anti-tuberculous therapy, frequent monitoring of drug blood levels and liver and renal biochemistry is essential, with appropriate omission or modification of drug dosages as required. The interpretation of blood levels of protein bound drugs is complicated by the reductions in circulating protein and presence of competing ligands (such as bilirubin or bile acids) that occur in liver failure. These tend to reduce the protein binding and increase concentrations of free drug and lead to a poorly predictable downward shift of the therapeutic range of blood levels.

Supportive care

The effective management of hepatic failure frequently requires levels of patient care that can only be provided in an intensive care unit (ICU) or high-dependency unit (HDU) setting. The maintenance of haemodynamic and metabolic stability is essential if hepatic function is to recover. Furthermore, the rapidity of development of life-threatening complications in patients with hepatic failure makes the close monitoring of conscious level and haemodynamic and renal function essential, so that prompt and effective treatment may be instituted.

Of particular importance is the protection of the airway in those patients with encephalopathy and a reduced conscious level; aspiration and respiratory failure may be rapidly fatal. Sedation of the encephalopathic patient outside an ICU/HDU environment is a potentially hazardous undertaking. Unpredictable effects or drug accumulation may result in sudden deterioration in conscious level and the loss of a safe airway. It is essential to maintain a low threshold for the endotracheal intubation and ventilation of these patients; only low doses of standard sedative agents may be required to enable patients to tolerate such ventilatory support.

Propofol, whose metabolism may be relatively unimpaired in patients with cirrhosis is of particular value in this setting, although its hypotensive effects may preclude its use in patients with haemodynamic instability. Other appropriate agents include infusions of benzodiazepines (midazolam or lorazepam) or opiates (fentanyl or alfentanyl); however, doses should be titrated to the minimum required and administration terminated as soon as the indication for intubation has been treated effectively. Prolonged sedative effects after stopping such infusions should be expected.

A second and often under-appreciated aspect of hepatic failure is the greatly increased susceptibility to infection. In patients with CLD, sepsis frequently precipitates or accompanies hepatic decompensation and the development of encephalopathy, and must be sought actively in any patient who becomes encephalopathic. In patients with CLD and variceal bleeding, short-term antibiotic prophylaxis reduces the frequency of respiratory or ascitic infection and improves survival.[1] Current evidence would therefore support the use of systemic antibiotic prophylaxis in CLD patients who are hospitalized with variceal bleeding. In patients with ALF, bacterial or fungal infection is extremely common, and often unaccompanied by conventional clinical signs of sepsis.[2] The use of appropriate prophylactic antimicrobial agents in ALF patients is therefore advisable. In all patients with hepatic failure, meticulous attention to detail in nursing and medical practice is mandatory for the prevention of hospital-acquired infection.

PATHOPHYSIOLOGY

Hepatic encephalopathy

Hepatic encephalopathy (HE) is a syndrome of global cerebral dysfunction that may accompany ALF, CLD, portosytemic anastamosis or inherited metabolic defects in the urea cycle. HE may be classified as *acute HE* accompanying ALF, or as *portosystemic encephalopathy* (PSE) in

CLD or portosystemic shunting. Syndromes of PSE include *acute episodic HE*, which is seen in the cirrhotic patient with a superimposed precipitating condition such as sepsis or gastrointestinal bleeding. *Chronic portosystemic encephalopathy* may develop without an obvious precipitant in patients with CLD or large portosystemic shunts and is characterized by a prolonged and sometimes progressive clinical symptoms. *Subclinical hepatic encephalopathy* may be detectable only on detailed neuropsychiatric testing but affects between 30–80% of patients with cirrhosis and may have marked adverse effects on quality of life.[3]

Several grading systems for HE exist, and the same systems may be applied to HE in both ALF and CLD. The modified Parson-Smith scale[4] assigns HE into five grades ranging from subclinical changes to frank coma (Table 14.1).

The diagnosis of HE is essentially clinical, since there are no specific biochemical or electroencephalograph (EEG) tests to confirm the diagnosis of HE. The use of EEG and sensory-evoked potentials remains predominately the domain of research trials or in the assessment of subclinical encephalopathy. Blood ammonia is elevated in the majority of patients, although, in CLD, circulating ammonia levels correlate only poorly with the grade of encephalopathy.[5] In patients with CLD and an altered conscious level, it is particularly important to consider alternative diagnoses such as other metabolic or toxic encephalopathies or intracranial lesions that may have similar clinical manifestations.

Encephalopathy in patients with chronic liver disease

Encephalopathy in chronic liver disease accompanies portosystemic shunting of blood, which arises either spontaneously as a result of portal hypertension or following portocaval anastomosis or transjugular intrahepatic portosystemic stent shunts (TIPS) aimed at relieving portal hypertension. PSE often presents insidiously with personality changes and altered sleep patterns. Shortened attention span, muscular inco-ordination and asterixis follow, progressing to stupor and coma. Many patients with CLD without other overt manifestations of hepatic decompensation have detectable defects in cognition[3] and thus PSE may be one of the most subtle and early signs of impending hepatic failure. The development of overt PSE in patients with cirrhosis carries a poor prognosis: 1-year survival after an episode of PSE is less than 50%.[6,7]

The exact pathogenesis of PSE in CLD is not well understood and it is likely that multiple

Table 14.1	Modified Parson-Smith scale of hepatic encephalopathy.		
Grade	**Clinical features**	**Neurological signs**	**Glasgow coma scale**
0/Subclinical	Normal	Abnormalities only on neuropsychometric testing	15
1	Trivial lack of awareness, shortened attention span	Tremor, apraxia, inco-ordination	15
2	Lethargy, disorientation, personality change	Asterixis, ataxia, dysarthria	11–15
3	Confusion, somnolence to semi-stupor, responsive to stimuli	Asterixis, ataxia	8–11
4	Coma	+/− Decerebration	<8

mechanisms are involved. It is accompanied by marked abnormalities of cerebral astrocytic and neuronal function and, consequently with derangement of multiple neurotransmitter systems.[8] Chronic liver failure or anatomical portosystemic shunting may result in the exposure of the brain to substances of endogenous or exogenous origin that are either directly neurochemically active (so called 'false neurotransmitters') or have toxic effects on cerebral function.

Ammonia is generally accepted as an agent that is central to the development of PSE, and there is currently no other single candidate toxin that can better explain the clinical and neurochemical features observed.[5,8,9] The primary source of circulating ammonia appears to be the gastrointestinal tract, either from bacterial degradation of protein and urea in the large intestine, or from glutamine oxidation by the small intestine.[10]

The liver is the main site of ammonia metabolism to urea and glutamine, while skeletal muscle also takes up ammonia to form glutamine. Hyperammoniaemia in CLD is promoted by decreased hepatic function and portosystemic shunting, and by the reduction in muscle uptake that results from the skeletal muscle wasting common in malnourished cirrhotic patients.[11] Ammonia taken up by the brain has numerous direct and indirect actions that disrupt cerebral function through alterations in multiple neurotransmitter systems and the altered permeability of the blood–brain barrier to other neurotoxic substances.[8,12]

Most treatment measures of apparent benefit are based upon the hypothesis that ammonia of intestinal origin is a major factor in the development of PSE, and aims to reduce cerebral exposure to ammonia either by reducing production and absorption in the intestine, or by enhancing endogenous metabolism and detoxification.

THERAPEUTIC APPROACHES

Seek precipitant

The development of PSE in patients with CLD is commonly the result of a clinically apparent precipitant, most commonly gastrointestinal haemorrhage, electrolyte disorder and sepsis.[6]

The precipitants of portosystemic encephalopathy are as follows:

- Sepsis
- Metabolic
  —Dehydration
  　Excessive diuretic therapy
  　Excessive fluid restriction
  　Excessive paracentesis
  —Uraemia
  —Hypokalaemia
  —Hyponatraemia
  —Alkalosis
  —Anaemia
  —Hypoxaemia
- Gastrointestinal
  —Haemorrhage
  —Constipation
  —Excess dietary protein
- Hepatic
  —Underlying disease progression
  —Drug hepatotoxicity
  —Ischaemia
  —Hepatoma development
  —Portosystemic shunting
  　Transjugular intrahepatic
  　Surgical
  　Spontaneous
- Psychoactive drugs

The key to the successful management of PSE is to identify and treat effectively the precipitating factor, appreciating that several factors may be operating simultaneously in a given patient at a given time.

Sepsis commonly complicates variceal haemorrhage and should be actively sought and treated. As already discussed, a role for antibiotic prophylaxis in this setting is becoming apparent.[1] Some CLD patients with recurrent episodes of PSE without an apparent precipitating factor may have large portosystemic shunts and, in such cases, occlusion of such shunts by radiologically guided embolization may be effective in controlling PSE.[13]

Diet

Dietary nitrogen, predominately contained in protein comprises a major source of ammonia in the body. PSE may be precipitated by increases in dietary protein, either from diet or from gastrointestinal bleeding,[14] and early uncontrolled trials in patients with chronic PSE reported benefits of dietary protein restriction. Restriction of protein intake long formed part of the management of hepatic encephalopathy, although there is little evidence to suggest that it is of any clinical benefit.[15] Current management of diet in PSE is based upon the increased appreciation of the nutritional requirements of patients with chronic or acute on chronic liver disease.[11]

Patients with chronic liver disease are commonly malnourished[16,17] and have a higher caloric and protein requirement than normal, particularly in the presence of acute inflammatory disease, such as acute alcoholic hepatitis or sepsis. Mortality is doubled in those patients with cirrhosis who are also malnourished,[16] and aggressive enteral nutritional support accelerates improvement without exacerbating the PSE.[18]

Current recommendations are that the daily intake of protein should be approximately 1–1.5 g/kg depending on the degree of hepatic decompensation.[19] If PSE fails to respond to this, a transient reduction in dietary protein to 0.5 g/kg/day has been recommended, with supplemental requirements achieved by giving branched-chain amino acids (BCAA). Dietary BCAA are proposed to reduce the input to the brain of aromatic amino acids, precursors of 'false neurotransmitters'; however, the role of BCAA supplemented feeds in PSE remains contentious, with inconsistent results from several randomized controlled trials.[20–22] Our current practice is to maintain protein intake at no less than 1 g/kg/day, without the use of BCAA, and to exploit other methods for the treatment of refractory PSE.

Supplementation with vegetable rather than animal protein may be of benefit; controlled trials have shown improvements in PSE when vegetable protein is compared with equivalent meat protein diets.[23,24] This may result from the increased fibre content of vegetable-derived feed, through increases in the rate of gut transit and the increased faecal excretion of nitrogen.[14,25] Such diets may, however, be unpalatable and poorly tolerated by patients.

DRUG THERAPY

Lactulose

The non-absorbed disaccharide lactulose is used widely for the treatment of PSE, although in common with other agents used in the treatment of PSE, clinical trials of its efficacy are limited by methodological problems. Trials frequently comprise only small numbers of patients and have, in many cases, failed to control for the effect of the removal or treatment of the factors precipitating PSE.

Pathophysiological studies nevertheless provide a rationale for the use of lactulose. It has a direct cathartic effect, removing endogenous and exogenous ammoniagenic substrates from the gut lumen by reducing gut transit time.[26] Its major effects are, however, more likely to be as a result of changes in colonic microflora. Bacterial mass and incorporation of nitrogen increase as the colonic flora metabolizes lactulose, with increased faecal nitrogen excretion and a reduction in portal ammonia absorption.[25] The increased bacterial production of organic acids within the colon by bacterial fermentation reduces stool pH,[4] such that the non-urease producing flora are favoured,[27] and reduces the breakdown of nitrogen compounds to ammonia and other potential cerebral toxins.[25]

Dose

Individual responses to lactulose vary greatly. The oral dose should be titrated such that patients pass two to four soft stools daily, requiring usually between 30–60 g daily (30–50 ml of lactulose solution three times daily initially). The measurement of stool pH is seldom practical but an acidic stool (pH <6) is ideal.

Adverse reactions

Diarrhoea, abdominal cramps and flatulence occur commonly.

Drug interactions

Decreased effect of neomycin and antacids may occur with lactulose.

Contraindications

Galactosaemia and intestinal obstruction are contraindications for treatment.

Lactilol

A more recent synthetic disaccharide, lactilol has been used in the treatment of PSE. Its mechanisms of action are likely to be similar to those of lactulose. Clinical trials and meta-analysis[28] have been unable to demonstrate a difference in efficacy between lactulose and lactilol, although its effects upon colonic microflora differ from those of lactulose.[27] It may be better tolerated than lactulose by patients, since it is less sweet and consistently causes fewer untoward abdominal side-effects. Flatulence, which may occur independent of the dose of lactulose, tends only to occur at doses of greater than 40 g/day of lactilol.

Dose

Orally 500–700 mg/kg/day is given in three divided doses to result in at least two soft stools daily.

Adverse reactions

Diarrhoea, abdominal cramps and flatulence may occur.

Contraindications

Galactosaemia and intestinal obstruction are contraindications to treatment.

Lactose

In populations where lactase deficiency is common, oral lactose at a dose of 100 g daily is effective in the treatment of chronic PSE,[29] and may be effective when administered rectally.[30]

Adjunctive agents

Non-absorbable carbohydrates should be regarded as the first-line treatments of PSE. When encephalopathy is refractory to this approach, second-line agents may be considered. Antibiotics active against urease-producing bacteria, such as neomycin and metronidazole may be of benefit. Neomycin alone has efficacy similar to that of lactulose,[31] and that of metronidazole similar to that of neomycin.[32] The side-effects of prolonged use of both drugs, in particular the ototoxicity and nephrotoxicity resulting from systemic absorption of neomycin and peripheral and central neural disturbances from metronidazole, limit their use.

There are limited data to support the use of combination therapy with both antibiotics and disaccharides for refractory PSE. It is possible that neomycin may lower ammonia by inhibition of intestinal mucosal glutaminase activity rather than by its antibacterial action alone[33] and thus there is potential for synergistic action. However, the activity of non-absorbed carbohydrates is dependant upon bacterial metabolism, and thus antibiotics that eliminate metabolizing gut flora may reduce the efficacy of disaccharides. The available data suggest that neomycin, in combination with lactulose, may have an additive effect in those patients who have failed to fully respond to lactulose alone.[25,34] A rise in stool pH, indicating a failure of disaccharide metabolism, should be an indication to re-evaluate the continued use of combination therapy

Metronidazole

(See Chapter 5, p. 94).

Neomycin sulphate

Dose
An oral dose of 1 g is given 6-hourly for maximum course of 14 days.

Adverse effects
Vestibular and auditory damage, nephrotoxicity are side-effects of neomycin sulphate. Antibiotic-associated colitis may occur.

Contraindications
Pregnancy, renal failure and intestinal obstruction are contraindications to treatment.

Zinc supplementation

Zinc deficiency, probably as a result of increased urinary losses and dietary deficiency, appears common in patients with cirrhosis.[35] There have been reports of HE precipitated by zinc deficiency and reversed by zinc supplementation.[36] Since two of the five enzymes for the conversion of ammonia to urea in the urea cycle are zinc-dependant, there has been interest in zinc supplementation as a treatment of PSE through the activation of this pathway to reduce blood ammonia.

A randomized, controlled study of zinc acetate 600 mg daily, increased serum zinc, reduced serum ammonia and improved PSE as assessed by psychometric testing.[37] Further studies using zinc sulphate at a dose of 600 mg daily have shown mixed results, with improvements in PSE reported by some studies but not others.[38–41] Zinc toxicity remains a theoretical hazard, consequently zinc supplementation should be reserved for patients with documented deficiency or whose PSE is refractory to other forms of therapy.

Other agents

Numerous other agents have been used for the treatment of PSE; on the basis of available data none can be recommended at present for routine use. Endogenous benzodiazepines and γ-aminobutyric acid have been proposed as important factors in the pathophysiology of PSE, and the benzodiazepine receptor antagonist flumazenil has been used in several controlled trials of the treatment of PSE. A recent large-scale double-blind placebo controlled trial in 527 intensive care patients with PSE showed that less than 20% of patients given infusions of the drug showed a transient improvement in neurological score only.[42]

Supplementation of metabolic substrates for the conversion of ammonia to urea and glutamine appear promising as treatments for PSE. Ornithine aspartate provides substrates for both these detoxification pathways and, at an oral dose of 9 g daily, had an efficacy similar to that of lactulose,[43] and two recent studies have shown benefit in overt PSE, shortening the time to resolution of an altered mental state.[44,45]

Sodium benzoate improves ammonia clearance by increasing nitrogen excretion through pathways other than that of urea synthesis.[46] At an oral dose of 10 g daily, it may be equally effective as lactulose[47] and also enhances the blood ammonia-lowering properties of lactulose.[48] This combination therapy may be of considerable future importance.[49]

TREATMENT REGIMENS

A sequential approach to the treatment of PSE in CLD is outlined below and illustrated in Fig. 14.1.

Chronic and subclinical encephalopathy

In all patients with alcohol induced chronic liver disease, cessation of alcohol consumption and vitamin supplementation is indicated. Following a nutritional assessment we recom-

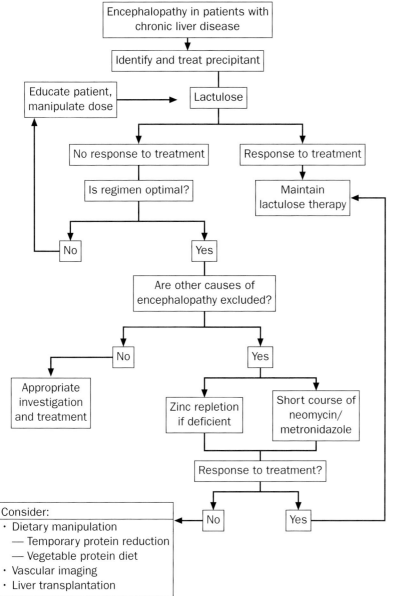

Figure 14.1 Schematic approach to the treatment of portosystemic encephalopathy in patients with chronic liver disease. Reproduced with permission from Mullen, Weber F 1991.[14] Copyright Thieme New York.

mend maintenance of protein intake to 1 g/kg/day, with small meals consumed often and eating a late evening meal.[50]

Lactulose therapy should be titrated to result in two to four soft stools daily, with education to ensure patient compliance. If the above fails then a trial of protein restriction to not less than 0.8 g/kg/day may be performed. If zinc deficiency is documented then supplementation with zinc sulphate, 600 mg daily, may be given. There is no place for the routine chronic administration of neomycin or metronidazole, however, limited courses of both of these agents may be beneficial in the management of chronic low grade portosystemic encephalopathy. Refractory chronic PSE alone may form an indication for liver transplantation, after exclusion of other non-reversible vascular or cerebral conditions. As already indicated, it is likely that new agents may be introduced in the near future following data from large controlled trials.

Acute episodic encephalopathy

Immediate measures for the treatment of acute episodic PSE in decompensated chronic liver disease should include the active detection and treatment of any precipitating factors. In patients in deep coma, where there is any question of airway compromise, endotracheal intubation and ventilation is indicated to prevent aspiration. Haemodynamic stability should be achieved and electrolyte abnormalities corrected. The recent observation that ammonia toxicity may be related to blood pH suggest that the normalization of acid–base status is of considerable importance.[51]

Lactulose delivery orally or via a nasogastric tube should be commenced, and titrated to achieve optimal effect. The placement of nasogastric tubes in patients who have had recent variceal haemorrhage should be deferred until at least 48 h after definitive endoscopic therapy. Where contraindications to oral or nasogastric administration exist, enemata should be employed.

In patients with acute decompensation of liver disease, protein intake is maintained at no less than 1 g/kg/day to ensure energy requirements are met, although active oral or nasogastric feeding should be deferred until variceal haemorrhage has been controlled.

The majority of patients with acute episodic HE will respond to the above measures, and it is uncommon for the supplemental use of zinc, metronidazole or neomycin to be necessary. If refractory HE continues despite these measures and withdrawal of sedative drugs, imaging of the portosystemic vascular architecture should be considered to exclude the presence of anatomical shunts that may be amenable to radiological or surgical intervention.

Encephalopathy and cerebral oedema in acute liver failure

The fundamental difference between encephalopathy in acute liver failure and that occurring with chronic liver disease is that cerebral oedema (CO) commonly occurs in the encephalopathy of ALF but has rarely been reported in patients with CLD.[52] HE in ALF may follow a much more rapid course than that seen in CLD, with progression over the space of a few hours from a normal conscious level to agitated aggressive confusion and eventually coma.

Ammonia is implicated as a causative agent in both acute HE and CO;[53] HE in ALF is characterized by higher circulating levels of ammonia than in decompensated CLD, with the highest levels observed in those ALF patients who develop CO.[54]

Multiple mechanisms probably operate in the pathogenesis of brain swelling in ALF but there is increasing evidence of the importance of the effects of glutamine, a product of cerebral ammonia detoxification.[53] Cerebral astrocytes play a central role in the regulation of cerebral extracellular fluid composition and volume and are the site of ammonia detoxification in brain. They lack a full complement of urea cycle enzymes and ammonia taken up by the brain is therefore eliminated via amidation of glutamate to glutamine, an action catalysed by glutamine synthetase. Glutamine contributes to abnormal neurotransmitter function,[12] but also acts as an osmolyte, promoting water entry into cells and cellular swelling. In patients with CLD, hyperammoniaemia may develop more gradually and compensatory mechanisms may have sufficient time to prevent the rise in intracellular osmolality, and hence the development of CO.[55] The incidence of CO thus probably relates to the rate of the development of hepatic failure.

There appear to be additional vasogenic

mechanisms involving permeability changes of the blood–brain barrier, and the acutely necrotic liver may release vasoactive substances. In patients with ALF who are awaiting transplantation, hepatectomy is associated with stabilization of systemic haemodynamics and intracranial hypertension.[56,57] Superimposed bacterial or fungal infection may precipitate the development of HE and CO in ALF,[2] perhaps as a consequence of the release of pro-inflammatory cytokines, which may have profound effects upon brain vascular and neuronal function.[58,59]

Currently no treatment modalities are able to specifically inhibit cerebral uptake and metabolism of ammonia, and thus the management of HE in ALF relies upon more general methods of reducing the propensity to develop CO and in its early detection and treatment.

Cerebral monitoring in acute HE

The cranial cavity forms a rigid container containing three relatively non-compressible components:

1. The brain substance
2. The CSF
3. The intravascular blood

The global intracranial pressure (ICP) represents the sum of the partial pressures of each of these components, related to their respective volumes. The major cause of raised ICP in ALF is an increase in brain water content[60] although, as a late event, cerebral vasodilatation may also contribute. Uncontrolled intracranial hypertension results in the compromise of cerebral perfusion and the development of brain ischaemia and, subsequently, compression of the brainstem, with uncal herniation as a terminal event.

The perfusion of the brain is determined by the cerebral perfusion pressure (CPP), which is equivalent to the mean arterial pressure (MAP) minus the ICP (CPP = MAP-ICP). The critical CPP for maintaining normal cerebral perfusion is about 50 mmHg, and the maintenance of adequate CPP forms the basis of management of

CO in ALF. This may be achieved by reduction of elevated ICP, or by increasing MAP as appropriate. In adults, the average ICP ranges from 0–10 mmHg, and pressures above 20 mmHg are considered elevated. Prolonged elevations of ICP over 40 mmHg or CPP lower than 50 mmHg are generally accepted as being associated with a poor neurological outcome,[61] although reductions in CPP below this threshold have been associated with full recovery.[62]

In all encephalopathic ALF patients monitoring to anticipate the development of raised intracranial pressure is necessary before irreversible neurological injury has developed. Several monitoring modalities have been advocated and of these, direct measurement of intracranial pressure is most commonly practised.

Intracranial pressure monitoring transducers may be placed extradurally, subdurally or directly within the brain parenchyma. Placement may be associated with a significant complication rate, particularly intracerebral haemorrhage.[63] Our current practice is to use the Camino extradural ICP monitoring system after correction of any coagulopathy but to defer insertion until there is evidence from clinical signs or other forms of less invasive monitoring of evolving intracranial hypertension. To this end, we utilize jugular venous oximetry, through the placement of a catheter within the jugular bulb via the internal jugular vein (IJV). The complications of this technique are similar to those of the placement of a routine IJV central line,[64] and permit the continuous or intermittent measurement of the oxygen saturation of the venous blood leaving the cerebral hemispheres.

An IJV saturation (SjO_2) of 55–75% is considered to be within the normal range and indicative of adequate cerebral perfusion. Reduction in SjO_2 may reflect inadequate substrate delivery or increased cerebral oxygen utilization, most commonly resulting from hypoperfusion or from increased metabolic activity occurring with seizures. Elevations in SjO_2 indicate cerebral hyperaemia, or reduced oxygen utilization as may occur during metabolic depression, cerebral infarction or brain death. In our experience, abnormalities in SjO$_2$ precede other clinical evidence of cerebral oedema and form an indication for the insertion of ICP monitors. Other clinical indications for placement include pupillary abnormalities, systolic hypertension and posturing, or for patients who are proceeding to transplantation.

Management of acute hepatic encephalopathy

A suggested treatment protocol for the management of encephalopathy and cerebral oedema in ALF is shown in Fig. 14.2.

Intubation and ventilatory support
The development of encephalopathy in ALF is characterized by rapid deterioration in the level of consciousness, and is an indication for endotracheal intubation to protect the airway. Ventilation strategies should optimize oxygenation, without the routine use of hyperventilation;[65] appropriate levels of arterial pCO$_2$ are between 4.5 and 5 kPa. In acute HE, cerebral oxidative metabolism is markedly deranged, with evidence of an underlying cerebral oxygen debt.[65,66] Treatment modalities, such as hyperventilation, that induce cerebral vasoconstriction are ineffective in preventing the development of cerebral oedema[67] and may worsen cerebral ischaemia.[65,68] We do not routinely administer muscle relaxants to encephalopathic ALF patients since this may mask signs of seizure activity and, in other ICU populations, they have been linked to the development of critical illness neuropathy and increased incidence of pulmonary infection.

Haemodynamic and metabolic stability
MAP should be maintained at least 60 mmHg through appropriate volume status monitoring, fluid replacement and the use of vasopressors. Rises in ICP may be precipitated by the use of intermittent haemodialysis[69] and thus continuous renal replacement therapies should be utilized where necessary. The development of

seizures may be prevented through the correction of disturbances in electrolytes, magnesium, calcium and glucose. Hyponatraemia may increase susceptibility to cerebral oedema[70] and the serum sodium should be maintained between 140 and 150 mmol/l.

Elimination of factors that increase intracranial pressure
Studies have suggested that CPP is usually optimal at a head elevation of 20°, and this is normally the standard nursing position, although position should be optimized for individual patients. Several factors may transiently increase ICP:

- Fever
- Seizures
- Agitation
- Jugular venous compression
- Head turning/angulation of neck
- Endotracheal suction

Nursing strategies should be employed to avoid or prevent these.

Treatment of cerebral oedema in ALF

Mannitol
Infusion of hypertonic mannitol solutions has been shown to reduce ICP rapidly in neurosurgical patients. Its effects are probably as a result of reduction in total brain water and from changes in the rheological characteristics of the blood. Its efficacy has also been demonstrated in patients with ALF, where it reverses clinical signs of cerebral oedema, reduces ICP and improves survival,[71] and constitutes the first-line agent for the treatment of CE in ALF.

Dose
Signs of cerebral oedema or sustained rises in ICP over 25 mmHg should initially be treated with intravenous bolus doses of 20% mannitol at a dose of 0.5 g/kg. The dose may be repeated to control further episodes of raised ICP, although maximum reductions in ICP may not occur until 20–60 min after commencement of the infusion.

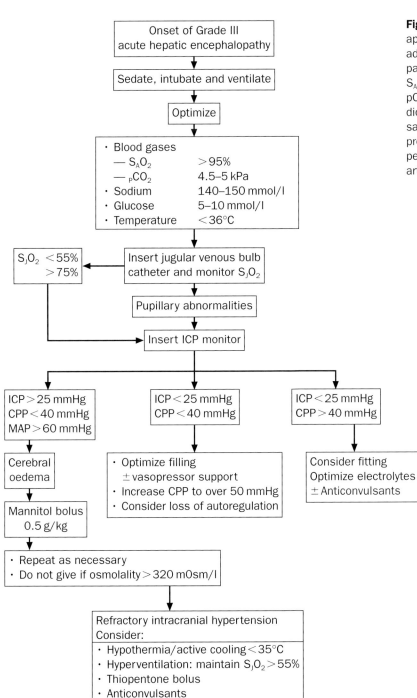

Figure 14.2 Schematic approach to the treatment of advanced encephalopathy in patients with acute liver failure. S_AO_2, arterial oxygen saturation; pCO_2, partial pressure of carbon dioxide, S_JO_2, jugular bulb oxygen saturation; ICP, intracranial pressure; CPP, cerebral perfusion pressure; MAP, mean arterial pressure.

Onset of Grade III acute hepatic encephalopathy

Sedate, intubate and ventilate

Optimize

- Blood gases
  — S_AO_2 >95%
  — $_pCO_2$ 4.5–5 kPa
- Sodium   140–150 mmol/l
- Glucose   5–10 mmol/l
- Temperature   <36°C

S_JO_2 <55% >75%

Insert jugular venous bulb catheter and monitor S_JO_2

Pupillary abnormalities

Insert ICP monitor

ICP >25 mmHg
CPP <40 mmHg
MAP >60 mmHg

ICP <25 mmHg
CPP <40 mmHg

ICP <25 mmHg
CPP >40 mmHg

Cerebral oedema

- Optimize filling
  ± vasopressor support
- Increase CPP to over 50 mmHg
- Consider loss of autoregulation

Consider fitting
Optimize electrolytes
± Anticonvulsants

Mannitol bolus
0.5 g/kg

- Repeat as necessary
- Do not give if osmolality >320 mOsm/l

Refractory intracranial hypertension
Consider:
- Hypothermia/active cooling <35°C
- Hyperventilation: maintain S_JO_2 >55%
- Thiopentone bolus
- Anticonvulsants

Pharmadynamics

Onset of diuresis is 1–3 h after administration and onset of reduction in intracerebral pressure is 15 min. Half-life is 1.1–1.6 h. Mannitol is excreted primarily unchanged in the urine by glomerular filtration.

Adverse reactions

Complications of mannitol therapy include dehydration and hyperosmolality, and thus monitoring of circulating volume status, arterial pressure and osmolality are mandatory during mannitol therapy. In patients with unimpaired renal function, a diuresis of twice the volume of mannitol infused should be seen within 1 h and, in anuric patients, this volume be removed with venovenous haemodiafiltration. Further boluses of mannitol should not be administered if osmolality is greater than 320 mOsm/kg since increases above this level may worsen renal failure and adversely affect cerebral function through increased permeability of the blood–brain barrier.[72]

Precautions/contraindications

Mannitol is contraindicated in severe renal disease (anuria), dehydration or active intracranial bleeding, and severe pulmonary oedema. Extravasation of mannitol causes inflammation and thrombophlebitis. Risks to the human fetus are unknown and, during pregnancy, potential benefits may outweigh the risks to the fetus.

Thiopentone

Barbiturates exhibit complex effects upon cerebral metabolism and may limit cerebral oedema through a combination of anaesthetic action and cerebral vasoconstriction secondary to reduced metabolic requirements.

Dose

In ALF, thiopentone bolus intravenous infusion at median doses of 250 mg over 15 min has been reported to control elevations in ICP refractory to mannitol therapy.[73]

Adverse reactions

Clinical use of thiopentone is limited by fre-quent side-effects of haemodynamic instability, necessitating the concurrent use of ICP monitoring to ensure adequate CPP. An apparent immunosupressant action may increase the risk of sepsis. Its use is therefore limited to only the most refractory cerebral oedema, and must be undertaken with appropriate monitoring and antimicrobial prophylaxis.

Precautions/contraindications

Thiopentone is contraindicated in variegate or acute intermittent porphyria, or known hypersensitivity to thiopentone or barbiturates. Laryngospasm or bronchospasm may occur so use with caution in patients with asthma or COPD. Extravasation or intra-arterial injection causes necrosis.

Other treatment modalities

N-acetylcysteine (NAC) is of proven benefit in ameliorating or abolishing the hepatotoxicty of acetaminophen when given early (under 24 h) after overdose. Later administration also appears to be of benefit and may reduce both the incidence and severity of cerebral complications and consequent mortality.[74,75] Such benefits may also extend to non-acetaminophen-induced ALF, and improvements in systemic and cerebral oxygen utilization following NAC administration have been reported (see Chapter 12, p. 283).[65,76] A recent placebo-controlled study of intravenous NAC versus placebo in 14 patients with advanced encephalopathy[77] found no significant effect upon systemic oxygen utilization, casting some doubt on the benefits of treating all ALF patients. Given the minimal side-effect profile of NAC, and its undoubted benefit in many patients, our current practice is to administer NAC by infusion at a dose of 150 mg/kg/24 h with paracetamol-induced ALF until the International Normalized Ratio (INR) is less than 2. The results of large-scale, placebo-controlled trials of NAC in ALF of non-paracetamol aetiologies are awaited.

Several other promising forms of treatment

of cerebral oedema in HE have recently been reported. Bolus infusion of 25 mg of intravenous indomethacin has been reported to be effective in controlling refractory intracranial hypertension in a single patient with paracetamol-induced ALF,[78] an effect attributed through its actions causing cerebral vasoconstriction. Such therapy may, theoretically, compromise cerebral oxygenation, and the risks of gastrointestinal haemorrhage in ALF patients with marked coagulopathies appear considerable.

A more promising approach is that of inducing moderate hypothermia with active cooling. In a series of seven patients with refractory elevations in ICP, cooling to a core temperature of 32–33°C reduced ICP, while maintaining CPP and reducing circulating ammonia and cerebral ammonia uptake.[66] Hypothermia may inhibit hepatic regeneration, which is a key process in recovery from ALF and thus the application of hypothermia might best be restricted to those patients who are listed for transplantation and awaiting a graft. The use of artificial liver support devices may, in the future, function as adjunctive treatment of HE in ALF but, at present, is restricted to limited experimental trials. Data from a trial of a porcine hepatocyte based bioartificial liver support device[79] demonstrated a fall in ICP and rise in CPP during treatment periods, suggesting a potential role as a future bridge to liver transplantation.

REFERENCES

1. Bernard B, Grange J-D, Khac E, Amiot X, Opolon P, Poynard T. Antibiotic prophylaxis for the prevention of bacterial infections in cirrhotic patients with gastrointestinal bleeding: a meta-analysis. *Hepatology* 1999; **29(6):** 1655–1661.
2. Rolando N, Philpott-Howard J, Williams R. Bacterial and fungal infections in acute liver failure. *Semin Liver Dis* 1996; **16(4):** 389–402.
3. Lockwood A. Early detection and treatment of hepatic encephalopathy. *Curr Opin Neurol* 1998; **11:** 663–666.
4. Conn H, Levy C, Vlahcevic Z, *et al.* Comparison of lactulose and Neomycin in the treatment of chronic portal-systemic encephalopathy. *Gastroenterology* 1977; **74(4):** 573–583.
5. Butterworth R. Alterations of neurotransmitter-related gene expression in human and experimental portal-systemic encephalopathy. *Metab Brain Dis* 1998; **13(4):** 337–346.
6. Bustamente J, Rimola A, Ventura P-J, *et al.* Prognostic significance of hepatic encephalopathy in patients with cirrhosis. *J Hepatol* 1999; **30:** 890–895.
7. Christensen E, Krintel J, Hansen SM, Johansen JK, Juhl E. Prognosis after the first episode of gastrointestinal bleeding or coma in cirrhosis. *Scand J Gastroenterol* 1989; **24:** 999–1006.
8. Hazell A, Butterworth R. Hepatic encephalopathy: an update of pathophysiologic mechanisms. *Proc Soc Exper Biol Med* 1999; **222:** 99–112.
9. Norenberg M. Astroglial dysfunction in hepatic encephalopathy. *Metab Brain Dis* 1998; **13(4):** 319–331.
10. Hawkins R, Mans A. Brain metabolism in encephalopathy caused by hyperammonemia. *Adv Exper Med Biol* 1994; **368:** 125.
11. Mizock B. Nutritional support in hepatic encephalopathy. *Nutrition* 1999; **15(3):** 220–228.
12. Jones E, Basile A. Does ammonia contribute to increased GABA-ergic neurotransmission in liver failure? *Metab Brain Dis* 1998; **13(4):** 351–360.
13. Sakurabayashi S, Sezai S, Yamamoto Y, Hirano M, Oka H. Embolisation of portal-systemic shunts in cirrhotic patients with chronic recurrent hepatic encephalopathy. *Cardiovasc Intervent Radiol* 1997; **20:** 120–124.
14. Mullen K, Weber F. Role of nutrition in hepatic encephalopathy. *Sem Liver Dis* 1991; **11(4):** 292–304.
15. Seymour C, Whelan K. Dietary management of hepatic encephalopathy. *Brit Med J* 1999; **318:** 1364–1365.
16. Lautz H, Selberg O, Korber J, Burgher M, Muller M. Protein-calorie malnutrition in liver cirrhosis. *Clin Invest* 1992; **70:** 478.
17. Italian Multicentre Study. Nutritional status in cirrhosis. *J Hepatol* 1994; **21:** 217–235.
18. Kearns PJ, Young H, Garcia G, *et al.* Accelerated improvement of alcoholic liver disease with enteral nutrition. *Gastroenterology* 1992; **102:** 200–205.
19. Plauth M, Merli M, Kondrup J, Weiman A, Ferenci P, Muller M. ESPEN guidelines for nutrition in liver disease and transplantation. *Clin Nutr* 1997; **16:** 43–55.

20. Charlton M. Branched chains revisited. *Gastroenterology* 1996; **111(1):** 252–255.

21. Morgan M. Branched chain amino acids in the management of chronic liver disease. Facts and fantasies. *J Hepatol* 1990; **11:** 133–141.

22. Fabbri A, Magrini N, Bianchi G, Zoli M, Marchesini G. Overview of randomised clinical trials of oral branched chain amino acid treatment in chronic hepatic encephalopathy. *J Parenteral Enteral Nutrit* 1996; **20(2):** 159–164.

23. Bianchi G, Marchesini G, Fabbri A, *et al.* Vegetable versus animal protein in cirrhotic patients with chronic encephalopathy: a randomised cross-over comparison. *J Int Med* 1993; **233:** 385–392.

24. Uribe M, Marquez M, Ramos G, *et al.* Treatment of chronic portosystemic encephalopathy with vegetable and animal protein diets: a controlled crossover study. *Digest Dis Sci* 1982; **27:** 1109–1116.

25. Weber F. Effects of lactulose on nitrogen metabolism. *Scand J Gastroenterol* 1997; **32 (Suppl. 222):** 83–87.

26. Riordan S, Williams R. Treatment of hepatic encephalopathy. *New Eng J Med* 1997; **357(7):** 473–479.

27. Ballongue J, Schumann C, Quignon P. Effects of lactulose and lactilol on colonic microflora and enzymatic activity. *Scand J Gastroenterol (Suppl)* 1997; **222:** 41–44.

28. Blanc P, Daures J-P, Rouillon J-M, *et al.* Lactilol or lactulose in the treatment of chronic hepatic encephalopathy: results of a meta-analysis. *Hepatology* 1991; **15(2):** 222–228.

29. Uribe M, Marquez M, Garcia-Rammos G, *et al.* Treatment of chronic porto-systemic encephalopathy with lactose in lactase deficient patients. *Digest Dis Sci* 1980; **25(12):** 924–928.

30. Uribe M, Berthier J, Lewis H, *et al.* Lactose enemas plus placebo vs. neomycin tablets plus starch enemas in acute portal-systemic encephalopathy. A double-blind randomised trial. *Gastroenterology* 1981; **81:** 101–106.

31. Atterbury C, Maddrey W, Conn H. Neomycin-sorbitol and lactulose in the treatment of acute portal systemic encephalopathy: a controlled, double-blind clinical trial. *Am J Digest Dis* 1978; **23:** 398–406.

32. Morgan M, Read A, Speller D. Treatment of hepatic encephalopathy with metronidazole. *Gut* 1982; **23:** 1–7.

33. Hawkins R, Jessey J, Mans A, Chedid A, DeJoseph M. Neomycin reduces the intestinal production of ammonia from glutamine. *Adv Exper Med Biol* 1995; **368:** 125–134.

34. Weber F, Fresard K, Lally B. Effects of lactulose and neomycin on urea metabolism in cirrhotic subjects. *Gastroenterology* 1982; **82:** 213–217.

35. Keeling P, Jones R, Hilton P, Thompson R. Reduced leucocyte zinc in liver disease. *Gut* 1980; **21:** 561–564.

36. Rijt CVD, Schalm S, Schat H, Focken K, Jong GD. Overt hepatic encephalopathy precipitated by zinc deficiency. *Gastroenterology* 1991; **100:** 1114–1118.

37. Reding P, Duchateau J, Bataille C. Oral zinc supplementation improves hepatic encephalopathy. *Lancet* 1984; **2:** 493–495.

38. Marchesini G, Fabbri A, Bianchi G, Brizi M, Zoli M. Zinc supplementation and amino acid nitrogen metabolism in patients with advanced cirrhosis. *Hepatology* 1996; **23(5):** 1084–1092.

39. Antoniello S, Auletta M, Cerini R, Cepresso A. Zinc deficiency and hepatic encephalopathy. *Ital J Gastroenterol* 1986; **18:** 27–31.

40. Bresci G, Parsi G, Banti S. Management of hepatic encephalopathy; results of a double-blind crossover trial. *Eur J Med* 1993; **2:** 414–416.

41. Riggo O, Aristo F, Merli M, *et al.* Short-term oral zinc supplementation does not improve chronic hepatic encephalopathy: results of a double-blind crossover trial. *Digest Dis Sci* 1991; **36:** 1204–1208.

42. Barbaro G, Lorenzo GD, Soldini M, *et al.* Flumazenil for hepatic encephalopathy grade III and IVa in patients with cirrhosis: an Italian multicenter, double-blind, placebo controlled cross-over study. *Hepatology* 1998; **28(2):** 374–378.

43. Herlong H, Maddrey W, Walser M. The use of ornithine salts of branched chain amino acids in porto-systemic encephalopathy. *Ann Int Med* 1980; **93:** 545–550.

44. Kircheis G, Nilius R, Held C, *et al.* Therapeutic efficacy of *L*-ornithine-*L*-aspartate infusions in patients with hepatic encephalopathy; results of a placebo-controlled double-blind study. *Hepatology* 1997; **25:** 1351–1360.

45. Stauch S, Kircheis G, Adler G. Oral *L*-ornithine-*L*-aspartate therapy of chronic hepatic encephalopathy: results of a placebo-controlled double-blind study. *J Hepatol* 1998; **28:** 856–864.

46. Brusilow S, Valle D, Bradshaw M. New pathways of nitrogen excretion in inborn errors of urea synthesis. *Lancet* 1979; **2:** 452–454.

47. Sushma S, Dasarathy S, Tandon R, Jain S, Gupta S, Bhist M. Sodium benzoate in the treatment of acute hepatic encephalopathy: a double-blind randomised trial. *Hepatology* 1992; **16**: 138–144.

48. Campollo O, Cortez R, Gutierrez M, *et al.* Sodium benzoate and lactulose in the treatment of hepatic encephalopathy. *J Hepatol* 1994; **21**: 1144–1157.

49. Conn H. A clinical hepatologist's predictions about non-absorbed carbohydrates in the early twenty-first century. *Scand J Gastroenterol* 1997; **32(Suppl. 222)**: 88–92.

50. Swart G, Zilkens M, Vuure JV, Berg JVD. Effect of late evening meal on nitrogen balance in patients with cirrhosis of the liver. *Brit Med J* 1989; **299**: 1202–1203.

51. Kramer L, Tribl B, Gendo A, *et al.* Partial pressure of ammonia versus ammonia in hepatic encephalopathy. *Hepatology* 2000; **31**: 30–34.

52. Donovan J, Schafer D, Shaw B, Sorrell M. Cerebral odema and increased intracranial pressure in chronic liver disease. *Lancet* 1998; **351**: 719–721.

53. Blei A, Larsen F. Pathophysiology of cerebral odema in fulminant hepatic failure. *J Hepatol* 1999; **31**: 771–776.

54. Clemensen J, Larsen F, Kondrup J, Hansen B, Ott P. Cerebral herniation in patients with acute liver failure is correlated with arterial ammonia concentration. *Hepatology* 1999; **29(3)**: 648–653.

55. Cordoba J. Glutamine, myo-inositol and brain edema in acute liver failure. *Hepatology* 1996; **23**: 1291–1292.

56. Bismuth H, Samuel D, Castaing D, Williams R, Pereira SP. Liver transplantation in Europe for patients with acute liver failure. *Semin Liver Dis* 1996; **16(4)**: 415–425.

57. Ringe B, Lubbe N, Kuse E, Frei U, Pichlmayr R. Total hepatectomy and liver transplantation as two-stage procedure [see comments]. *Ann Surg* 1993; **218(1)**: 3–9.

58. Seikyama K, Yoshiba M, Thomson A. Circulating proinflammatory cytokines (IL-1$_{beta}$, TNF$_{alpha}$ and IL-6) and IL-1ra in fulminant hepatic failure and acute hepatitis. *Clin Exper Immunol* 1994; **98**: 71–77.

59. Rolando N, Ellis A, Groote DD, Wendon J, Williams R. Correlation of serial cytokine levels with progression to coma (grade IV) in patients with acute liver failure (ALF). *Hepatology* 1995; **22(4)**: 1038.

60. Cordoba J, Blei A. Cerebral edema and intracra-nial pressure monitoring. *Liver Transplant Surg* 1995; **1**: 187–194.

61. Donovan JP, Shaw BJ, Langnas AN, Sorrell MF. Brain water and acute liver failure: the emerging role of intracranial pressure monitoring [Editorial]. *Hepatology* 1992; **16(1)**: 267–268.

62. Davies M, Multimer D, Lowes J, *et al.* Recovery despite impaired cerebral perfusion in fulminant liver failure. *Lancet* 1994; **343**: 1329–1330.

63. Blei A, Olafsson S, Webster S, Levy R. Complications of intracerebral pressure monitoring in fulminant hepatic failure. *Lancet* 1993; **341**: 157–158.

64. Mata B, Lam A, Mayberg T, Shipera Y, Winn H. A critique of the intraoperative use of continuous jugular venous bulb catheters during neurosurgical procedures. *Anaesth Analg* 1994; **79**: 745–750.

65. Wendon JA, Harrison PM, Keays R, Williams R. Cerebral blood flow and metabolism in fulminant liver failure. *Hepatology* 1994; **19(6)**: 1407–1413.

66. Jalan R, Damink S, Deutz N, Lee A, Hayes P. Moderate hypothermia for uncontrolled hypertension in acute liver failure. *Lancet* 1999; **354**: 1164–1168.

67. Ede R, Gimson A, Bihari D, Williams R. Controlled hyperventilation in the prevention of cerebral odema in fulminant hepatic failure. *J Hepatol* 1986; **2**: 43–51.

68. Strauss G, Hogh P, Knudsen G, Hansen B, Larsen F. Regional cerebral blood flow during mechanical hyperventilation in patients with fulminant hepatic failure. *Hepatology* 1999; **30**: 1368–1373.

69. Davenport A. Renal replacement therapy for patients with acute liver failure awaiting orthotopic hepatic transplantation [Letter]. *Nephron* 1991; **59(2)**: 315–316.

70. Cordoba J, Gottstein J, Blei A. Chronic hyponatraemia exacerbates ammonia-induced brain edema in rats after portocaval anastomosis. *J Hepatol* 1998; **29**: 589–594.

71. Canalese J, Gimson A, Davis C, Mellon P, Davis M, Williams R. Controlled trial of dexamethasone and mannitol for the cerebral odema of fulminant hepatic failure. *Gut* 1982; **23**: 625–629.

72. Paulson O, Hertz M. Blood–brain barrier permeability during short-lasting intravascular hyperosmolality. *Eur J Clin Invest* 1978; **8**: 391–396.

73. Forbes A, Alexander G, O'Grady J, *et al.* Thiopental infusion in the treatment of intracranial

hypertension complicating fulminant hepatic failure. *Hepatology* 1989; **10(3):** 306–310.

74. Keays R, Harrison P, Wendon J, *et al*. Intravenous acetylcysteine in paracetamol induced hepatic failure: a prospective controlled trial. *Br Med J* 1991; **303:** 1026–1029.

75. Makin A, Wendon J, Williams R. A 7-year experience of severe acetominophen-induced hepatotoxicity (1987–1993). *Gastroenterol* 1995; **109:** 1907–1916.

76. Harrison P, Wendon J, Gimson A, Alexander G, Williams R. Improvement by acetylcysteine of haemodynamics and oxygen transport in fulminant hepatic failure. *N Engl J Med* 1991; **324(26):** 1852–57.

77. Walsh T, Hopton P, Phillips B, Mackenzie S, Lee A. The effect of N-acetylcysteine on oxygen transport and uptake in patients with fulminant hepatic failure. *Hepatology* 1998; **27(5):** 1332–1340.

78. Clemmesen J, Hansen B, Larsen F. Indomethacin normalises intracranial hypertension in acute liver failure: a twenty-three-year-old woman treated with indomethacin. *Hepatology* 1997; **26(6):** 1423 1425.

79. Chen S, Hewitt W, Watanabe F, *et al*. Clinical experience with a porcine hepatocyte-based liver support system. *Internat J Artific Org* 1996; **19(11):** 664–669.

15

Adverse effects of drugs on the gastrointestinal tract

Michael JS Langman

INTRODUCTION

Adverse effects of drugs on the gastrointestinal tract are common, although epidemiological data demonstrating overall frequency and impact are limited. Thus, lack of data arises because general estimates of frequency for well-established adverse effects are seldom established. Confident attribution is also difficult in the absence of data from control populations. Such difficulties are particularly obvious in examining the risks of functional symptoms such as diarrhoea, vomiting and constipation, because they are common in the general public. However, they also pose difficulty in assessment of disease burden related to most organic conditions, particularly when other causal factors are inadequately understood and possible interactions even less so.

Although adverse effects on the liver, gall-bladder and pancreas necessarily occur in response to absorbed drug, or to the metabolites once absorbed, it must not be assumed that epithelial damage in the gut arises as a direct effect of drug present at the mucosal surface. Thus, anti-inflammatory drug-induced damage can be demonstrated with parenteral as well as oral preparations.

Within the gut adverse effects may also be indirect, notably, in the case of antibiotics, through the selective advantage conferred on the growth of bacteria.

CASE REPORTS

Reports that are published in medical journals will tend to emphasize unusual patterns, often of severe disease. Assumptions of causality may be founded insecurely because most drug-associated disease mimics naturally occurring disease. In addition, mechanisms are often unclear. Thus, the occurrence of, say, acute pancreatitis in takers of, say, diuretics may represent simple coincidence, or a causal association. When examining the risks of adverse effects, the strengths and weaknesses of data must be understood clearly.

When assessing the significance of these adverse effects several factors must be taken into account. They include timing, dose relationship, possible mechanisms, resemblance to and possible confusion with, spontaneously occurring disease, and re-occurrence with challenge.

Collections of spontaneously submitted adverse reaction reports suffer from all these problems. In addition, the reasons why reporters report are unclear. It is known that reporting is more common for new than old drugs (a trend that is actively encouraged), and that publicity given to particular possible adverse effects will generate more reports of the same type.

When attempting to assess possible causality, regulatory agencies compare report numbers for compounds used with similar clinical indications at similar stages following release commercially. Secondly, comparative profiling is carried out so as to contrast the relative proportions with, say, digestive, cardiovascular and neurological complaints, or subsets of special interest. Although the information obtained is useful in signposting and giving early warning it is seldom definitive.

Controlled trials

Adverse effects reported in good randomized double-blind trials, or where assessment, although not blind, is reasonably objective, can provide valuable evidence.

Thus, the risks of azathioprine-induced acute pancreatitis were shown clearly in such studies. The strength of the data lies particularly in the securing of evidence suggesting causality because the act of randomization of subjects treated should 'factor out' extraneous complicating, and potentially causal, influences. The weaknesses derive from the inability to relate the data clearly to risks in general populations who may be more susceptible by reason of coincident disease, extreme age or other factors.

Case-control studies

The validity of data obtained in such studies where risks are contrasted between disease in cases treated or not treated with a specific drug will stand or fall by the security of the contrasts. Were the controls appropriate? If the patients were hospital attenders then what biases will be engendered? What are the effects of types of systematic exclusion? Could bias derive from inevitable knowledge of whether individuals were cases or controls? Despite these, and other

difficulties, case-control studies are powerful methods, particularly in assessing the causation of rare diseases. Thus non-steroidal anti-inflammatory drug (NSAID)-associated ulcer complications are rare relative to the total numbers of prescriptions issued, and case-control studies clearly indicated clinically important increased risks.

Cohort studies

These have strength in that biases in selecting cases and controls are eliminated; however unless existing databases form the framework they are slow to conduct and expensive, because it takes time for the end-points under scrutiny to appear. Large databases exist in the UK, notably the General Practitioner Research Database (GPRD) or Mediplus, where general practitioners agree to contribute data on prescriptions written and diseases diagnosed in their patients. GPRD has been used successfully, for instance, to examine the risks of NSAID-associated peptic ulcer, and has given substantially the same results as case-control studies. Database studies have disadvantages, however; demographic and social data are often lacking, and they cannot usually be applied where drugs are prescribed in hospitals rather than in the community. Thus databases may correctly identify smokers but may not identify ex-smokers from non-smokers.

GASTROINTESTINAL TRACT

Mouth

Glossitis is a not uncommon sequel of broad-spectrum antibiotic treatment owing to fungal overgrowth. Treatment with metronidazole can result in altered taste perception, as a metallic taste, while use of the antifungal drug terbinafen can result in loss of perception of taste.

Emepromium bromide has repeatedly been shown to cause mouth and oesophageal ulceration. Stomatitis is also associated with treatment with gold salts, penicillamine and griseofulvin.

Tetracyclines are well-known to cause yellow/brown discoloration of the teeth; this may be associated with enamel defects, and maternal exposure during pregnancy is a known risk for the child. Staining of teeth by liquid iron salts reverses on stopping exposure. Gingival hyperplasia is described with nifedipine and verapamil use, as well as phenytoin.

Oesophagus

Most adverse effects probably manifest as symptoms associated with reflux, or as oesophagitis or oesophageal ulcer.

Ulcer

Retention of tablets in the oesophagus, characteristically in the elderly, can lead to ulceration. NSAIDs are known to cause this problem, probably because tablets taken late at night tend to be retained in the oesophagus if swallowed without water while recumbent. Epidemiological data suggest that the risk of stricture is increased several fold. Effects appear to be direct. Oesophageal ulcer is also a known risk of treatment with the bisphosphonate, alendronic acid.

Drug treatment that increases the chances of developing gastro-oesophageal reflux may be of long-term importance, given the possibility of predisposing to oesophageal adenocarcinoma, now increasing in frequency in the Western World.

Helicobacter pylori eradication therapy has been claimed to be associated with the precipitation of reflux symptoms through enhanced acid secretory output as the organism is eliminated. Others have denied such effects. Reduced oesophageal sphincter tone is also associated with anticholinergic drug treatment, and it is pharmacologically likely that the same is true for tricyclic antidepressant use, the drugs being intrinsically anticholinergic.

Chest pain, which is possibly of oesophageal origin, occasionally can be induced by use of the triptans used for the treatment of migraine.

Stomach

Peptic ulceration

Anti-inflammatory drug treatment, whether non-steroidal (NSAIDs and aspirin) or corticosteroid, is associated with increased risks of peptic ulceration and its complications.

NSAIDs and aspirin

There is compelling evidence that associations are causal. The increased risks have been demonstrated consistently in case-control and cohort studies; indeed, acute ulceration is induced in humans and animals by NSAID and aspirin treatment. Effects are dose-related, and there is a plausible mechanism in inhibition of production of protective prostanglandins.

NSAID damage was considered initially to be a gastropathy but there is good evidence from studies of risks of ulcer complications that both duodenal and gastric ulcer are involved. Large case-control and cohort studies have shown differential risk, with ibuprofen and diclofenac associated with lesser risk and piroxicam, azapropazone and probably, ketoprofen with high risk.[1-3]

Risk is increased for all non-selective drugs by three- to four-fold by increments of dose within the normally recommended range. In addition, risk is greater in older individuals, reflecting a greater propensity to suffer from ulcer disease whether NSAID treated or not. Other risk factors for ulcer complications add to those of NSAIDs. Those of particular strength include a prior ulcer history, treatment for heart disease or diabetes, use of corticosteroids, anticoagulants or aspirin and, to a lesser extent, smoking and alcohol consumption.

The fundamental mechanism, namely, inhibition of cyclo-oxygenase (COX) leading to reduced prostaglandin production, appears to be caused by inhibition of COX-1. This enzyme is expressed constitutively in the gut mucosa, and elsewhere, notably in platelets. By contrast, COX-2 is an inducible enzyme associated with inflammatory states. The recent development of drugs that are selective COX-2 antagonists has allowed the development of anti-inflammatory and analgesic agents that have reduced propensities to cause mucosal damage,[4] and maybe no greater effects than base expectation. It should be noted, however, that COX-2 antagonists do not inhibit platelet COX as it is a COX-1 enzyme.

Aspirin

This is a non-selective inhibitor of COX-1 and COX-2, but inhibits platelet COX-1 irreversibly, making it a valuable drug in managing cardiovascular disease. Aspirin because of its low pKa is absorbed in the stomach, whereas most drug including non-aspirin NSAIDs, are absorbed by passive diffusion in the small bowel. Not all aspirin-induced damage is, however, necessarily direct, and it is known, for example, that systemically administered non-selective COX antagonists can damage the stomach. Whether enteric coating reduces the likelihood of aspirin-induced gastric damage is unclear.

Although analgesic doses of aspirin of 300–900 mg one or more times a day are well-known to cause endoscopically visible gastric damage, it has been less clear whether cardio-protective doses of 75 and 150 mg daily have the same effect. Case-control study shows that the risks of gastric or duodenal ulcer bleeding are increased, by approximately two-fold for doses of 75 mg daily, and three-fold for doses of 150 mg daily (Table 15.1).[3] The burden of imposed disease is substantial and, although aspirin as a tablet is cheap, its real costs are significantly enhanced by the consequential burden of gastrointestinal disease owing to adverse effects. Convincing evidence is lacking that reformulation in enteric or slow-release form reduces the risk of peptic ulceration.

Corticosteroids

The general pattern of evidence now indicates that oral corticosteroid treatment raises the risk of peptic ulceration and its complications. Overall, the effects are moderate but are likely to be dose-related, and may be substantial in high-risk sick patients who, for example, have multisystem inflammatory disease, or have illnesses related to transplant rejection.

Other drugs

Confirmation is required as to whether calcium-channel antagonists and selective serotonin reuptake inhibitors (SSRIs) increase the risk of peptic ulcer bleeding. Evidence may often lack conviction through limited attention being paid to potential confounding factors.

Altered gastric emptying

Anticholinergic drugs (whether simple antimuscarinic agents such as atropine or synthetic variants, or tricyclic antidepressants) can retard gastric emptying, which may be critical in patient with pyloric canal disease associated with peptic ulceration.

Small and large bowel

Anti-inflammatory drugs

Following case reports suggesting that NSAID treatment might cause colonic ulceration, bleeding and perforation, formal epidemiological case-control studies showed a two- to three-fold increased risk of colonic perforation or bleeding. It is unclear whether risks are greater with one NSAID or another. It is also unclear whether slow-release formulations present special risks, although the problem was partly brought to light by the description of colonic perforation during treatment with slow-release indomethacin. However, that preparation incorporated a potassium-driven osmotic pump, and it is known that enteric-coated potassium chloride alone can cause ileal ulceration.

Fibrotic strictures are also described in the ileum and colon, presumably reflecting healing responses.[5] Damage may be related to two mechanisms. Firstly, studies with synthetic sugars have shown that NSAID treatment increases intestinal permeability. Secondly NSAIDs can alter cell kinetics; this is well-illustrated in cancer cell lines in which apoptosis is increased

Table 15.1   Calculated risks [as odds ratios] associated with use of some commonly prescribed NSAIDs and with prophylactic aspirin for cases with gastric and duodenal ulcer complications.[1-3]

	Agent	Database	UK Case control	Spain Case control	Italy Case control
Drugs	Azaproprazone	23.4	31.5		
	Diclofenac	3.9	4.2	7.9	4.4
	Ibuprofen	2.9	2.0		
	Indomethacin	6.3	11.3	4.9	9.2
	Ketoprofen	5.4	23.7	2.6	
	Naproxen	3.1	9.1	6.5	
	Piroxicam	18.0	13.7	19.1	7.7
	Aspirin (prophylaxis)				
	75 mg	2.3			
	150 mg	3.2			
	300 mg	3.9			

and this effect may be related to the protective effects of NSAIDs against large bowel cancer.

High-dose pancreatic enzyme supplements
Initial case reports suggesting that use of high-dose pancreatic enzyme supplements could cause a fibrosing colonopathy in patients with cystic fibrosis of the pancreas were followed by descriptions of case series in the UK and elsewhere. Risk does not appear uniform. A UK national case-control study compared 14 cases (all but four were notified previously to the UK Committee on Safety of Medicines) occurring in 7600 patients with cystic fibrosis and matched controls (four per case). Cases had taken, on average, twice as much daily treatment as controls. Risks appeared greater in boys, in those with more severe cystic fibrosis and in those taking laxatives concomitantly. Nutrixyn 22 and pancrease HL were associated with risk whereas Creon 25000 was not. Creon 25000 is released by a different mechanism, and lacks the methyl methacrylate coating of the other preparations. Nutrizym GR, a standard dose supplement, has also been associ-

ated with the development of colonopathy. Following these reports, the Committee on Safety of Medicines has recommended that pancrease HL, Nutrizym 22, and Panzytrat 25000, which have similar release mechanisms, should no longer be used, and doses of any supplements should be limited to 10 000 units of lipase/kg/day.[6] Subsequently, case reports have ceased.

Exacerbation of colitis and Crohn's disease
Anecdotal evidence indicates that takers of NSAIDs may be prone to exacerbation of ulcerative colitis; it is presumed that the mechanism relates to altered prostaglandin production although this has been poorly defined. Rare hypersensitivity reactions associated with exacerbations of colitis are also described for sulphasalazine. Oral contraceptive use appears to increase the chances of developing Crohn's disease and of suffering from relapses.[7,8] Suggestions that use of the measles-mumps-rubella (MMR) vaccine is associated with an increased risk of inflammatory bowel disease have not been confirmed.[9]

Constipation

Morphine and its analogues, central and peripheral, all cause constipation; this effect is utilized therapeutically in diarrhoea with drugs with lesser or no central agonist actions such as codeine and loperamide. Loperamide is to be preferred because of its peripheral action without central effects. Use of any of these compounds in acute severe colitis can precipitate toxic megacolon, and they should, therefore, be avoided.

Antimuscarinic agents are also common causes of constipation. The range includes not only atropine but also drugs, which are intrinsically anticholinergic, such as tricyclic antidepressants, used for other purposes. Others include oxybutinin hydrochloride, which is used for the treatment of bladder instability, and anti-Parkinsonian drugs with anti-cholinergic actions such as benserazide, and the antiarrhythmic agent disopyramide.

Obstruction

The tendency of NSAIDs, the bisphosphonate alendronate, and high-potency pancreatic enzyme supplements to cause fibrotic strictures, presumably on a basis of healed ulceration, is well known.

Recent evidence indicates that rotavirus vaccines are associated with intussusception, which is thought to be due to hypertrophied and prolapsed lymphoid tissue. Infantile hypertrophic pyloric stenosis has also been associated with treatment in pregnancy with erythromycin.[10] The mechanism is unclear but may be related to its agonist actions on intestinal motility.

Paralytic ileus is occasionally produced by the anticholinergic effects of tricyclic antidepressants and the morphine-like peripheral agonist loperamide.

Diarrhoea

Drugs may cause diarrhoea by a variety of mechanisms. These include altered bacterial flora, secretory efflux into the colon, prostaglandin-like activity, the excessive effects of standard or overdoses of known purgatives, and direct motor stimulation.

Osmotic diarrhoea

Excessive treatment with the synthetic sugar lactulose, with simple salts used in managing constipation, and with magnesium-based alkalis will inevitably cause diarrhoea. Sorbitol and any other non-absorbed sugar would be expected to be as likely to cause diarrhoea as lactulose. Acidification of the faeces through bacterial fermentation may contribute to the diarrhoea.

Increased motility

Any drugs stimulating motility will tend to cause diarrhoea; selective serotonin reuptake inhibitors (SSRIs) are classic examples, which can also induce other non-specific gastrointestinal symptoms. Parasympathomimetics, and cholinergic drugs, such as the anti-cholinesterase, neostigmine, can cause diarrhoea, which may be counteracted by atropine or another antimuscarinic agent.

Prostaglandins have natural stimulant effects on gut motility, well-exemplified in the synthetic prostaglandin misoprostol. As expected, these actions are dose-related.[11]

Erythromycin is a motilin receptor agonist with the expected effect of enhancing gut motility. This side-effect has been utilized in the treatment of gut paresis of diabetic patients when other treatments have failed.

Secretory and idiopathic diarrhoea

Mefanamic acid, often used in treating menstrual pain, can occasionally cause diarrhoea. Symptoms may appear malabsorptive or colitic and reverse on stopping the drug. The mechanism is unclear but since mefanamic acid is NSAID-like it would be expected that constipation would occur rather than diarrhoea. 5-aminosalicylate, although used to treat inflammatory bowel disease is an occasional cause of diarrhoea, and exacerbation of diarrhoea during its use may indicate drug toxicity rather than an exacerbation of inflammation. Olsalazine, which has two 5-aminosalicylate molecules linked through a diazobond, is particularly likely to cause diarrhoea. The symptom may be secretory in origin.

Malabsorptive diarrhoea

Drugs given specifically to induce malabsorption, such as the α-galactosidase inhibitor, acarbose, will inevitably be prone to cause diarrhoea, since unabsorbed carbohydrate poses an osmotic load in the colon. In the same way, binding of bile acids by cholestyramine will tend to induce fat malabsorption.

Occult laxative consumption

Attempts to lose weight by bulimic individuals through laxative intake can induce hypokalaemia, hypoalbuminaemia and, in some patients, finger clubbing. The hypokalaemia is presumed to be caused by excessive secretion and the hypoalbuminia to excessive protein loss; the cause of finger clubbing is, however, unknown.

Spurious diarrhoea

Faecal retention with overflow can lead to inappropriate administration of constipating drugs, and exacerbation of the base problem.

Infective diarrhoea

Antimicrobial treatment can commonly favour the growth of particular organisms resulting in acute diarrhoea.[12] Clindamycin, broad-spectrum penicillins, cephalosporins, and a variety of other antibiotics are well recognized to precipitate diarrhoea owing to *Clostridium difficile* infection. Disease is diagnosed by bacteriological culture and detection of toxin in the stools. It is characterized by watery diarrhoea, the typical pseudomembranous lesions at endoscopy and by rectal biopsy appearances of volcano-like lesions generated by polymorphonuclear leucocytes erupting from mucosal crypts. Infection responds to oral vancomycin or metronidazole. It is transmitted by the faecal–oral route, which is facilitated by it being a spore-forming organism. Asymptomatic carriage is common.

Overgrowth of other organisms, including other *Clostridia* spp. and *Escherichia coli*, is common during antibiotic treatment, which responds to discontinuation of the antibiotic.

Staphylococcal enterocolitis is rare but is characterized by severe diarrhoea developing during treatment with antibiotics.

Treatment with antisecretory drugs, proton pump inhibitors (PPIs) or histamine H_2-receptor antagonists, by removing the gastric acid barrier, will approximately double or triple the risk of infection by classical diarrhoea-causing micro-organisms.[13] Whether all spontaneous adverse reports of diarrhoea during treatment with PPIs are attributable to this cause is uncertain.

Gallstones

Alterations in the ratio of secreted cholesterol to bile salts (the former raised, the latter reduced) favours microcrystallization and gallstone formation. Treatments well-described as having such efforts are oral contraceptives,[14,15] and the lipid-regulating agent, clofibrate. Somatostatin and its analogues predispose to gallstones by reducing gall-bladder contractility.

Pancreatitis

In clinical practice, most cases of acute pancreatitis are attributable to alcoholism or are associated with gallstone disease. Certain groups of drugs, notably the 5-aminosalicylates, used in the treatment or prophylaxis of inflammatory bowel disease, azathioprine, the nucleoside reverse transcriptase inhibitors (such as zidovudine) and the anti-epileptic drug, sodium valproate are well-described causes. There is also epidemiological evidence to suggest that diuretic treatment may significantly increase the risk.

The particular circumstances under which disease may be precipitated are unclear. Overall risks are difficult to quantify because evidence largely derives from published case reports, often with recurrence on rechallenge, and from spontaneous adverse reaction reports but not from formal studies.

Drug causes of pancreatitis categorized by strength of evidence are listed in Table 15.2.[16] Much of the uncertainty arises because evidence is limited.

Table 15.2   Risks of acute pancreatitis occurrence associated with drug treatment.[16]

Definite risk	Likely risk
Azathioprine and 6-Mercaptopurine	Combined cancer chemotherapy
Loop and other tubular diuretics	Cimetidine
Oestrogens	Corticosteroids
Sulphonamides	Diphenoxylate
Sulindac	Metronidazole
Tetracycline	Nitrofurantoin
Valproate	Piroxicam
	Procaineamide

DRUG INTERACTIONS IN THE GUT

Within the gut there is the potential for interactions through altered absorption patterns. Motility stimulants or retardants, by modulating gastric emptying can influence the rate of drug absorption because most absorption takes place by passive diffusion in the small intestine. Such actions are seldom clinically important, although metoclopramide is often deliberately used to speed absorption of drugs used for the treatment of migraine.

Binding resins, cholestyramine being the exemplar, can reduce the bioavailability of warfarin. Antacids can have modest effects inhibiting drug absorption.

REFERENCES

1. Langman MJS, Weil J, Lawson DH, *et al*. Risks of bleeding peptic ulcer associated with individual non-steroidal anti-inflammatory drugs. *Lancet* 1994; **343**: 1075–1078.
2. Henry D, Lim L L-Y, Garcia-Rodriguez LA, *et al*. Variability in risks of gastrointestinal complications with individual non-steroidal anti-inflammatory drugs. Results of a collaborative meta-analysis. *Brit Med J* 1996; **312**: 1563–1566.
3. Weil J, Colin Jones DG, Langman M, *et al*. Prophylactic aspirin and risk of peptic ulcer bleeding. *Brit Med J* 1995; **310**: 827–830.
4. Emery P, Zeiderler H, Kvien TK, *et al*. Celecoxib versus diclofenac in long-term management of rheumatoid arthritis: randomised double-blind comparison. *Lancet* 1999; **354**: 2106–2111.
5. Bjarnason I, Hayllar J, MacPherson AJ, *et al*. Side-effects of non-steroidal drugs on the small and large intestine in humans. *Gastroenterology* 1993; **104**: 1832.
6. Committee on Safety of Medicine. Fibrosing colonopathy associated with pancreatic enzymes. *Curr Prob Pharmacovigilance* 1995: **21**: 11.
7. Vessey M, Jewell D, Smith A, *et al*. Chronic inflammatory bowel disease, cigarette smoking and use of oral contraceptives: findings in a large cohort of women of child-bearing age. *Br Med J* 1986; **292**: 1101–1103.
8. Timmer A, Sutherland LR, Martin F, *et al*. Smoking, use of oral contraceptives and medical induction of remission were risk factors for relapse in Crohn's disease. *Gastroenterology* 1998; **114**: 1143–1150.
9. Committee on Safety of Medicines. The safety of MMR vaccine. *Curr Probl Pharmocovigilance* 1999; **25**: 9–10.
10. Honein MA, Paulozzi LJ, Himelwright IM, *et al*. Infantile hypertrophic pyloric stenosis after pertussis prophylaxis with erythromycin: a case review and cohort study. *Lancet* 1999; **354**: 2101–2105.
11. Silverstein FE, Graham D, Senior JR, *et al*.

Misoprostinol reduces serious gastrointestinal complications in patients with rheumatoid arthritis receiving non-steroidal inflammatory drugs. A randomised, double-blind placebo-controlled trial. *Ann Intern Med* 1993; **123:** 241–249.

12. Committee on Safety of Medicines. Antibiotic-associated colitis. *Curr Probl Pharmacovigilance* 1994; **20:** 7.

13. Nwokolo CU, Loft DE, Holder R, *et al.* Increased incidence of bacterial diarrhoea in patients taking gastric antisecretory drugs. *Eur J Gastroenterol Hepatol* 1994; **6:** 697–699.

14. Murray FE, Logan FRDA, Hannaford PC, Kay CT. Cigarette smoking and parity as risk factors for the development of symptomatic gall bladder disease in women: results of the Royal College of General Practitioners' oral contraceptive study. *Gut* 1994; **35:** 107–111.

15. Thijs C, Knipschild P. Oral contraceptives and the risk of gallbladder disease: a meta-analysis. *Am J Public Health* 1993; **83:** 1113–1120.

16. Bergholm U, Langman M, Rawlins M, *et al.* Drug-induced acute pancreatitis. *Pharmacoepidemiol Drug Safety* 1995; **4:** 329–334.

Index